# A pathway to NVQs in care: an underpinning knowledge

# To Pat, David, Paul and Moss

*'You cannot teach a man anything; you can only help him to find it within himself'*
*Galilei Galileo (1564–1642)*

# A PATHWAY TO NVQs IN CARE:
## *An underpinning knowledge*

*by*
***N Okon Ironbar***
***RMN RGN BTA Cert Dip N (Lond) RNT Cert Ed (Leeds)***
***Director of Studies***
*Inservice Education (Nursing) Consultancy Service*

NLA/B.

(E9PD3)

610.730693

IRO

Quay Books, Division of Mark Allen Publishing Group
Jesses Farm, Snow Hill, Dinton, Salisbury, Wiltshire, SP3 5HN

© Mark Allen Publishing Limited 1998

Reprinted 2002

ISBN 1 85653 062 0

British Library Cataloguing-in-Publication Data
A catalogue record for this book is available from the British Library

All rights reserved. No part of this material may be reproduced, stored in a retrieval system, or transmitted in any form, or by any means, electrical, mechanical, photographic, recording or otherwise, without the prior permission of the publishers.

Printed and bound in the United Kingdom by The Bath Press, Bath

# Contents

Acknowledgements — vii
Preface — viii
Foreword — x
Guidance on how to use this book — xii

## Section I: Introduction: an overview

The care assistants — 3
Care establishments — 8
The elderly person — 14

## Section II: Essential supporting skills

Caring skills — 21
Appendages for care — 34

## Section III: The delivery of care: mandatory units

Unit 1: Foster people's rights, beliefs and equality — 63
Unit 2: Promote effective communication and relationships — 80
Unit 3(a): Health, safety and security in the workplace — 89
Unit 3(b): Assist in the control of infection — 113
Unit 4: Contribute to the protection of individuals from abuse — 136

## Section IV: The delivery of care — option group A

Unit 5: Assist clients adjust to changes in care — 145
Unit 6: Promote communication in care through physical contact — 157
Unit 7: Enable clients to achieve physical comfort — 170
Unit 8: Enable clients to eat and drink — 184
Unit 9: Assist clients to access and use toilet facilities — 208
Unit 10: Assist clients with personal hygiene and appearance — 227
Unit 11: Assist clients to move, exercise and maintain desirable posture — 243

## Section V: The delivery of care — option group B

Unit 12: Assist in clinical activities: investigations in care — 267
Unit 13: Assist in clinical activities: delivery of care — 284

| Unit 14: | Assist clients to participate in leisure activities | 304 |
| Unit 15: | Health education and promotion | 319 |
| Unit 16: | Assist clients to express sexuality | 327 |
| Unit 17: | Community care | 330 |
| Unit 18: | Support clients in the activity of dying | 336 |
| Unit 19: | Special care needs (mental health) | 348 |

## Section VI: Personal development

| Unit 20: | Vocational qualifications | 377 |

## Section VII: Appendices

| Appendix A — Flow chart: A pathway to NVQs in care | 405 |
| Appendix B — Level 2 qualifications | 407 |
| Appendix C — Useful information | 409 |
| Index | 413 |

# Acknowledgements

No book of this kind could possibly be written without the help and encouragement of others and I particularly want to express my grateful thanks to the following:

- for writing the foreword AV Atkinson, Principal, Atkinson's Nursing Homes; Malcolm P Laryea, Principal Lecturer, Thames Valley University; Christine E Hutchman, IV Co-ordinator, Royal County Assessment Centre
- Vivienne Perkins whose sketches depict the problems of elderly people in various settings
- Pat for her patience and support in preparing the final typescript
- The Institute of Health and Care Development (IHCD), Bristol for permission to reproduce Overview of the Awards in Care NVQs/SVQs — Level II Qualifications,
- All the course members who acted as 'guinea pigs' by participating in the Development Course, and commenting on handouts presented during the course. Collectively, these form the basis of this book
- All the proprietors, managers and matrons of care establishments for their support and involvement with Inservice Education (Nursing) Consultancy Service, in its innovative ON-SITE staff training schemes.

# Preface

Vocational qualifications are a national topic relating to all aspects of the care industry. They are concerned with maintaining standards which require a wide variety of skills and resources in the process of restoring deficits in an individual's care needs. The private sector of health care is a complex and expanding business, where clients have the right to expect the highest standards and quality of care, value for money and quality service. This ideal service cannot be delivered without proper knowledge, skills and understanding, and failure to achieve these objectives means the loss of customers, reputation and status. Good standards of care are the work of a team and require every member to play his or her part. Team members should be able to depend on each other's support, trust and contribution. In the health care industry, particularly in nursing homes, a greater proportion of the work force is unqualified, and they are valuable members of the healthcare team. Qualified practitioners who always remain accountable for total client care needs, rely on the support of their unqualified partners, the care assistants, without whom the service would come to a standstill.

The role of care assistants is that of assisting and supporting professionally qualified practitioners in providing high standards and quality of care in a variety of settings. Care assistants are a diverse group of people from a wide range of cultural, educational and social backgrounds. Some have no previous experience in this type of work. Nevertheless, they bring a multiplicity of attributes and life experience to the care team. There is a fundamental need to build upon these attributes and provide carers with the means to acquire the information, knowledge and skills necessary to become competent, and grow in the profession.

The process of NVQ places emphasis on the assessment of candidates performing to nationally agreed standards in a real-work situation. Assessment is based on skills and experience gained via on-the-job training schemes provided by employers. However, skills and enthusiasm on their own are not enough. The worker also has to show that he or she understands how and why the procedure is done in a particular way which implies displaying evidence of possession of basic knowledge.

Caring for people is based on a framework of theory and practice, both of which are inseparable. Theory underpins knowledge which involves principles of care. Practice is the repetition of procedures based on hands-on-experience under the guidance and supervision of qualified staff, in nursing homes and in hospital settings. In some situations a planned programme of training is offered, while in other places there is little or no training, and learning takes place by trial and error combined with suggestions from colleagues. Attendance at a course of preparation is not a pre-requisite to the process of work-based assessment. It follows that there is disparity in the procedures available for carers to gain the relevant underpinning knowledge and practical skills necessary to support the quality and quantity of evidence essential to become competent.

*A Pathway to NVQs in Care* offers care assistants a realistic link and a broad foundation on which to prepare themselves for vocational or professional roles (see *Appendix A*). As a research-based book, it provides them with a degree of relevance to underpinning knowledge, skills, and understanding. It also offers candidates an incentive to learn and experiment with their newly acquired knowledge and skills under supervision.

# Foreword

I am delighted to add my thoughts to those of the author of this book. I have worked closely with Okon for many years as he developed his **on-site training programme**. I would commend him as a diligent teacher committed to imparting knowledge to those who seek it in order to deliver proper care to the elderly. He is enthusiastic in this field, efficient in delivering and simplifying structures to his learning audience. Indeed he has taught a great number of staff to levels and qualifications commendable to any caring setting in the British Isles.

*A pathway to NVQs in care* is designed specifically for care assistants, to equip them to undertake duties that are expected in the growth of individualised care, combined with the training to fulfil this role. It is well set out, covers the topics adequately, is easy to read and gives succinct guide-lines on aspects of care. It provides texts that encourage carers to accept responsibility for their own learning as a discipline and as a practical skill. It helps to provide understanding of the basis and principles of care of the elderly, and to this end, provides a wide range of resources which the learner can draw upon to enrich and reinforce the learning experience

It is a practical guide because the work of care assistants is practically orientated. However, underlying every practice is theory and it is increasingly important in the complex care of the elderly that theory is well developed. The author of this book has tried to do just this.

More importantly, it provides a basic standard on which anyone who wishes to enter the field of care, can begin to build their skills and expertise after they have properly read this book and followed its practical modules. *A Pathway to NVQs in Care* can be used as a reference book for those who do not pursue the whole course to NVQs and can also be used as a guide for those who wish to gain NVQ qualifications.

I whole heartedly recommend this book to all who seek knowledge in care of other people.

**A V Atkinson, Principal**
**Atkinson's Private Nursing Homes,**
**Camberley, Surrey.**

During the last few years, there has been a rapid growth in the uptake of National Vocational Qualifications within the care/health care sector, and the requirement to meet various needs for more related education and training is increasingly apparent. Many care assistants seeking NVQ awards do so in the context of a structured learning programme which provides opportunities for them to acquire and demonstrate achievement of all the required outcomes.

*A pathway to NVQs in care* provides care assistants with a coherent learning experience and adopts a flexible approach, giving opportunities for learning at the most appropriate time and place. It recognises the need to widen learning opportunities and choices for care assistants and enriches the quality of the learning experience.

This book is expertly designed with high quality material and has relevance to the wide ranging needs of care assistants working in community, health and social care settings. All data are clearly structured and explained, with each section guiding the care assistant through achievable objectives. There is a close cross reference to practice and it provides a contribution to learning in a realistic way.

A variety of relevant learning approaches are used, aimed at providing a unique and invaluable underpinning knowledge to support the evidence requirements for assessment. It answers some of the criticisms of the lack of rigour in the knowledge and understanding domain.

Written in a jargon-free, user-friendly manner, it enables care assistants to reach the level of national occupational standards required for competent practice.

This book is about personal growth and development. It is practically designed to help facilitate the acquisition of knowledge and understanding which underpins practice in the delivery of quality of care.

I wish the book well.

**Malcolm P Laryea, MA, B Ed (Hons), Cert Ed, PGD in Mngt. Studies, RMN, RNT, RCNT, Principal Lecturer, Thames Valley University**

This book gives a very comprehensive and full account of the various problems likely to be faced by care assistants in their day-to-day role as carers. Care staff in nursing and residential homes need to be able to have access to training courses and training material which will inform them, in the most practical way possible, about common illnesses associated with care of the elderly.

Staff need to learn how to recognise these disorders and when to refer for an opinion or assessment, and in particular when they, themselves, can help the resident. Carers need to understand the different types of behavioural problems some of which can be associated with often treatable disorders, and which should not necessarily be regarded as part of the normal ageing process. Behavioural problems usually have an understandable cause. The book provides this information in a concise, readable and understandable format.

The majority of older people are in reasonably good health, do not suffer from physical or mental illness and live a full, happy and contented life. With the help and guidance of this accessible, practical and well-written book, care staff will gain the necessary underpinning knowledge and skills to carry out their roles confidently and with a sense of achievement.

This book helps to provide a framework for practice and a source of readily available information and advice in an easy-to-follow guide for care staff. It covers a wide range of topics and problems which are faced daily by carers carrying out their roles. It will undoubtedly assist staff in achieving their NVQ qualification.

I was pleased to be given the opportunity to comment on the contents of this book in relation to the underpinning knowledge required for NVQ. Much time and effort have been spent in mapping the contents against the units within the standards, which will be of enormous help to the candidates and their assessors.

I recommend this book.

**Christine E Hutchman, Internal Verifier Co-ordinator,**
**Royal County Assessment Centre, Theale, Reading, Berkshire**

# Guidance on how to use this book

## The candidate

*A pathway to NVQs in care* offers you the unique opportunity of being in control of your study. You are required to learn in your own time and at your own pace, and prepare for your *Workbased Assessment of Competence*. In order to help you, information is presented in a concise and synoptic format for easy reading. It covers relevant underpinning knowledge for the revised care standards and qualifications, based on mandatory units which are common to all qualifications at that level. It also deals with basic underpinning knowledge to practice for option units groups A and B at level 2, with guidelines on the number of units to be assessed from each option group (see *Appendix B*). You will have to choose the units best fitted for your role and specific care group, together with its relevant underpinning knowledge as set out in the text.

Guidance is given on the action to be taken in certain situations. This is only a recommendation, and it is meaningful if you are familiar with, and follow agreed practice in the area of your work. Specific assignments appear at the end of some units of learning which you should attempt as suggested. It is crucial that you should try and integrate your knowledge and skills with your practical work. Always seek clarification from your mentor. This approach should help you to develop confidence and prepare you for your workbased assessment. However, it is important that you should register with, use and seek the services of your local public lending library.

## Vocational trainers and assessors

The contents of this book form the basis of a development course designed to provide candidates with underpinning knowledge, and prepare them for NVQs in Health and Social Care. It is based on units of learning, each offering guidance on the basic principles of care, together with an opportunity for use as a tool for refreshing knowledge, skills and attitude. Emphasis is placed throughout, on the development and maintenance of good interpersonal relationship skills, which form the hallmark of care delivery. As the work of candidates is practically orientated, it is important for them to work and gain supervised hands-on-experience under the support of a mentor, within the culture and agreed practises of their respective care settings. The framework is a participate relationship approach whereby mentors work alongside candidates and share their knowledge, skills and attitudes with them. It is hoped that this approach will support candidates' development and help them to gain confidence and competence, and grow within the profession.

The questions for assignments which candidates are asked to attempt and submit, are specimens only. Please feel free to formulate your own questions. However, experience has shown that motivation for learning is enhanced if the candidates are given an immediate acknowledgement of the correctness of their homework.

# Section I: Introduction: an overview

At the end of this section, candidates should be able to have a general overview of the following:

**The care assistants** 3

- *Background to role* 3
- *Functions of care assistants* 4

**Care establishments** 8

- *Registered nursing and residential care homes* 8

**The elderly person** 14

- *Human ageing process* 14

# The care assistants

## Background to the role

Since the inception of the National Health Service, hospitals and privately owned care establishments have relied upon the services of unqualified staff working under the guidance of professionally qualified practitioners, in the delivery of total care to their clients. These are likely to be men, school leavers, and more importantly, women who have taken time out to raise a family and would now like to play a major role in the basic care of people. Some have no professional qualifications, but they all bring various attributes and skills, and valuable experience of life to the health care team of which they are a part.

There are about 150 000 unqualified staff employed as nursing assistants or auxiliaries in all care settings. They constitute a greater proportion of the total workforce, including people from black and ethnic minority groups, and a majority undertake a more demanding role in specialist areas. Some have an initial induction program, while others have no basic training at all. Quite often their experiences go unrecognised and learning takes place by trial and error, by imitation of others and suggestions from colleagues. The whole area of service would be unable to function without their indispensable contributions, both in the public and private sectors.

During the last ten years, a number of factors have forced the training and development of care assistants to appear on the planned national agenda. At one level this was a political question when it became apparent that British workers would not be able to compete in the European Community, due to lack of training and development in relation to the national standards defined by employers. As a solution to this problem, vocational qualifications emerged, with the establishment in 1986 of the National Council for Vocational Qualifications (NCVQ), now known as the Qualifications and Curriculum Authority (QCA).

In the health care sector, the idea of support workers was first mentioned in the DHSS (1987) *Review of Nursing Skill Mix*, where it was suggested that some nursing duties could be delegated to non-professionals. Secondly, it related to the Project 2000 proposals in which students have supernumerary status, thus leaving a deficit of manpower in the clinical setting as well as a need to address skill mix issues.

As the implementation of Project 2000 gathered pace, the need to train support workers to be skills-based became apparent, and tasks and activities needed to be defined and supervised on that basis. When trained they should be able to support professionally qualified nurses, midwives, health visitors, physiotherapists, occupational therapists, speech therapists, chiropodists and other qualified health care workers. In the nursing care setting, they fill the gap left by student nurses who no longer form part of the total workforce. It then became government policy that all staff should have access to vocational qualifications within the context of the Care Sector Consortium. It was agreed that the term *Health Care Assistant* should apply to all unqualified staff who are closely involved in the provision of care, in direct support of a professional group. The use of this term is interchangeable with *care assistants*, *health care workers* and *professional carers* throughout this book.

## Role of care assistants

Role is defined as the part one is called upon to play or do within the organisation. It is a pattern of behaviour expected to be seen in the position which the individual holds, and how he or she relates to other people. In this context, the prime commitment of care assistants is to assist professionally qualified practitioners in providing high standards and quality of care to users of the service. This involves assisting in a systematic assessment, planning, implementation and evaluation of total care, in relation to the client's physical, psychological, social and spiritual needs under the guidance of qualified practitioners

## Functions of care assistants

Functions are the range of duties the care assististant is called upon to do in order to perform his or her role effectively. They are a range of duties, usually performed under the supervision of qualified staff, who remain at all times accountable for the care of clients. A *job description* should provide information on the range of these duties in both flexible and more specific terms, to allow for local variations in accordance with the needs of the service. The range of duties may include the ability to:
- support and act as an advocate for clients
- assist in all aspects of care as may be delegated using relevant knowledge and skills
- maintain health, safety and security of the total care environment
- act as a member of the health care team.
- attend personal and vocational development courses and keep up-to-date
- participate in research.

### Membership of the health care team

Traditionally, care is provided by a multi-disciplinary team comprising doctors and nurses, and paramedical staff, such as social workers and occupational therapists. The care team looks after the total well-being of each person, and those receiving care are the most important people. Every member of the team has a responsibility to contribute his or her professional expertise and to communicate with other members in a recognised setting or case conference. However, in nursing home settings, the use of expertise is based on the needs of individual residents. Care assistants are members of this team and are required to set high standards for themselves in a professional way, and to earn the trust and respect of everyone. All members of the care team should understand the organisation's:
- philosophy and structure
- policies and practices, including reporting mechanisms.

### Factors which may influence roles and functions

The role and function of care assistants may be influenced by:
- clients' care needs, eg. advocacy, rights, beliefs and demands
- personal needs, eg. social, financial, vocational training, new experiences, skills
- rules and regulations, eg. statutory and non-statutory
- local expectations of colleagues and members of the health care team
- those in authority, eg. the manager or matron
- availability of resources, eg. personnel, equipment

- new knowledge, personal development, participation in research
- care environment, eg. loyalty, teamwork.

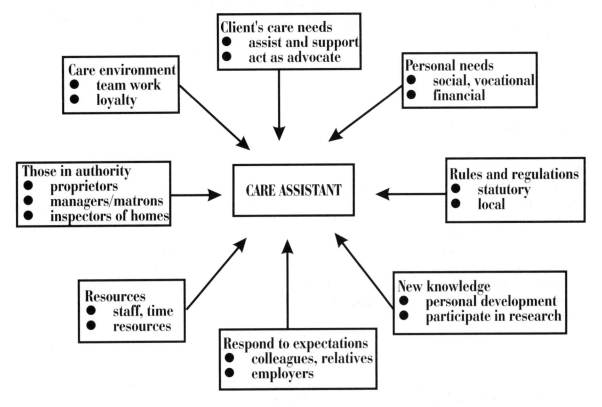

Factors which influence the role of care assistants

## Essential attributes

It is often difficult to define or prescribe the 'ideal qualities' expected of a worker. Generally, the degree of excellence or attributes expected are governed by many factors, such as society, statutory demands of the service, speed of change and local rules and regulations currently in operation in individual care establishments, including the individual's attitudes. In order to function effectively, care assistants should be able to:

- develop and maintain good interpersonal relationship skills, eg. communication, social and assertiveness
- demonstrate knowledge of the principles of good health care, with in-depth knowledge of individual clients, helping to maintain their personal beliefs, independence, respect and dignity
- encourage clients to express their personal beliefs, preferences, opinions provided that these do not affect the rights of others. Be aware of the effects of prejudice, stereotyping, institutionalisation, and ways in which these may be challenged or overcome
- demonstrate a sense of loyalty, dedication and sensitivity to the needs, rights, choices, wishes and views of those receiving care, their own needs and those of employers and colleagues
- support the aims, philosophy and objectives of the organisation
- observe and work within the legal and organisational policies relating to confidentiality of information, anti-discriminatory practices and support the individual at all times

- demonstrate at all times basic human attributes, eg. empathy, respect, tolerance, flexibility, honesty and trustworthiness, responsibility and integrity in dealing with people.

In carrying out their duties, care assistants who disobey orders, use verbal or physical abuse, neglect their duties, lie, steal or wilfully damage property, alter or falsify records, smoke or are found to be under the influence of drugs or alcohol will usually be liable to instant dismissal and will probably find clauses forbidding such behaviour in their contracts of employment.

It must be remembered that users of the service have individual desires, fears and anxieties, and all actions should be aimed at accommodating such feelings and helping the clients to maintain their individual *self-respect, dignity* and *independence*.

## Preparation for the role

Training is the recognised means by which staff acquire the necessary information, knowledge and skills to become competent. It is by no means the only, or the best way of helping people to learn; and it is important to keep in mind that care staff are a very mixed group of people from a wide range of educational and social backgrounds. There can be no simple solution to the multitude of training needs which this represents. What is required is the means whereby people are able to learn immediately and continuously from the point of entry to a new job.

Towards this end, NVQs emphasise the assessment of performance and accumulation of credits. It is believed that attendance at a course of preparation is not a prerequisite, and that any training for a particular area of work should be provided by qualified practitioners. This is based on supervision of defined activities, leading to the accumulation of credits towards an NVQ. This is similar to a 'block-building' approach whereby candidates work to build up an aggregate of units in their personal portfolio of credits. The process usually involves assessment of the training needs of individual candidates, recognition and accreditation of prior experience, skills, and achievements which are brought into the care team. The existing and experienced staff do not necessarily need to be taught what they already know, but will be able to gain access to work-place assessment immediately, and start building up credits for NVQ.

## References

Anon (1990) Why all the fuss? *Nurs Stand* **4**(2): 43
Bush T (1991) Who supports whom? *Nurs Times* **87**: 18
COHSE (1990) *NCVQ and You — A Guide to The Story So Far*. COHSE, Banstead
Flack M, Johnson M (1986) *Handbook for Care*. Beaconsfield Publishers Ltd, Beaconsfield
IHCD (1989) *The Way Forward: The Role, Recruitment and Training of Support Workers*. IHCD, Bristol
Johnston C (1991) Who support the worker? *Nurs Times* **85**(7): 26–28
Kemp V, Thornton B (1989) Training in the private sector. *Nurs Times* **85**(20): 60–62
Malby R (1990) Vocational support. *Nurs Times* **86**(16): 81–83
Manthey M (1991) Primary partners. *Nurs Times* **87**(25): 27–28
Mersey Regional Health Authority (1989) *But Who Will Make the Beds?* A research report on assessment of nurse staffing and support worker requirements for acute general hospitals. Nuffield Institute for Health Service Studies and Mersey Regional Health Authority
Nichol DK (1990) *Health Care Assistants*. Management Executive, Department of Health, London
Scoullar K (1991) A constant source of support. *Nurs Times* **87**(25):29–30
Oxford University Press (1987) *The Pocket Oxford Dictionary*. OUP, Oxford

Thomas LH (1993) Comparing qualified nurse and auxiliary roles. *Nurs Times* **89**(38): 45–48

United Kingdom Central Council for Nursing, Midwifery and Health Visiting (1988) *Position Paper on the Development of Support Worker Role*. UKCC, London

United Kingdom Central Council for Nursing, Midwifery and Health Visiting (1992) *Code of Professional Conduct*. UKCC, London

# Assignment

The purpose of this homework is to assist you in preparing for your Workbased Assessment of Competence. As there is no pressure on you, feel free to work in your own time and pace, but avoid the temptation to procrastinate. After you have read your notes and suggested references, submit your work for correction. The completed work becomes part of your Personal Portfolio.

## Introduction: The care assistants

1. Write a short note about your work as a Care Assistant touching on:
   a) Reasons for your choice of this type of work
   b) Why you continue to do this work?
   c) How much other people influence your work. For example:
      - needs of your clients or patients
      - those in charge, colleagues, family and others.

2. Discuss your role and functions and list:
   a) What you consider to be the important part of your job and which gives you most satisfaction
      - the things you like to do most.
   b) Three aspects of your job which give you least satisfaction
      - the things you do not like doing
   c) Two obstacles which might impede your current job performance
   d) Changes which might make your job performance better if made by:
      - your immediate manager
      - yourself
      - proprietor or owner of the care establishment.

4. How you hope to see your career develop, say in two years time.

# Care establishments

## Registered nursing and residential care homes

The concept of health care homes as an alternative to geriatric hospitals has been in existence for well over 70 years. In the 1980s, there was a shift of emphasis from hospital to community, following the closing down of long-stay geriatric wards and the sale of local authority old people's homes. This led to a rapid development of privately-owned nursing and residential care homes. These homes are developed and staffed by different groups, such as housing organisations, voluntary organisations or charitable trusts, and private individuals. The larger homes are owned and run as multi-national limited companies, while others are run by independent operators. In spite of unfavourable publicity from the media and public outcries about the quality of care in some homes, the majority provide excellent facilities in a warm, cheerful and sympathetic environment.

In recent years, the number of elderly people has steadily increased as a result of demographic changes. As they grow older and more frail, they will require skilled nursing care. It is estimated that by the year 2000, there is likely to be two million people over 85-years-old, and 800,000 of these will need care facilities. It is not always possible for an elderly person in need of care, to live alone in the community or with his family or close relations. This may be due to inadequate accommodation, the burden of caring for an elderly person or tension within the family. As a result, the elderly person may seek to live elsewhere. With the introduction of the Community Care Act 1993, it is believed that a majority of the elderly will be cared for in their own homes, although a proportion will still need nursing and residential care home services.

### Inspection and registration

Historically, nursing homes have been required to be registered since 1927. In 1975 the Registered Homes Act was passed, setting out new standards and requirements for registration and inspection. During the intervening years, various amendments were made, which led to the repeal of the 1975 Act. The current legislation is the Registered Homes Act 1984, in which the Secretary of State for Health delegates the inspection and registration of all homes to district health authorities and departments of social services.

The Act talks about 'adequate' standard without actually defining it, and is more about basic protection of the public. Although registered homes are meeting their legal obligations, the standards vary widely because the legislation is open to interpretation, and health authorities have their own varying guidelines. It is anticipated that the duties of inspection and registration will, in future, be undertaken by one authority. It remains to be seen how this will work.

Current reports, on inspectors' visits to residential care homes, are available to the public in public libraries or by contacting the local social services registration and inspection units.

### Nursing homes

The Registered Homes Act 1984 defines a nursing home as 'any premises used or intended to be used for the reception of, and the providing of nursing care for persons suffering from any sickness, injury or infirmity'. The term embraces a wide variety of establishments, from maternity nursing homes, mental nursing homes, to a large acute general hospital. Under the Act, all homes offering services for four or more people must be registered and inspected at least twice a year by district health authorities. Nursing homes are high dependency homes and provide clinical care in which qualified nursing staff cover is obligatory at all times.

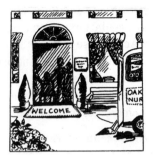

A majority of these homes are members of the Registered Nursing Home Association, which sets standards of care for its members, provides training manuals and carries out periodical inspections. Members display a blue plaque on their premises. As the number of nursing homes has grown, so has the workload.

## Residential care homes

These are low dependency homes defined in the Act as 'any establishment which provides, or intends to provide, whether for reward or not, residential accommodation with both board and personal care to persons in need of personal care by reasons of old age, disablement, past or present dependence on alcohol or drugs or past or recent mental illness or mental handicap.' Under the Act, social services departments accept delegated responsibility to assess and meet needs for care in the community, and will inspect and register these homes. Residential care homes are usually small and provide a more homely atmosphere, with a wide variation in cost, according to the staff and facilities provided. The care is provided by skilled staff 24 hours a day, who give their residents a high level of care. Members belong to the British Federation of Care Home Proprietors. There is a movement towards the provision of qualified nursing staff in the residential care homes.

## Dual registration

Under the Registered Homes Act 1984, there is provision for homes to have dual registration by offering both nursing and personal care with a two-tier system. It is inspected by both the local authority and the health authority.

## Other regulations

### 1. Conduct of Nursing Home Regulations

All care establishments are required to maintain the following records:
- register of patients to include: name and address, date of admission, discharge or transfer, time of death
- records on residents to include: diagnosis of acute illness, a daily statement of the client's health, a periodical statement of health, staff records.

### 2. Town and Country Planning Act 1971

The provision of independent health care is governed by other statutory regulations defined within various acts of parliament. For example, planning permission is required for any development, including making structural alterations to the building.

### 3. Employment Protection (Consolidation) Act 1978

The regulation refers to the provision of:
- terms and conditions of employment
- rules and disciplinary procedures
- grievance and appeal procedures
- holiday entitlement and conditions of service

- sickness benefit, record of absence, etc.
- general working arrangements, such as redundancy or retirement policies.

### 4. Health and Safety at Work Act 1974
This legislation governs health, welfare and safety of all employees and their responsibilities under the Act. These include:
- safe lifting and handling of clients
- first-aid procedures
- infection control and management
- procedures to be followed if a resident is found to be missing.

### 5. Fire Precaution Act 1971
Each care establishment is required to have its own fire prevention equipment, such as smoke detectors and fire extinguishers, and procedures to be followed in case of fire.

### 6. Equal Opportunities Commission's Code 1985
Employers are required to formulate local policy which must accept the principles of equal opportunities as being an essential part of good employment practice.

### 7. Non-statutory regulations
In order to maintain a high standard of professional practice, care establishments should aim to issue their own individual policies on:
- wearing a uniform, jewellery, shoes or cosmetics when on duty
- nursing procedures relating to standards and quality of care
- continuing education of qualified nurses
- training and development of health care assistants, eg. NVQs in care, levels 2 or 3.

## National Health Service and Community Care Act 1993

The Act, which came into being in April 1993, aims to look at the needs of clients in their individual settings, and offer quality and choice of care. Emphasis is placed on a corporate working relationship between health authorities, social services and the independent sector for the provision of care. It is hoped that government money will be put into a single fund to be used where needed.

One of the main recommendations of the NHS and Community Act requires employers to plan for 'the best way of doing things' and set standards of care in specific areas of the service being offered. These areas include:
- philosophy of care
- accommodation and general service
- staff levels and continuing education and training
- admission procedures
- activities, such as leisure, social, religious and provisions for visitors
- complaints procedures
- residents' Contracts of Care and financial affairs
- health care standards in relation to:
  - choice, privacy and dignity of care
  - care of pressure areas, restraint, promotion of continence
  - management and administration of drugs
- grief and loss
- nursing, personal, day care and respite care plans

- information on The Patient's Charter of Rights and Responsibilities
- daily routine, use of community services
- health and safety, eg. first aid procedures, infection control, safe lifting of residents, no smoking policy and procedure on a missing person.

Most homes are now providing a local 'Patient's Charter' setting out the philosophy of care, complaints procedures and approaches for monitoring consumers' satisfaction.

## Monitoring

The standards and quality of care having been set, they must be continuously monitored on a regular basis, through:

- an internal system covering all those involved in care, eg. staff, users of the service and relatives
- external and objective assessment by inspectors of homes, representatives of colleges of nursing (auditing for suitability of placement of student nurses for specific experience) and interested consumer groups.

This process involves maintaining a variety of records of meetings with residents, dates of inspectors' visits, staff rota and turnover of staff.

## Staff training and development

Both nursing and residential care homes provide an option to be involved in acute care for many nurses, care assistants and other health professionals working in the private sector of health care. In 1986, the Department of Health figures showed that the independent sector was employing 24,683 full-time and 28,062 part-time nurses and care assistants.

The 1984 Act recognises the value and importance of staff training and development, and recommends that health authorities consider inviting nurses in registered nursing homes to participate in NHS nurse education programmes. Contrary to popular belief, few proprietors genuinely believe in feeding their staff with the same inservice educational diet as their counterparts in the National Health Service. Training is the key to changing the regimental attitudes to institutionalisation that is found in some of these establishments.

However, some managers seem to have difficulty in reconciling the needs of the service with the training needs of their staff. In most cases, staff training and development is considered a luxury and an optional extra which puts financial constraints on the overall expenditure of the establishment. Although there is, as yet, no statutory requirement for staff training, the idea is hovering on the horizon with the introduction of National Vocational Qualifications.

## References

Anon (1988) Independent ways. *Nurs Standard* **2**(2): suppl 4

Booth T (1985) *Home Truths — Old People's Homes and Outcome of Care*. Grower Ltd, Aldershot

Bowling A (1992) Hospital and nursing home care. Care of the elderly in an inner city health district. *Nurs Times* **88**(13): 51–54

Department of Health and Social Security (1981) *Health Circular HC(18)8 LAC(81)4: Health Service Management: Registration and Inspection of Private Nursing Homes and Mental Nursing Homes. (including Hospitals)*. HMSO, Lancashire

Goodwin S (1992) Freedom to care — nursing homes debate. *Nurs Times* **88**(34): 38–39

Heywood-Jones I (1989) Home from home. *Nurs Times* **85**(17): 43–44

Ineichen B (1992) Managing residential care. *Nurs the Elderly* May/June: 29–30

Mangan P (1993) Home rules. *Nurs Times* **89**(40): 18

Mounce R (1989) There's no place like home. *Nurs Times* **85**(16): 36–38

National Association of Health Authorities (1985) *Registration and Inspection of Nursing Homes*. NAHA, London

*Private Health Care* (1987) Key Note Report: An Industry Sector Independent Hospitals Association Statistical Report

Ramdhaine P, Robinson I (1992) Registering support, registration and inspection. *Nurs Standard* **4**(3): 42–43

Registered Nursing Homes Association (1981) *Manual: Conditions of Admission to Nursing Home and Terms of Business*. Mawers Printers, Darlington

Robinson I (1992) Registering support, nursing the elderly. *Comm Care Iss* **4**(3)

Royal College of Nursing (1996) *Nursing Homes: Nursing Values*. RCN, London

Royal County of Berkshire Social Services Department (1993) *Care Specification for Nursing Homes for Elderly People*. Social Services Department, Reading, Berks

Swafield L (1990) Nursing homes monitoring muddles. *Nurs Times* **86**(45): 31–32

United Kingdom Central Council for Nursing, Midwifery and Health Visiting (1992) *The Scope of Professional Practice*. UKCC, London

United Kingdom Central Council for Nursing, Midwifery and Health Visiting (1994) *Professional Conduct — Occasional Report on Standards of Nursing in Nursing Homes*. UKCC, London

The Wager Report (1988) *Residential Care — A Positive Choice*. HMSO, London

Winter D (1990) Nursing homes buyers beware. *Nurs Times* **86**(45): 26–28

### Audio visual aids

#### Format: VHS Video

BBC Horizon: *In the Last Resort*. BBC London

RCN Nursing Update: *Life in a Nursing Home: Nursing Older People*. RCN, London

# ASSIGNMENT

The purpose of this homework is to assist you in preparing for your Workbased Assessment of Competence. As there is no pressure on you, feel free to work in your own time and pace, but avoid the temptation to procrastinate. After you have read your notes and suggested references, submit your work for correction. The completed work becomes part of your Personal Portfolio.

## Care Establishments:

1. Describe briefly the care establishment in which you work:
   a) its name and address and location.
   b) responsible registration authority.
   c) the number and kind of patients or clients, men and women and their age range.
   d) how many patients are admitted or discharged each year.
   e) how many move to other homes, hospitals or go back to their own homes in the community in a year, following admission.
   f) model of nursing care currently being used in the home.
   g) facilities available for the care of patients/clients.
2. List the different types of policies and notices on display, and classify them as local or national.

3. Find out whether there is an induction programme for new staff and an orientation programme for the existing staff.
4. Make a list of various textbooks, professional journals and magazines that are available in your home.
5. What would you do to prepare the home for an inspection visit?

# The elderly person

## Human ageing process

In modern society, ageing is viewed as a logical extension of a full life-cycle beyond the normal reproductive and parental phase in terms of chronological age. It is not a passive process dictated by hereditary, but influenced by an individual's own perception of old age, lifestyle, occupation, personal experience and ability to cope. Man is said to be old from a pre-retirement period (55–65 years of age) and definitely old at 70 years of age.

In 1982, the United Nations International Plan of Action on Ageing Problems, identified the 'aged' as those over 60 years. And according to the International Council of Nurses, there are about 488 million people in the world age 60 years or over, with nearly one million crossing the 60 year barrier every month.

During this century, life expectancy has greatly increased due to progress in public health measures, housing conditions, medical and social care and improved nutrition. The outcome is a proportional increase of elderly people in relation to the number of younger people within the population. For most people, ageing is a slow and variable process that periodically impinges upon one's consciousness, especially when it involves situations in which the person actively compares himself with others. At times one's age has a significant outcome or effect in relation to retirement, bereavement and, more importantly, to being excluded from various pursuits for being 'too old'. It is believed that the population is increasing not because of increased birth rate, but because of decreased death rate.

## Human ageing process

There are many theories of human ageing and its mechanisms, but growing old is a normal process and forms part of the cycle of human existence and experience. The study of the process is known as gerontology. It concerns the biological, psychological and social health of the individual, and includes motivation, perception, emotion and intelligence. Every aspect of human nature undergoes some changes.

### 1. Biological aspect

This aspect is genetically linked and people vary in the rate at which they age. The effects and responses to the demands of ageing can differ widely in the same age group, eg. climacteric period (menopause in women: 45–50 years and in men: 50–55 years). These biological changes tend to influence lifestyle and personal habits and can result in increased health problems. Significant changes may affect the following systems of the body:

**Nervous system**: the loss of brain cells and reduced blood flow to the brain and body may cause brain and bodily disturbance. The onset of confusion may be an indication of physical illness in the elderly. Confusion may also be due to the effects of drugs, such as hynoptics or tranquilisers.

**Circulatory system**: coronary arteries and veins narrow resulting in a reduction in blood flow and oxygen.

**Respiratory system**: there are more lung deposits, it is harder to breathe and the lungs lose elasticity.

**Muscular system**: weakening of the muscular system may cause atrophy and loss of height. The person may be at greater risk of hyperthermia and more likely to feel the cold.

**Skeletal system**: joints become less flexible and brittle bones can be caused by a less efficient metabolism. Falls and immobility are common and are the most frequent reasons for admission to nursing homes and hospitals.

**Digestive system**: metabolism slows and body heat is reduced; swallowing is difficult with a loss of taste and appetite. Indigestion and constipation are frequent complaints. Some elderly people have an impaired sense of thirst. They become too weak and apathetic to drink and may refuse food. This can lead to dehydration.

**Urinary system**: functions of the kidney are impaired resulting in a reduction in bladder control. This can cause incontinence in some elderly people.

**Reproductive system**: men become sexually impotent and there is reduced vaginal lubrication in women.

**Endocrine system**: decreased hormone levels cause malfunction of the endocrine glands. This may cause dehydration and weight loss.

**Sensory network**: as a result of the ageing process, people can experience failing eyesight, hearing loss, a decrease in their sense of taste and smell, and voice muscles may slacken. There may be a loss in sensations of touch resulting in a reduced ability to feel pain. This loss of the pain reflex increases the risk of injury and even serious injuries such as fractures, may not be obvious.

**Epidermal system:** there is reduced elasticity and the skin becomes wrinkled and dry, and marked with age spots. The sensation of touch is diminished. Temperature increases in response to infection are less severe.

## 2. Psychological aspect

Eccentricity is more pronounced with age, and can precipitate psychological changes which may influence an individual's personality. These changes can have the following effects:

**Memory**: this begins to fail and there may be difficulty in remembering recent events; but long-term memory usually remains intact.

**Intelligence**: the ability and motivation to learn decreases and elderly people are less likely to undertake new study; the ability to retain new knowledge lessens with age.

**Behaviour**: Some elderly people are more quarrelsome, irritable and overactive and may indulge in antisocial behaviour because of their frustration.

Mental health problems, such as confusion, disorientation and depression may develop. These may be existing disorders or a recurrence. In other cases these problems are a result of the ageing process. Elderly people tend to be inflexible and are frequently unable to modify their behaviour or adapt to new ideas.

### 3. Social aspect

Many people dread growing old. There are many negative attitudes and prejudices towards the elderly that can isolate them from normal social activities. Although some elderly are unable to contribute much to society, others continue to enjoy life and benefit from the social sphere in which they live, sometimes to an advanced age.

## Factors influencing old age

### Physical state

The presence of chronic and painful conditions, particularly those which limit mobility and increase dependency, and the inability to cope with daily living activities can have a detrimental effect on the physical state. Good physical health usually relates to good mental health.

### Social state

As people grow older, their social needs change and hectic social activities give way to more settled habits. Instead of chasing after new pursuits they prefer to establish and maintain contacts with old friends. But in some cases, loneliness and a reduction in the amount of social interaction may make it difficult for the person to accept some of the limitations and expectations of social behaviour. For those who still consider themselves young, in spite of advancing years, remarks such as 'be your age' or 'dirty old man' are very damaging. This antogonistic attitude from younger family members or companions can lead to social isolation, loneliness and loss of status, and may have negative effects on mental health.

However, in the presence of supportive relationships and regular contact with others, elderly people have the potential to continue their social life, develop new relationships and will make a worthwhile contribution to their family and community as a whole.

## Problems in maintaining social contacts

- Personal interests: the ability to meet leisure needs and develop meaningful activities generates a sense of purpose and avoids boredom. Inability to continue activities that give meaning to life leads to frustration and despair
- Housing conditions: higher numbers of the elderly live in the poorest housing conditions, ie. those which are cold, poorly maintained and with limited hygiene facilities. A warm, safe and clean environment gives a sense of security and promotes good physical and mental health
- Income: elderly people with reduced income can live in abject poverty. Therefore financial security is an important resource that helps to avoid money worries and gives the person a sense of freedom, control and choice
- Stress experienced: bereavement, specific worries and adverse life events are distressing but not always avoidable. The ability to develop a stable, forceful personality to cope with stress is particularly important in the maintenance of mental health
- Self-esteem: it is important for the older person to develop a strong internalised sense of self-worth and to accept his or her own ageing process.

Other factors which can influence a person's attitude to the ageing process include life-style, occupation, life experiences, illness, trauma and death.

## Categories of elderly people

Elderly people in hospital or nursing homes may be categorised as follows:
- Geriatrics: a branch of medicine covering old age and its associated disorders
- Psychogeriatrics: this is a branch of psychological medicine concerned with psychiatric disorders which develop in elderly people over the age of 65 years. The majority of confused elderly people are cared for at home

by their spouses and relatives. Others are cared for in hospitals, old people's homes, registered nursing homes and Social Services Part 3 Accommodations. This category is generally known as 'elderly mentally infirm' (EMI)
- Well-preserved: This grade relates to those who could look after themselves, manage their affairs, but are in residential care homes due to social problems.

## Admission to institutions for care

The number of elderly people in the community is growing and the majority live in their own homes, enjoying normal healthy lives and contributing to community life. When there is a breakdown of health, many will continue to be cared for in the community within the National Health Service and Community Care Act 1990/95. Reasons for admission to institutions for care may include:

### Inability to cope

- The recent death of a loved one or a close friend may cause feelings of hopelessness and increase the elderly person's level of dependence, necessitating short-term admission to care. In some cases, spouses or family are unable to cope and a long-term admission to the hospital or nursing home is the only alternative. Elderly people are usually forced to take this action because they too are frail and unable to meet the personal needs of their relatives without help. The elderly person may be unable to cope with the home environment and this may result in damage to the caring relationship.

### Specific disease

- In addition to problems relating to performance of activities of daily living, some elderly people also suffer from chronic ill health, physical conditions associated with poor nutrition and diabetes, medical conditions, such as pneumonia or psychological conditions, such as dementia.

## Care of the elderly

Caring for the elderly is an extremely demanding and often stressful experience. The situation is made worse by deterioration in physical, psychological and social health. The carers will need to develop and extend their skills. For example, by training as a health educator, counsellor or support person for the client and his/her family or by acting as an advocate or a spokesperson.

## Aims of care

Generally the three main aims are to: promote independence; identify and achieve a realistic outcome and establish a key support.

## Framework for care

The ideology of care is directed to maintaining a client's independence, self-respect and dignity. The person is helped to maintain his or her lifestyle and use his/her remaining skills to enjoy as high a standard and quality of life as possible. The implementation of care is based on a comprehensive assessment of physical, psychological, social and spiritual needs of all individual elderly people upon admission, and planning care to meet those needs. Access to care involves the use of an Individualised Care Plan (Nursing Process) based on Activities of Daily Living. This important aspect of care is based on the concept that individual clients will be given a choice and be involved in decision-making and the control of their care and lives.

# References

Faulkner N (1996) *Nursing: The Reflective Approach to Adult Nursing*. Chapman and Hall, London

Harper M (1991) *Management and Care of the Elderly. Psychological Perspectives*. Sage Publications, London

Ironbar NO, Hooper A (1988) *Self-instruction in Mental Health Nursing*. Bailliere Tindall, London

Kyriazis M (1994) Age of reason. Theory of ageing, ageing mechanisms. *Nurs Times* **90**(18): 61–3

Laurent C (1992) The heart of ageing. *Nurs Times* **88**(20): 18–19

MacGuire J (1993) *Primary Nursing in Elderly Care*. King's Fund Centre, London

Shukla R (1994) *Care of the Elderly*. HMSO, London

Schulman J (1989) Informing the patient. *Nurs Elderly* 1(1): 142

Roper N, Logan W, Tierney A (1997) *The Elements of Nursing*, 3rd edn. Churchill Livingstone, Edinburgh

Tyler J (1992) Travesties of care: rights of elderly people. *Nurs Elderly* **4**(3): 24–25

Wynn M, Wynn A (1993) Catering concerns: Older people — nutrition. *Nurs Times* **89**(20): 61–64

## Audio visual aids

### Format: VHS video

Ref: *For Old Time's Sake (Killing Time)*. Concord Film Council

Ref: *Ten Million People* (VHS Video). BBC Enterprises Hire Library

Ref: CNE 3634: *Healing Handbook: Myths of Ageing*

Ref: CME 5334: *Principles of Geriatrics*

Ref: CME 5730: *NIH Update: Ageing*

Oxford Educational Resources Ltd

# Assignment

The purpose of this homework is to assist you in preparing for your Workbased Assessment of Competence. As there is no pressure on you, feel free to work at your own pace, but avoid the temptation to procrastinate. After you have read your notes and suggested references, submit your work for correction. The completed work becomes part of your Personal Portfolio.

## The elderly person: human ageing

1. Discuss the concept of the human ageing process.
2. Give a brief description of the three main categories of elderly people generally found in a care institution.
3. What are the reasons that may be given for the first admission of an elderly person to a care institution?
4. Discuss the factors that may influence the health of an elderly person in later life.
5. State briefly the aims and principles of care of the elderly.

## Section II: Essential supporting skills

Skill is defined as 'ability, talent, cleverness, proficiency, practised ability and facility in an action' (*The Pocket Oxford Dictionary*, 1987). Skills are the most significant tools and when used in various combinations can be a formidable force in bringing about total client care. These include interpersonal relationships, problem solving, counselling, observation, social and communication skills. But observation and reporting skills are the hallmark of a high standard and quality of care, and should be developed by every member of the care team.

As front line workers, care assistants should develop these skills so that they can recognise and prevent serious problems from worsening, and earn the respect of their colleagues. Other members of the care team depend upon accurate information based on observation and reporting in order to manage each client's care programme effectively. It is therefore essential to bring your observations to the attention of those in charge, no matter how trivial these may appear.

At the end of this section, candidates should be able to understand the importance of developing and using the following skills and knowledge in care:

|  | Units and Elements of Learning | |
|---|---|---|
| **Caring skills** | | 21 |
| o Observation and reporting (monitoring) | OD2 | 21 |
| o Problem-solving and decision-making | CU8: 1–2 | 24 |
| o Counselling skills | CU8: 1–2 | 28 |
| **Appendages for care** | | 34 |
| o Standards and quality of care | NC4: 1–4, NC11: 1–3 | 34 |
| o Models of care | NC4: 1–4, NC11: 1–3 | 38 |
| o Research appreciation | CU7.2, CU8.1 | 44 |
| o Advocacy for clients | Z2: 1–4 | 50 |
| o Effectiveness of team-work | CU9: 1–3, CU10: 1–2 | 54 |
| o Management of change | NC2: 1–2 | 57 |

# Caring skills (OD2, CU8)

## Observation and reporting (monitoring) (OD2)

Today, the concept of total client care is based on the belief that an individual is a functional whole, ie. there is a constant interaction between physical, psychological, environmental, social and spiritual well-being of the person. The outcome of this interaction affects the person's ability to cope and live independently. It also forms the basis upon which the needs of the person are assessed for care.

Some members of the decision-making team, especially doctors, see their clients for one hour a day. Consequently, unless specifically brought to their attention, they are unaware of events and relationships which take place during the remaining 23 hours, events which may be relevant to care. Information with respect to a client's ability to function independently is important when planning the treatment and care necessary to meet his/her total care needs.

**Observation skills**

This is the ability to 'examine, take note and remark' on clients' conditions. It is a conscious mechanism through which we see and recognise things as they are, through our senses and experience.

| 1 | Eyes | are used for sight (watching) |
|---|---|---|
| 2 | Nose | is the organ which recognises smell |
| 3 | Tongue | used for tasting; bitter, sweet, sour, salt |
| 4 | Ears | are organs for hearing |
| 5 | Skin | the sense of touch, ie assessing temperatures |
| 6 | Intuition | or extra sensory perception (ESP). This may be a feeling or 'hunch' and is often developed through experience. It is a combination of conscious and unconscious skills used in assessing a situation which prompts further investigations. This awareness can help the development of insight, a useful attribute in the care environment |

In order to observe and report objectively, it is necessary to have a holistic knowledge of the person, ie. what to look for, and how to recognise indications, such as signs and symptoms of common conditions. For example, redness of the skin and swelling of the legs could indicate oedema. Lack of knowledge, inattention or distraction may result in symptoms which present and then fail to be recognised. Constant vigilance is necessary to avoid missing such signs of ill health or mental disorder.

## Clients' needs

These are caring problems which are generally known as individual clients' total care needs. They are the outcome of the assessment which forms the basis of the care plan. They vary from person to person in intensity and may not be readily apparent. Some develop in a few days, others take months to appear; they may be imagined or real and some may be a reaction to drugs, such as rashes or salivation (dribbling of saliva). Clients should be observed discretely and continuously. Observation and reporting should be recorded in individual clients' care plans as follows:

### 1. *Physical well-being*
- safety: poor eyesight, bumps and falls, risk of burns
- eating and drinking: nutrition and warmth: weight loss, malnutrition, dehydration
- elimination: incontinence, constipation, menstruation (eg. elderly ladies on HRT)
- skin: scratches, rashes, pressure sores, wounds, bruises, hot and clammy
- mobility: poor mobility may be due to swollen and painful joints, ingrowing toe nails, corns, poor fitting shoes, problems associated with the use of walking aids
- breathing difficulties: due to bronchitis, coughs, alcohol, acetone in diabetes.

### 2. *Sleep, rest and relaxation*
- insomnia, sleep-walking, nightmares, dreams, noise, restlessness.

### 3. *Social well-being*
- isolation and loneliness
- sexuality and sexual identity
- interest in occupational or diversional therapies, leisure and social activities, age-related games and activities, coach outings, listening to the radio, watching TV, reading
- contact with relatives, significant others, pets
- lifestyle, confidence, self-respect, dignity, independence.

### 4. *Spiritual well-being*
- interest in attending church services, receiving the Holy Sacraments.

### 5. *Psychological well-being*
- communication: slow and deliberate, rambling, incoherent speech or mute
- depression, forgetfulness, confusion, delusion, hallucination, paranoia
- expression of self-harm, suicidal or homicidal talk — report to the person-in-charge
- behaviour, for example overactivity, violence, aggression, manipulation, bad language.

### 6. *Environmental influences*
- inability to settle in
- independent living and ability to look after self and personal belongings
- awareness of new environment and desire to socialise with other residents.

### 7. *Special investigations*
- results of investigations, eg. TPR, blood pressure, urine tests.

## Reporting skills

Accurate and objective accounts of changes and management in the total care needs of individual clients, their conditions, complaints and other relevant data should be recorded. This information is written on official records, such as report books, care plans or computers. Personal computerised information is maintained in accordance with the requirements of the Data Protection Act 1984. All health care records are confidential documents that must be accurately written, jargon-free, signed and handed over at the end of each shift of duty.

**Written reports**

### *Guidance*
- follow organisational policy, guidelines and practices on reporting on clients
- demonstrate knowledge of methods of obtaining information, the purpose for which it may be required and the necessary details
- check the sources of information
- write notes on paper first, then check for accuracy and spelling. Consult the person-in-charge and transfer the report on to the care plan
- write clearly, neatly and legibly, using ink in accordance with organisational policy
- be aware of legal requirements on reporting and maintenance of records, eg. Data Protection Act 1991, Mental Health Act 1983
- correct errors by drawing a single line through the error and signing it. **Never** erase on a record
- write the date and time, and sign every new entry in the care plan
- demonstrate good practice by maintaining security of records, especially where these are being transferred to another home, or taken to a hospital
- keep all information confidential, and be aware of ways in which confidentiality may be breached. Report any violation to the proper authority
- on completion of procedures, write down only those procedures which you have done
- refuse to provide information of a confidential nature to unauthorised persons, but remain polite and helpful
- **watch, look, listen, develop and trust your skill.**

**Legal requirement**

Daily statements about clients should be made in accordance with the requirements of the Nursing Homes Act 1984. These statements should include response to treatment, information on drugs, ie. types, dosages, frequency of administration and any side-effects. Reports should also be made about special visits and clients' functional ability in relation to the part that these play in activities of daily living. All hand-written health care records are not legal documents, but may be required in a court of law.

# References

Barber B (1992) Security screening. *Nurs Times* **88**(49): 50–52

Bryant N, Griffths G (1985) Caught in the act? *Nurs Times* **81**(6): 16–17

Data Protection Registrar (1989) *Guidelines 1–8*. Office of the Data Protection Registrar, Winslow

Flack M, Johnson M (1986) *A Handbook for Care: Practical Guidelines for Care Assistants*. Beaconsfield Publishers Ltd, Bucks

Robertson B (1992) *Study Guide for Health and Social Care Workers*. First Class Books Inc, USA

**Audio visual aids**

***Format: VHS video***
Ref: *Interpersonal Communication Skills* (VHS/Cassette)

Ref: *Professional Telephone Skills*
Career Track Inc

# Assignment

The purpose of this homework is to assist you in preparing for your Workbased Assessment of Competence. As there is no pressure on you, feel free to work at your own pace, but avoid the temptation to procrastinate. After you have read your notes and suggested references, submit your work for correction. The completed work becomes part of your Personal Portfolio.

## Observation and reporting (OD2)

1. What do you understand by the term 'observation and reporting'?
2. Discuss the importance of observation and reporting in care.
3. Mr Andrew Jones, an 87-year-old gentleman is one of the residents in your Primary Nursing Team, and you are assigned responsibility for his care. What report would you give to the leader of your team at the end of your shift of duty on:
   a) his personal cleanliness
   b) nutritional needs
   c) how you spent your time with him.
4. Discuss how you would deal with an infuriated man, who claims to be the husband of one of your clients, and asks for telephone information about the condition of his wife?

## Problem-solving and decision-making (CU8: 1–2)

Problems are met daily when a prescribed course of action needs to be taken to alter the situation. The issue may involve changes in work routines or difficulty in empathising with colleagues. Resolving these problems depends on your experience and your ability to relate and communicate effectively. In caring for people, difficult situations are encountered daily. The demands of these situations require flexibility of ideas, attitudes and judgement to enable you to find solutions.

As professionals, we are required to accept responsibility for the decisions and actions we take in the course of our work. It follows that every action or decision we make regarding clients' care has possible outcomes which may or may not be desirable, but we must accept that responsibility. Frequently, decisions taken to solve problems contain element of risks, and so every member of the health care team should be equipped with strategies for solving problems and making informed decisions.

### Advantages of problems

Most problems challenge our intellect and understanding, and our ability to investigate, report and work as a team on difficult issues. We are continually faced with situations in which we have to make a decision. For example, a client may ask a question which you have difficulty in answering, eg. 'nurse, what is this tablet for?' You must reply but may not immediately know the answer. The advantage of problems is that they provide us with a learning situation that can be used to find answers and to reinforce our confidence. As individuals we use our natural inborn abilities, and process the information available to us within the environment. This process is known as a *problem-solving* approach.

## Problem-solving

Basically, this is a general term for an experience in which the individual, faced with a complex situation, uses initiative and his/her intelligence to achieve the goal and learn new skills. Problem-solving is influenced by our beliefs, values, culture and attitudes. For example, at work we may prefer to spend more time with one client rather than another, or at home we may spend money on our children or pets and not on ourselves. Decisions for these actions may be due to our culture, beliefs and commitment to the needs of others based on our experiences. The process, therefore, emphasises the need for an individual or group to take responsibility for seeking solutions to the problems, and learning from experiences generated, rather than believing that an inimical force is working against them or that the problems are insoluble.

## A problem-solving cycle

The key to problem solving begins with a systematic assessment of needs and proceeds to making decisions. It involves a series of stages which enables an individual or a group to examine a problem systematically and choose the best possible solution from a number of correct answers, committing themselves to act upon it in future. The approach is designed to reveal relevant information for each step, and then move to the next stage as appropriate. Each stage is given a time allocation beginning with experience.

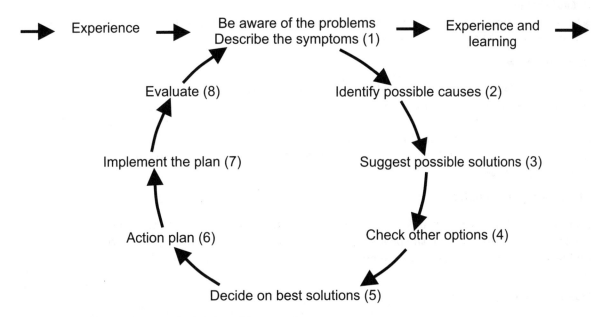

**A simple problem-solving cycle (Klob and Fry, 1975)**

## The approach

An individual or a group of people may be asked to carry out the following steps and learn from the experience gained.

### 1. Be aware of symptoms
- describe the event in detail, including the specific concerns which brought the problem to light.

### 2. Identify possible causes
- detect possible causes. A brainstorming exercise may be used.

### 3. Suggest possible solutions
- list likely solutions, if necessary using a brainstorming exercise. Be aware of barriers which may hinder progress, eg. staff attitudes or resources.

### 4. Check other options
- examine the advantages and disadvantages of each option, assessing their usefulness for short or long-term solutions.

### 5. Decide on the best solution
- decide which solution is most likely to succeed.

### 6. Devise an action plan
- design an action plan and identify the steps needed to achieve success; check the resources required
- set a target for achieving the goal and select methods for evaluating the outcome.

### 7. Implement
- put the plan into action.

### 8. Evaluate the outcome
- assess the overall results. Review each stage taking into account the resources and action produced. Reflect and reinforce the plans made and learn from the experience gained.

## Brainstorming

This is a simple means of producing ideas. Each member of the group is required to generate as many ideas as possible about the problem under discussion, without pausing to think or evaluate them. One member makes a list of all the ideas generated and, at the end of this exercise, the group evaluates them for their suitability for implementation, ranking them in order of priority. Some ideas may be bizarre and impractical, but others may be innovative and nothing suggested is considered useless.

## The role of care assistants

As members of the decision-making team, care assistants should be able to assist in all stages of the process. They help to define the problems, devise measures which will help to overcome the issues and learn through the experiences generated. The person-in-charge should be able to facilitate and lead the group.

## Decision-making in care

The idea of involving residents and their relatives in the decision-making process in care was considered controversial until recently, partly because of the 'whistle-blowing' possibilities. The advent of rights, choice and justice in care based on an individualised care approach (Nursing Process) has abolished this argument, and clients are now taken into partnership in their care. This involves consulting them on all aspects of care, through the use of a modified version of the decision-making process that is based on their needs and ability to participate. The aim is to involve them and their relatives in the process, although there are no guarantees that a correct decision will be made. Methods used are similar to those of democratic leadership and include combinations such as 'tell', 'sell', 'consult' or 'involve'.

The idea of 'selling' involves 'telling' the person what has been decided by the health care team, and seeking the person's co-operation as feedback. This involves giving information or explanation on the care topic which has been decided by the health care team, through the skilful use of the 'questions and answers' technique. Some elderly people often feel more secure with a firm leadership approach, and will accept the decision more readily if it is based on the premise that he or she had been consulted, and so contributed to the decision-making process. However, others may be unable to express their wishes or make their feelings known due to the nature of their condition, eg. confusion or frailty. In this case, next of kin should be consulted or the person's advocate. The outcome should be that the decision taken will be in the best interests of the person concerned. But it is important that when opportunities arise, those involved socialise with the client and use such moments to gain an insight into his or her wishes.

The act of 'selling' really means counselling and persuading the individual to accept changes in his or her treatment and care. This is usually carried out by the doctor who is responsible for the person's treatment along with the person-in-charge. Generally, clients will accept advice which is given with respect to their current anxieties, particularly when they are a party to the decision-making process.

# References

Aspinall MJ, Tanner CA (1981) *Decision-making for Patient Care*. Appleton-Century-Crofts, New York

Broom A (1990) *Managing change. Essentials for Nursing Management*, Macmillan Education, London

Carson D (1988) Taking risks with patients: Your assessment strategy. *Prof Nurse* **3**(247): 247–50

Heron J (1973) *Experimental Training Techniques*. Human Potential Research Project, University of Surrey

Kilty J (1982) Feelings: learning from practical experience. *Nurs Times* **2**(4 educ suppl): 1–5

Klob DA, Fry D (1975) Towards applied theory of experiential learning. In: Cooper CL (ed) *Theories of Group Process*. J Wiley & Sons, Chichester

Macklin D (1982) Just imagine. *Nurs Times* **2**(4 educ suppl): 5–7

Miers M (1990) Developing skills in decision-making. *Nurs Times* **86**(30): 32–3

United Kingdom Central Council for Nursing, Midwifery and Health Visiting (1989) *Exercising Accountability*. UKCC, London

## Audio visual aids

### Format: VHS video
Ref: DEC: *Decisions, Decisions*. Video Arts Production, London
Ref: CEM 8187: *Decision Exercises. Dealing with Difficult Situations*
Ref: CEM 6311: *Communication. How to Manage Conflict*
Ref: CEM 8443: *Communication for Results*
Oxford Educational Resources Ltd

# ASSIGNMENT

The purpose of this homework is to assist you in preparing for your Workbased Assessment of Competence. As there is no pressure on you, feel free to work at your own pace, but avoid the temptation to procrastinate. After you have read your notes and suggested references, submit your work for correction. The completed work becomes part of your Personal Portfolio.

## Problem-solving and decision-making (CU8: 1–2)

1. Define the what you mean by 'problem-solving and decision-making'.
2. Discuss how the acquisition of this knowledge and skill could be useful in your:
    a) Place of work
    b) Personal life.
3. Give two examples of the part you personally played in solving a problem relating to the care of one of your clients.
4. A client is reluctant to accept a decision made on his behalf. Discuss how this problem could be resolved in order to protect his wishes and best interests.

## Counselling skills (CU8: 1–2)

The term 'counselling' is difficult to define as it involves the use of special skills which make it possible for people to gain a deeper understanding of their situation. It is concerned with people finding solutions to their own problems without advice from outside. Counselling is a specialised subject in which counsellors undergo a recognised training. It provides and develops in them an insight into their own individual personal problems, beliefs, attitudes, prejudices and emotional needs.

The practice of counselling is based on mutual trust, respect and good relationships. Carers and other professionals use similar skills to support their clients and improve the standard and quality of care in their individual practices. It is generally known as an 'emotional walking stick'. Communication, observation, social listening, befriending, supporting and paraphrasing are the skills widely used. Goldberg (1986) believes that because carers are people in emotional need, they can understand and recognise the need for personal help themselves. However, the use of these skills by carers does not make them counsellors.

### Care assistants

These are the front-line workers, who use various life and counselling skills in their daily contact with residents for the purpose of carrying out specific tasks. They dress, undress and bathe clients, and while carrying out these tasks, they use the opportunity to talk and establish a good rapport and friendship with residents. During this period of close contact, a carer may notice that the resident appears unwell, or may be heard to remark that he/she is feeling sad or distressed. The carer can then offer the client the 'counselling' and support which he or she needs. Start by trying to find out what the problem is and offer help. Even if time is limited, the carer should ensure that the client is allowed to communicate his/her distress.

## Personal support

Carers who use counselling skills in their work must ensure that they have access to adequate personal support system themselves. They should know the limits of their ability and if the help needed exceeds the carer's capabilities, he/she should refer residents to the person-in-charge who will arrange for specialist help. If the client is crying and expresses intentions of self-harm, it is crucial to discuss the matter with the person-in-charge, but explain your decision to the resident concerned before doing so.

## Counselling skills

The ability to communicate effectively offers a chance for expression of feelings, giving and receiving of information and assessment of the situation. Being a good listener, expressing things in your own words, allowing other people to express their feelings, reflecting back to them and at times challenging their belief, is also useful. Munro (1991) states that becoming skilled in counselling techniques, involves taking risks by revealing parts of yourself to others (self-disclosure). At the same time, you should learn to ask for, and accept feedback from others about the effects of your behaviour on them. An ability to build a trusting and confidential relationship over a period of time is good, but the use of counselling skills requires special training.

## Other skills

These include:
- supporting, empathising and sharing clients' feelings
- honesty, flexibility, showing respect and helping the person to set goals
- being non-judgmental and using self-disclosure where appropriate
- establishing a secure atmosphere which encourages free expression
- treating as highly confidential the other person's confidences
- facilitating catharsis, ie. freeing repressed feeling.

## Specific skills include:

### 1. Active listening
- give your full attention and provide feedback to what has been said.

### 2. Social
- receive and greet the person to affirm his or her identity with a handshake, or an embrace.

### 3. Friendship
- demonstrate affection in recognition of the other person's uniqueness. It is a an expression of companionship and emotional attraction.

### 4. Communication
- convey ideas and feelings effectively, in order to achieve a positive action or reaction.

## Using counselling skills

There are many ways of using counselling skills, but the most suitable method is a one-to-one, non-directive approach which is based on the belief that the individual can, with help, resolve his or her own difficulties over a period of time. In the course of providing personal care, you may see a resident who is usually happy appear to be sad and distressed. It is important to encourage the person to talk about his or her anxieties and feelings. But do not give opinions or advice. The approach should be as follows:

## Guidance
- find a quiet room where you will not be disturbed for about half an hour. If you are in the resident's room, close the door. Always provide appropriate conditions and privacy in a comfortable environment
- ensure that the person is comfortable, either sitting in a chair or lying down
- sit comfortably opposite the client; lean slightly forward and relax
- maintain effective eye contact but do not stare.

### 1. Assess and identify symptoms of the problem
Ask questions only if you need to clarify a point you do not understand. Start by giving the client an opportunity to talk by using open ended questions to find out how the client sees his or her situation — use words, such as 'what', 'how' 'where', 'when'.

**Example:** 'You seem to be upset. What is happening to you to make you feel that way?'

Ask the person to clarify a situation. Having given him/her the opportunity to explore his/her feelings, listen attentively.

*Allow time to think and respond*

**Example:** The resident may say to the nurse, 'I don't feel well, am I dying'?

The response could be 'what makes you ask that question? What is happening to you to make you to ask that question?' Encourage the person to talk more about his/her problem or difficulty, by occasionally breaking in. Demonstrate verbal listening skills by saying:
- 'could you tell me more about that'
- 'how did you feel when that happened' or 'you felt depressed?'
- 'tell me more — go on', 'give an example of what you mean by that'

*Allow time to think and respond*

It is believed that, by allowing the person to talk about him or herself, then the healing process will begin.

### 2. Identify possible causes of the problem
The carer helps to identify the causes or meaning of the problem by asking: 'what is the meaning of it' or 'what do you think that might be?' The carer then reflects back to the client the fact that he/she seems distressed and offers an opportunity for him/her to explore the issues further.

*Allow time to think and respond*

When he/she has finished, ask him/her to reflect and think of what to do — but do not give advice. Instead:
- summarise and reflect back to the individual what he or she has said, with emphasis on important points which have been learnt
- encourage the person to try to identify the changes or new skills he or she may need to reach his or her goal, and report any changes.

*Allow time to think and respond*

The person may be able to express feelings about his or her problems, and accept responsibility by saying 'I suppose it was my fault and I think I'll do X, Y, Z'.

### 3. Planning — setting the goal

Once the problem has been identified and clarified, help the resident to set a realistic goal by asking 'what are you going to do now?' or 'what is happening here?' It is important to spend time with the person so that he/she finds the right goal without you giving advice. It is possible to consider many choices, but the client must be helped to select a realistic goal which can be achieved and not to attempt too much, for example, 'I suppose I have to think about it'.

### 4. Implementation

This is a stage in which the person decides what action he or she wishes to take in order to achieve the goal, in response to the question, 'what are you going to do about it?' Both parties may enter into a moral contract in which the carer trusts the client to do what was agreed. Neither should expect miracles as attitudes cannot be changed overnight. The person should be able to identify the changes or new skills he or she needs to reach a goal.

### 5. Evaluation

This is the summary of the overall results, which may not take place immediately. Progress is continually reviewed and reinforced, and any resources used are reviewed. The client's motivation is a major factor.

## Catharsis

This is a release of repressed feelings, generally by spoken words, and at times accompanied by the shedding of tears. This may be the result of the death of a loved one, an accident, or other traumatic events in a person's life. It is hoped that through the shedding of tears the client may be able to gain an insight, resume self-control and regain the capacity to love and understand, and thus choose to allow healing to take place.

## A helping approach

The carer should allow catharsis to continue until the client experiences false shame, embarrassment and laughter. At this point the client reaches down into the hidden place of hurt emotion (distress) and accepts and honours these painful experiences. This is followed by the release of pain itself. He or she may grieve and sob, tremble and express fear, anger, and may even scream. During this phase the carer has the scope to intervene by touching or echo-posturing, and by making practical suggestions. But the decision to 'take' belongs to the individual client. The carer may ask 'What are you thinking?' 'How do you feel about it?'

> ### Guidance
> - show your genuine concern and caring
> - advise the client to be patient and not to expect too much from him/herself, and not to impose any self-coercion
> - talk about the special, endearing qualities of the lost companion/friend/pet
> - reassure the client that he/she did everything that he/she could
> - do not say you know how he/she feels, unless you have had a similar experience yourself
> - do not tell him/her what he/she should feel or react with tactless phrases, such as 'pull yourself together'
> - do not make comments which may suggest that the problem was his/her fault.

## Stress

This is a demand on mental resilience by passing events and the strain experienced in response to them. Stress is an invisible pressure and an integral part of human existence. It is closely related to anger, fear, grief, embarrassment and we react to it in different ways. A moderate amount is essential for effective functioning. A person's behaviour and feelings must be organised into an acceptable mode to enable him or her to minimise the potential for emotional distress.

### Coping mechanism

The aim is to build up a defence against feelings of strong emotion, and there are many ways of doing this. Some people may laugh, cry, shout or scream, blame other people (projection) or make an excuse for a personal reaction.

#### 1. Immediate
- reflect on the situation, think through possible causes and identify your feelings
- accept your feelings and shortcomings and try to come to terms with them
- express appropriate feelings, have a good cry, scream, laugh or shout
- examine and direct your feelings to something else, eg. active work or humming a tune.

#### 2. Long-term
- talk to a friend about your problem; remember a problem shared is a problem halved
- seek information, modify your feelings, develop a decision and problem-solving skill
- network and attempt to change a difficult situation by being assertive
- explore alternatives, learn new skills, eg. relaxation and develop coping mechanisms.

### Usefulness of counselling skills

Counselling skills are useful in every life situation, for the exploration of fear, bitter feelings, resentments, frustrations, hopelessness and anger. In most cases it is a one-to-one meeting in which confidentiality of information is respected. Summarising, the discussion, will enable you and the client to confirm and grasp what the difficulty is, and understand each other. If you have not practised counselling before, it is advisable that you try it out with someone you can trust. It is important to recognise that counselling has its limitations, and it is necessary to report to the person-in-charge the need of clients for counselling.

### Silence

This is the ability to keep quiet without speech or making any sound, and many people feel uncomfortable or awkward with silence. It has its place in counselling sessions, as it allows time for clients to gather their thoughts and reflect on what had been said and what they need to say.

# References

Armstrong E (1994) *Best Practice in Counselling Skills*. RCN Update. Learning Unit 049. Nursing Standard, RCN, London
British Counselling Association (1989) *Training Directory*. BCA, Rugby.
Heron J (1990) *Helping the Client. A Creative Practical Guide*. Sage Publications, London
Macleod-Clark J, Hooper J, Jensen A (1991) Progression to counselling. *Nurs Times* **87**(8): 41–43
Munro A, Manthei B, Small J (1991) *Counselling: The Skills of Problem Solving*. Routledge, London
Tschudin V (1992) *Counselling Skills for Nurses*. Bailliere Tindall, London

## Audio visual aids

**Format: VHS video**

Ref: CNE 4373: *Stress Management for Nurses*
Ref: *Best Practice in Counselling*. RCN Nursing Update on BBC 1
Ref: CEM 8528: *Workplace Stress*
Oxford Educational Resources Ltd

# ASSIGNMENT

The purpose of this homework is to assist you in preparing for your Workbased Assessment of Competence. As there is no pressure on you, feel free to work at your own pace, but avoid the temptation to procrastinate. After you have read your notes and suggested references, submit your work for correction. The completed work becomes part of your Personal Portfolio.

## Counselling skills (CU8: 1-2)

1. What is 'counselling'?
2. Differentiate between 'befriending' and 'counselling' someone.
3. Identify three situations in which the use of this skill might be appropriate in your area of care.
4. Give an example of a situation in which you would report the need of a client for counselling to the person-in-charge.

# Appendages for care (CU5, CU7, CU8, CU9, CU10, NC2, NC4, NC11, Z2)

## Standards and quality of care (NC4: 1–4, NC11: 1–3)

Elderly people enter hospitals, nursing homes and residential care homes because they are ill or old and need personal care. The need for these services is universal, and clients who use them are known as *consumers* of the service to receive care.

The Patient's Charter (1995) sets out standards which the public should expect in various public services, including public expectations in health care. It means that as consumers, elderly people are entitled to fundamental rights — to choice, to information, to have their voice heard, to be treated with dignity; and to have their rights and beliefs respected at all times. They also have the right to take risks, to entertain their friends, the right of access to health facilities, and to live their life as they choose within reason. In other words, they are entitled to a good quality and value-for-money service, and any breach of these rights may incur a complaint and/or litigation.

### Standard of care

There is a right and a wrong way of doing things, and the consequences of using the wrong approach may, indeed, be serious. 'Standards' describe an agreed quality and level of performance workers have to achieve, in relation to knowledge, skills and attitude. They are the outcome of what we must do to bring about customers' satisfaction. In the health care sector, every employer has the right to set their own individual standards. But the National Occupational Standards set out an agreed level of performance for care assistants. The standard should be achievable, observable and measurable. In order to ensure standards and quality of service, it is important that everyone should consider their own attitudes, values and beliefs to ensure that decisions taken on standards of care are based on research knowledge.

### Quality of care

In recent years people have become more conscious of the need for a high quality of care, and associate this with their rights to maintain personal lifestyle, dignity and independence. The NHS and Community Care Act (1993) requires purchasers and providers of services to have an interest in the quality of the service that they provide. Quality relates to the ability of the company to find out what their customers need, and to be able to deliver a service to meet these needs. In health care settings, it means delivering care to meet physical, psychological and social needs. The care must be acceptable from the point of view of the service users, individual practitioners, the care team, the medical or health care profession, health care organisations and the government. It is not easily achievable, and requires the right people, equipment, environment, attitude of mind and training.

### Duty of care

This means an average care, carried out by competent carers taking reasonable care and precautions against accidents. The care should be given, when carrying out the duties one is employed to perform, without causing material loss or damage to the employers or unnecessary risk or injury to clients or colleagues. Care assistants should try to do their best at all times to meet a reasonable standard of care. If they are required to take on new duties, they must be satisfied that they can do the work competently or should seek guidance and/or refuse to carry out duties that are incompatible with their level of competence. The consequence of accidents in care could give rise to lawsuits if incompetence is suspected.

### Assault

This is an unfair personal attack which causes a person to believe that he or she is going to suffer immediate and unjust harm or violence. For example, a carer who shakes a fist under the nose of a client or points a pen at the person in anger, is guilty of an assault. Restraining someone without consent is unlawful and may also constitute assault.

### Battery

This is a deliberate or reckless act of outrage on another person, such as delivering a blow to any part of the body.

### False documentation

This involves making statements or entries that are not true or altering information in a client's record. No attempt should be made to erase a record. Errors should be corrected by drawing a single line through the mistake, then signing or initialling it.

### Negligence

Ignoring the consequences of your actions can be construed as carelessness. Negligence may also be construed as a failure to carry out a duty (omission) or carrying out duties incorrectly. It could be the result of poor delegation, bad management or failure to observe and report on clients' care. Every duty carries the risk of a charge of negligence but, in order to prove an oversight, the allegation must show that:
- the carer owes the client a duty of care
- there has been a breach of this duty of care
- the client has suffered harm or damage as a result of the action or omission.

Negligence is a way of establishing liability so that clients can sue the person who caused the damage or his/her employers. The boundaries between neglect and assault may not always be apparent to hard-pressed staff in an emergency. However, in English law, although the carer may be at fault, it is employers who are liable for negligence, because they should be aware of what their employees know and do. In theory, employers could recover an 'indemnity' from a negligent or careless employee.

### Defamation

This is making a statement which lowers or damages the reputation or credibility of a person, and causes the individual to be shunned by others. Defamation may be:
- libel — a written statement
- slander — a spoken statement.

Care assistants should not give any information or make statements to anyone outside the immediate circle of the health care team. All requests for information should be directed to the person-in-charge in accordance with organisational policy. Care must also be taken to ensure that what we do or say does not cause harm or injury to anyone.

**Complaint code**

Dissatisfaction by users of the service or with employees that is made known to any member of staff can result in a complaint. This may be a real grievance, expressed verbally or in writing, that relates to tangible objects, such as loss of money or wedding rings. Complaints are often the outcome of a failure in communication that causes the client hardship or distress. It can also be an expression of feelings such as, 'it is too hot or too cold' or 'I asked for a drink ages ago, and I'm still waiting' or 'I can't see to read'. These are all complaints and must be reported in accordance with the policy of the home, together with any suspicions of abuse.

**Making complaints**

This can be extremely difficult and, as a result, the staff member concerned may face victimisation from colleagues and/or management. There is no doubt that many cases go unreported for these reasons. Another type of 'whistle-blowing' is a staff complaint about poorly maintained standards of client or patient care that are due to extenuating circumstances, such as inadequate staffing levels or resources. All complaints must be reported and recorded, including those from visitors and relatives. In order to maintain high standards and quality of care, complaints should be dealt with swiftly and thoroughly.

**Gifts from clients**

The question of gifts is linked with professional behaviour towards clients and their relatives, and relates to ethics of care or moral judgement. Care assistants should refuse any gift from clients. Small gifts may lead to embarrassment, and substantial ones may be challenged in the court of law by relatives. Therefore, it is important to follow local policy on gifts from clients.

**Good faith**

The duty of good faith concerns honesty and integrity in carrying out duties. Care assistants must not act in a manner that is likely to prompt other people or clients to resort to litigation in order to redress malpractice, or give a rival home the opportunity to damage the reputation of their current employer.

**Living wills**

It is difficult to draft a will that is clear and legally binding. Avoid offering help in the making or signing of a client's will. Report all requests for this service to the person-in-charge.

**Equal opportunities and anti-discrimination**

It is the duty of care that no client should be treated less favourably than others on the grounds of race, ethnic origin, colour, sex, social status, religious or political persuasions, or because he or she has contracted an infectious disease, such as HIV. All employers are required by law to set out policy stating their commitment to developing equal opportunities and anti-discriminatory practices. However, research has shown that where race is concerned, equal opportunity in employment is still far from being achieved.

## Monitoring standards of care

The background for maintaining standards of care is based on a system which should be included in the organisation's policy on risk-taking and quality of care. Employers should make sure that this policy is understood and agreed by everyone, including residents and their relatives. Managers should then devise and monitor procedures for using it. But the act of monitoring the policy is the work of a team in which care assistants play an important role. They have more contact with clients than any other member of the health care team and it is important that they are trained and supervised in the implementation of the policy.

### *Guidance:*
- develop and maintain good interpersonal relationship skills
- be aware of your organisation's philosophy on risk-taking and quality of care
- observe, monitor and report all activities which focus on client or patient care to the person-in-charge or at the primary care team's meetings
- be aware of local policy on Complaints Procedures and Management of Risk
- demonstrate knowledge of agreed procedures and practices for care, and bring any changes you would like to make to the attention of the person-in-charge or the team meetings
- inform or report to the appropriate person any lack of resources or faulty equipment
- question any aspect of care with which you are unsure or unhappy
- seek guidance if you are required to take on new duties for which you have not received training to carry out satisfactorily
- examine your own attitudes, values, beliefs and role in the organisation
- seek and maintain a personal support system; seek counselling if you experience stress
- be assertive; act as advocate to your clients
- attend training programmes designed to develop your knowledge, skills and attitudes
- beware of participating in activities or procedures that are not in the best interests of those in your care, such as restraining them without their consent
- ensure that the care you provide is documented in individual clients' care plans.

Successful monitoring of the practice of delivery of care to ensure satisfaction, especially client's satisfaction, includes dissemination of information, access to care and continuity of care. Therefore, it is important that you know what part you play in the care setting and also, where and what information is available.

## References

Care Sector Consortium (1992) *National Occupational Standards for Care*. HMSO, London

Department of Health and Social Security (1995) *The Patient's Charter and You*. HMSO, London

Docherty A (1995) Welcoming the challenge to provide quality care. *Caring Times* October 1994. Hawker Publications, London

Handy C (1989) *Age of Unreason*. Business Books, London

Mensah J (1996) Everybody's problem. *Nurs Times* **92**(22): 25–7

Rowdwen R (1990) Colouring attitudes. Racism in nursing. *Nurs Times* **86**(24): 47–8

Speller SR (1972) *Law Notes for Nurses*. RCN, London

Tate CW (1996) Race into action. *Nurs Times* **92**(22): 28–30

Tingle J (1990) Responsible and liable. *Nurs Times* **86**(25): 42–3

Tingle J (1990) A duty of care. Nurses and the law. *Nurs Times* **86**(30): 60–61

Tingle J (1990) Nurses and the law. Ethic ways. *Nurs Times* **86**(43): 60–1

Windup M (1973) The nurses' duties. Occasional papers. *Nurs Times* **69**(32): 125–128

### Audio visual aids

*Format: VHS video*

Ref: CNE 9920: *Nursing Quality Assurance — Define Quality*

Ref: 1137: *The Professional Nurse in Court*

Ref: CNE 4268: *Nursing — Expanding the Quality of Caring*

Ref: CEM 6312: *Motivating People*

Oxford Educational Resources Ltd

## Assignment

The purpose of this homework is to assist you in preparing for your Workbased Assessment of Competence. As there is no pressure on you, feel free to work at your own pace, but avoid the temptation to procrastinate. After you have read your notes and suggested references, submit your work for correction. The completed work becomes part of your Personal Portfolio.

### Standards and quality of care (NC4)

1. What do you understand by the following terms?
   a) quality of care
   b) standards of care
   c) negligence.
2. Describe a situation in which you would help a client to make a complaint, and how you would go about it?
3. Discuss how you would help to monitor the standards and quality of care in the area of your work.

### Models of care (NC4: 1–4, NC11: 1–3)

The aim of this section is to look at the background of the care profession's attempts to deliver quality of care in a more structured way. Although the word 'nurses' is used, it applies equally to care assistants whose role is to support professional qualified practitioners and who are members of the health care team.

For many years, what nurses 'do' has been the subject of discussion at seminars and conferences throughout the world. Nursing authors have tried to define and introduce points of view for consideration. Henderson (1966) coined the phrase 'nursing process', familiar in most care establishments, in an attempt to explain what nurses actually do. She believed that 'nursing is primarily assisting the individual (sick or well) in the performance of those activities contributing to health, or its recovery (or to a peaceful death) that he would have performed unaided if he had the necessary strength, will or knowledge, and to do this in such a way as to help him gain independence as quickly as possible'. This viewpoint sets the initial scene for the development of the *Model of care*.

## Model of care

In the past, caring for sick people has been linked with the medical model, ie. curing diseases, and many tasks were aimed at fulfilling this goal, ignoring the care of the person as a whole. This situation led to a search for a 'map' of care which would strongly emphasise 'wholeness' of the individual and promotion of health. After much examination the idea of 'wholeness' was accepted and led to an identification of **needs**, and to planning and delivering care to meet the needs of the whole person, known generally as a *holistic concept of health*.

## Holistic concept of health

This is a belief in which the person is considered as a functioning whole rather than a composite of several systems. It means that everything the person does or comes in contact with, aims at meeting his or her needs, lifestyle and well-being, eg. good housing, job training and education. However, a serious deficiency in any of these needs could bring about ill-health These needs are broadly classified as follows:

1. **Physical** — this is concerned with the function of the body.
2. **Social** — this is the ability to develop and maintain relationships with other people.
3. **Psychological** — this relates to mental health and an ability to think clearly and reasonably; the ability to recognise and respond to emotions, such as fears, grief, anger, and to express and cope with stress and stressful situations.
4. **Spiritual** — this is concerned with the individual's religious beliefs and practices, and ways of achieving peace of mind according to his/her beliefs.

A model of care, should be consistent, reliable, predictive, measurable and flexible enough to allow the person to exercise a certain degree of risk to support his or her remaining skills, independence and lifestyle as far as possible. The most important requisite is a constant flow of information and choices for those who provide care to make informed decisions that are best suited to their clients' needs. Although there are many forms of models from which to choose, 'nursing process' seems to be the most widely accepted and used in the United Kingdom.

## Nursing process

The term relates to a systematic way of planning and delivering care, using a problem-solving approach and available resources, to meet individual client's total care needs. It is *an action research* in which clients and their relatives are taken into partnership. It succeeds by using professional knowledge, skills, experience and attitude in planning and delivering care, based on what everyone does daily, what Roper (1983) called 'activities of daily living'. These are outlined below:

- maintaining a safe environment
- communicating
- breathing
- eating and drinking
- eliminating
- personal cleansing and dressing
- controlling body temperature
- mobilising
- working and playing
- expressing sexuality

- sleeping
- dying.

The main purpose of this approach is to help clients or patients to stop, resolve, relieve or deal with their problems.

**Individualised care programme**

The process of delivering care starts immediately the doctor diagnoses that the person is in need of care, and continues throughout his or her stay either in a hospital or a registered nursing or residential care home. Planning the programme is the work of a team, and once information has been obtained, it is entered into a problem-solving cycle. Care assistants should be able to make a valuable contribution by demonstrating their ability, skill, knowledge and attitude to assist in each of the following stages of the process.

**Guidance**

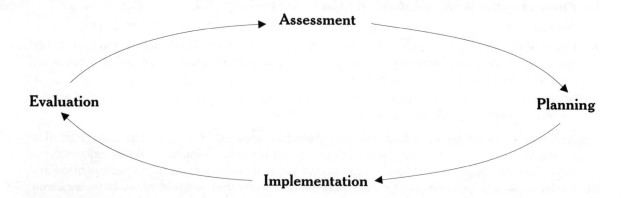

### 1. Assessment

This stage relates to identification of the needs of individuals clients. It involves collection and analysis of 'historical' information about the person in order to:

- establish what is his or her normal pattern of living, lifestyle, interests, likes and dislikes
- identify problems relating to his or her physical, social, psychological and spiritual well-being. Some of these problems may be imagined or possible (potential) while others may be real (actual)
- provide information on *risk taking* and *restraint*
- make decisions about the *care plan*
- identify the changes or new skills the person will need to reach his or her own goal.

**Types of needs or problems**

Once these needs have been identified, decisions will be made about the care plan on whether these problems are:

- immediate — requiring instant attention, eg. difficulty in breathing
- medium or long-term — those which do not require immediate attention.

### 2. Planning

Involves setting goals and the steps necessary to achieve them. The process will aim to:

- rank care needs or problems in the order of priority

- formulate a care plan to meet individual clients' total care needs
- decide methods, procedures to be used in solving the problem
- ensure that there are adequate resources available for the care plan
- agree on methods of evaluation of care and the client's progress.

## A specimen of a care plan

### Nursing care plan

Patient's name: ............................  D.o.b................................................

Doctor:.......................................  Room no:...........................................

| Date | No | Problem/need | Expected outcome/goal (if relevant) | Nursing action | Initial | Discontinued | | Final evaluation |
|------|----|--------------|-------------------------------------|----------------|---------|--------------|--------|------------------|
|      |    |              |                                     |                |         | Date | Initial |          |
|      |    |              |                                     |                |         |      |         |          |
|      |    |              |                                     |                |         |      |         |          |
|      |    |              |                                     |                |         |      |         |          |
|      |    |              |                                     |                |         |      |         |          |
|      |    |              |                                     |                |         |      |         |          |
|      |    |              |                                     |                |         |      |         |          |
|      |    |              |                                     |                |         |      |         |          |

### 3. Implementation

This is the actual delivery of care, ie. putting the care plan into action to meet clients' total care needs, based on ability to select, adopt/use appropriate resources, eg. equipment, skills and knowledge

### 4. Evaluation

This is a continuous monitoring of standards and quality of care given. It involves critical examination of the following:
- the status of client's health and progress in achieving the desired goals
- effectiveness of intervention and quality of care practice, including resources used
- all the four stages of the process, ie. assessment, planning, implementation and evaluation.

The process of evaluation involves everyone in the delivery of care including patients' or clients' relatives in specific circumstances.

## A framework for delivery of care

The purpose is to keep everyone informed about changes in a client's or patient's care. Quite often care assistants and part-time staff do not know what changes have taken place even on the shift of duty. There are basically three systems for delivering care and their application varies considerably from one care establishment to another. These are mentioned below.

### Primary nursing

This is a framework for organising care to promote independence, with the emphasis on the client as a whole person. The 'primary nurse' is responsible for day-to-day planning of care, and on his or her days off-duty, care is carried out by an 'assistant', who follows the care plan developed by the 'primary nurse'. This type of co-operative working relationship is designed to provide continuity and to focus on the individual client's care. The person's rights of choice, dignity, independence and lifestyle are respected at all times.

### Team nursing

This approach requires the appointment of a team and a leader to be responsible for a group of clients. The team leader gives total care to some clients in her group, while supervising the work of other team members, eg. care assistants caring for other clients. All members of the team have a particular interest in all clients in the group. The advantage is that the staff have detailed knowledge of care plans for each of their clients, and care assistants give planned care rather than undertaking isolated tasks for their clients. This approach offers an opportunity for members of the team to constantly observe, assess, identify problems and discuss the care being given. Moreover, it provides an opportunity for teaching and learning.

### Task orientation

This method of care means that certain allocated tasks are linked with the regular pattern of care routine. For example, one care assistant may be assigned the responsibility for bathing a group of residents, while another takes on the task of feeding another group. The carers initiate and assume the responsibility of 'doing things' for those in their care. The problem is that carers see their clients as 'tasks' and so cannot build up any meaningful type of relationship with them. Obviously, flexibility is necessary in carrying out these tasks. Residents should be given the opportunity of using their remaining skills to tackle problems themselves and, as far as possible, to stay independent. The following guidance is useful in transferring responsibility to residents and in helping to develop and maintain good interpersonal relationships.

### *Guidance*
- decide on the problem, set goals and break these down into simple and manageable steps
- initiate action by demonstrating to the client each step of activity
- take the client's hands and guide them to the task, thus 'teaching' him or her how it can be tackled
- allow the client plenty of time to perform the task
- gradually withdraw assistance as the client's confidence increases and he/she gains control
- talk to and encourage the client to express his or her needs and thoughts at all times
- praise the client for trying as well as completing the task
- use touch gently to show your gratitude and reward the person with a hug and a smile.

## Essential skills

The success of an individualised care plan depends upon the carers' in-depth knowledge of the total care needs of individual clients, a sound basis of accurate information on specific needs and risks outlined in the care plan and the ability to demonstrate the following skills:
- essential support, eg. counselling, interpersonal and problem solving skills, advocacy, observation and reporting
- interviewing — use of the words 'when', 'where', 'how', 'what', eg. 'how or where are you?'
- Teamwork
- management, especially economical use of resources

- professional knowledge, experience and a positive attitude.

### Risk-taking

On admission, a care plan should be designed for each client, agreed by everyone who has an interest in the client's care and reviewed frequently. The care plan should include details of risk-taking agreements so that members of the care team, clients and their relatives are fully aware of the details. This awareness should extend to their expectations of each other. It is important that a checklist related specifically to risk taking and restraint, should be included in the care plan. Under each heading, there should be detailed discussion to determine the way in which the home will undertake to meet residents' own wishes concerning their life style.

### Assessment of risk

The framework concerns every member of the care team. Appropriate methods to determine the risk involved should be in place with the outcome being recorded in the care plan. A problem-solving approach, including brainstorming exercises may be used. In order to avoid accidents, the care team should devise their own checklist so that a more accurate decision can be made on how to plan activities safely. Decisions on why restriction is necessary are essential as are the methods for imposing such restriction, which should only be used as a last resort. In this way risk assessment can be based on staff and relatives' solicitude, rather than residents' aims.

### Guidance:
- identify and discuss the risk involved in the care plan and agree on use of restraint
- list activities, their advantages and benefits to be gained from taking the risk, eg. increased self-esteem, retention of independence, value of taking own decision
- discuss these activities in terms of the disadvantages and possible harm which may occur if the risk is taken, eg. physical danger, possibility of attack, losing his/her way or failure to achieve which could cause loss of self-esteem. Agree on restrictions with respect to the choice of activities
- consider the gains/losses and balance these against the degree to which they are life-threatening
- decide on the likelihood of each gain or loss occurring.

The decision will be based on a balance between the right of choice and the resident's competence in undertaking an activity. This should ensure that he or she is not being unduly protected from an extremely unlikely occurrence. The role of the carer is, therefore, to seek ways to enhance, or compensate for a lack of competence. It may also involve offering extra support to make it possible for the resident to undertake an activity with an acceptable degree of risk. This extra support may mean additional staff.

## References

Cole A (1994) A problem shared. *Nurs Times* **90**(43): 16

Dickinson S (1982) The nursing process and the professional status of nursing. Occasional paper. *Nurs Times* **78**(16): 61–64

Docherty A (1994) Welcoming the challenge to provide quality care. *Caring Times* October 1994: 8–9

Henderson V (1966) *The Nature of Nursing*. Collier Macmillan Ltd, London

Kendell H (1990) Monitoring standards of care. *Nurs Standard* **4**(37): 32–33

McKenna H (1993) The effects of nursing models on quality of care. Occasional paper. *Nurs Times* **89**(33): 43–46

Malby R (1988) Primary nursing: All you need is thought. *Nurs Times* **84**(51): 47–48

Pearson A (1988) *Primary Nursing. Nursing in the Burford and Oxford Development Units, Beckham.* Croom Helm, London

Roper N, Logan W, Tierney A (1987) *The Elements of Nursing.* Churchill Livingstone, Edinburgh

Singleton P, Gamlin R (1989) A primary change over. *Nurs Times* 85(40): 39–41

**Audio visual aids**

*Format: VHS video*

Ref: 427/1CT: *The Nursing Process: Part 1— medical ward* (cassette tape)

Ref: NT 45/2: *Planning Care*

Ref: NT 44/1: *Planning Care*

Ref: CNE7619: *Primary Nursing*

Oxford Educational Resources Ltd

## Assignment

The purpose of this homework is to assist you in preparing for your Workbased Assessment of Competence. As there is no pressure on you, feel free to work at your own pace, but avoid the temptation to procrastinate. After you have read your notes and suggested references, submit your work for correction. The completed work becomes part of your Personal Portfolio.

## Models of care (NC4: 1–4, NC11: 1–3)

1. What do you understand by the terms 'nursing process' and 'risk assessment'?
2. List four stages of the nursing process.
3. Describe what you understand by the word 'client's needs'. How would you help the person-in-charge to identify these needs?
4. Discuss how you would help the person-in-charge to identify the needs of a newly admitted client.
5. Discuss how you would transfer responsibility of care to clients in the environment in which task orientation is practised.
6. Name seven skills which are necessary for the implementation of the nursing process.
7. State briefly how you would help to identify clients at risk.

## Research appreciation (CU7.2, CU8.1)

Research is a word that we hear nearly everyday in the media. Sometimes it is mentioned in our place of work, whether that is in the community, health care homes or hospitals. Research is a planned, systematic search for information for the purpose of increasing the total body of knowledge. It involves looking for information which is not readily available or for which there is no generally accepted evidence. In this respect information means data collected and analysed in the course of investigation.

Research is responsible for the emergence of new knowledge in the fields of medicine, science and technology. It also shows that changes in our lifestyle can alter the pattern of disease, and adds more to the body of existing knowledge. More importantly, it shows that changes in the structure of society, eg. increases in the size of the elderly population, can bring about new habits and customs and create fresh health problems. All these new discoveries and changes make demands on health care, and so the use of research becomes imperative in order to enhance standards and quality of care. Brotherston (1960) says that awareness of research should be developed at all levels, in order to maintain professional competence. This means that every member of the health care team should be helped to develop an attitude of inquiry.

## Care assistants

As front-line workers care assistants spend a greater proportion of their time on duty in direct and close contact with residents, and assist qualified practitioners in delivering care to meet the residents' total care needs. This is based on a **problem-solving** approach, ie. asking a question about a problem in a client's care, collecting information, however elementary, and analysing it realistically. This is research processes at a clinical level. Being members of the care team, care assistants should be encouraged to take a closer look at what they are doing, how and why they do it and **ask** questions. In this way, they are able to provide useful information on the nature of the individual resident's problems they encounter when providing care. Many research projects were started in this way, eg. personal hygiene, mouth care, sleep, promotion of continence.

## The need for research

The need for research often begins when a person takes a closer look at all aspects of his/her work and focuses on issues that challenge him/her, asking the question 'why the problem'. Obviously, anyone can ask 'why', which may be an outcome of observation on how things are done, or an untested idea (hypothesis) in which the person sets out to find the answer. The aim is to increase the body of knowledge, in that carrying out the study may result in sharing information with a number of people so that they, too, may take a closer look at what they are doing and how they are doing it.

At times we find ourselves in a situation where a resident may ask a question which may be difficult to answer. This may be because our existing knowledge and practice are out-of-date. Therefore, it becomes necessary to reflect on these difficult questions and make a personal decision to learn and acquire some skills and contribute to the growth of research. The acquisition of these skills will, of course, depend on our interest and the source of **knowledge**.

## Sources of knowledge

Everyone has personal qualities, different types of knowledge and life experiences, which they bring into the caring profession. But, it is necessary to develop and use these attributes in carrying out research projects. The sources of such attributes may be classified as follows:

- **Academic knowledge**: knowledge which is acquired from learning subjects, such as biology, arithmetic, science, history, humanities from qualified tutors
- **Personal experience**: this is the sum of a person's life experiences. It is said that experience is the best teacher. A person's character and knowledge develop through a variety of experiences, ie. through interaction with others, loss of a loved one or travelling round the world.
- **Group knowledge**: a common knowledge which is shared with other members of a social group, eg. peer group
- **Vocational knowledge**: most people have acquired vocational knowledge which they bring into the care team from working in a variety of vocations since leaving full-time education. This is a special kind of knowledge and relates to previous work experiences

- **Special skill:** this is a complex type of knowledge which relates to experience gained in carrying out certain aspects of practice and procedures in specific field of care, eg. mental health, the elderly, paediatrics. The carers acquire 'specialist' knowledge which they can be relied upon to use under supervision.

In practice, all these different types of knowledge are continuously being used in our daily lives and work situations. Carers usually interact and share their life experiences with clients and, by doing so, demonstrate empathy, ie. putting themselves in their residents' shoes when dealing with their needs.

## Other sources of knowledge

Apart from the knowledge that is gained from personal experiences, there are other sources which are equally useful in carrying out a research project. These include learning from our parents, friends, brothers and sisters, teachers and other people with whom we come into contact. In addition, other sources of knowledge are from television, the Internet, radio, newspapers, magazines, videos and journals, research reports, articles and textbooks.

Occupational knowledge develops by watching people at work, such as matrons, sisters, nurse tutors, student nurses, colleagues, doctors, paramedical staff, and from nursing procedures and policy, nursing journals, specialist nurses, eg. infection control officers, patients and relatives. It is important that the care environment should encourage and support the undertaking of research.

## Types of research

There are different kinds of research in which care assistants may assist or undertake in health care, depending on what questions are asked and which methods are used to find an answer. It is difficult to classify the different types as they often overlap, but any of the following methods may be considered.

### *Action research*

Action research is essentially an on-the-spot procedure designed to investigate aspects of clinical care, analyse and solve problems or improve standards of care. It is a key approach for promoting high standards and quality of care and deals with changes in health care. The process involves constant monitoring of the situation over varying periods of time, and using a variety of devices such as questionnaires, computers, diaries, interviews and case studies.

The aim of the researcher is to provide answers to practical problems, and increase understanding of the issue, through feedback and participation during the project. It is a form of experiment in an everyday setting, because the researcher can introduce changes and assess the outcomes.

### *Critical essays*

This is a careful examination of evidence to decide what should be accepted and what should be rejected. It involves citing the findings of several researchers in the field, and offers new findings in relation to a particular view, analysis, or a new integration of previously unrelated work. A review of literature and an understanding of theory in the field to be studied enables the researcher to place his or her question in perspective.

### *Project work*

This is a means of studying a particular topic, eg. care of the elderly. It encourages a questioning attitude and the application of research findings to care by the care team. The topic may be suggested by the work-based assessor, course tutor or left completely to the candidate. Quite often project work is a group activity but may be undertaken by individuals.

## Case studies

This is a very popular form of inquiry in which students can make studies of the clients or patients they have nursed. They are asked to give an account of how they contributed to an aspect of the person's care, drawing on their own individual experiences. The studies involve gathering background data about their clients, approaches to management of their problems, evaluation of outcome and conclusions reached.

Although work of this kind may not be research in the sense of extending knowledge, it can be a valuable exercise in directing students' attention to factors they might otherwise overlook. It also offers training in guided observation, and encourages the testing of hypotheses rather than the expression of personal opinions.

### Preparing a case study

#### *Guidance*
- establish and maintain good interpersonal relationship with colleagues and clients
- consult your mentor or a qualified member of staff regarding the choice of a suitable topic
- preserve the confidentiality of the information on the client by using a fictitious name
- cover adequately the issues under consideration with reference to the client as an individual
- recognise the individuality of the client by assessing and identifying his or her personal needs in relation to physical, social, psychological and spiritual well-being
- provide information on the various skills and activities used in managing the problems, including information on any outside specialist care and investigations
- mention the outcome of the care, eg. client was discharged home or is now living in the community with relatives.

#### *Content*
- emphasise how the client's problems were resolved, and the decision making process, including your own contribution to care
- provide some diagrams or illustrations — remember that a picture is worth a thousand words
- give ample references with an acknowledgement of those who supported your effort.

#### *Presentation*
It is better to present the study in a story form and as simply as possible, bearing in mind that 'the story' is about a human being. In doing so, you are expected to give an account of the part you played in providing the care.

#### *Guidance*
- keep to the suggested length of the study, preferably typewritten in double line space
- include relevant details and sources of information, eg. client, doctors, nurses, community nurses, paramedical staff, ccupational therapists, clients' relatives
- submit an appropriate project file.

### Carrying out a project

Research does not necessarily have to be carried out by trained researchers. There are, however, certain procedures which students should observe, beginning with the choice of topics for their research work. Once a topic has been decided, each candidate is allocated a mentor or facilitator who is responsible for supervising the study. A submission date is usually set, and it is essential to seek the help and support of librarians from local public lending libraries, work-based assessors, matrons, qualified staff and colleagues. Basic knowledge in research methodology and prior attendance at a research appreciation course or membership of a local research interest group may be helpful.

Whatever the purpose of the investigation or the method, the sequence is often used synonymously with a problem-solving approach, ie. assess, plan, implement and evaluate. But research is more precise than problem-solving as the latter does not necessarily involve research.

## Guidelines for project work

It is important to keep to the stipulated word limit probably 15000 words, but basically the eight steps are as follows:
- choose something that really interests you
- agree the topic including its scope with your work-based assessor
- define the subject and purpose of the study in relation to the aspect of care investigated
- decide on a suitable structure. Your mentor or facilitator will give you guidelines
- draw up a timetable, setting dates by which you intend to have reached certain stages
- summarise the findings relating to the aspect of care investigated, and suggestions for improving care based on the investigation
- provide references and acknowledgements for your work.

## Preliminary preparation of the report

### Draft
The work should be presented in a draft form. Number all pages and ask someone with sufficient knowledge of the subject to read and criticise the work at each stage. Sub-headings are helpful and make reading easier. Edit and refine your work until you are happy.

### Manuscript
Present the work in a formal but creative way. Keep the length within the agreed word limit. Submit the manuscript for typing, preferably typewritten in double line spacing on A4 size paper. Check carefully for spelling and correct any errors. Fasten together firmly for presentation.

### Illustrations
Diagrams and tables should be numbered and titled. They should be inserted in the text so that the reader can understand them without having to search through the text for information. Data which has been collected should be included where appropriate in the body of the text.

### Bibliography/references
These are all the relevant works to which reference has been made in the course of the study. Give proper references to all articles mentioned and list them alphabetically, according to the authors' names. References in the body of study should be author's name followed by date of publication in brackets, eg. Brown (1978). No work should be cited if not actually used.

## How to write a reference for a book:

| Author's name | Initials | Year of publication | Title of book | Publisher | Country |
|---|---|---|---|---|---|
| Brown | R | 1978 | Care in Action | Penguin Books | London |

## How to write a reference for an article from a journal:

| Author's name | Initials | Year of publication | Title of article | Title of journal | Volume/issue number | Page numbers |
|---|---|---|---|---|---|---|
| Tyler | J | 1992 | Travesties of care | Nurs Standard | 4(3) | 24–5 |

### Appendix or appendices

An appendix completes the study. It should contain acknowledgements, copies of any supplementary material which are relevant to the study, but which cannot be conveniently included in the body of the report, eg. profiles of famous people, assessment criteria and findings, recommendations and charts.

### Conclusion

It is both unwise and discourteous for an individual to make arrangements for research in a care environment without first obtaining the consent of the matron, owner of the residential care home, and local ethical committees in the area in which they work. Under the Patient's Charter, it is also necessary to obtain the consent of clients or their relatives to research work. It is important that a research worker is honest. It can be tempting to slant results to make them fit the arguments presented. Objectivity about one's own work is necessary however hard this may be.

### Presentation of project

An attempt should be made to invite members of the health care team to attend and participate in the presentation and learn from it. Trainees should be encouraged to use audio-visual equipment and to view the exercise as a valuable experience in the development of their own skills.

#### Guidance
- include audio visual aids
- type your script and use double line spacing
- leave triple line spaces between paragraphs
- number your pages and use one side only.

Copies of the project could be provided and used as a source of reference in the care setting.

## References

Altschul A (1974) Beginning and end. Nursing research. *Nurs Times* May 9, 1974: 718–9

Beard R (1970) *Teaching and Learning*. Penguin Books, London

Brotherston JH (1960) *Research Mindedness and the Health Profession. Learning to Investigate Nursing Problems*. Report of International Seminar on Research in Nursing. International Council for Nurses, London.
Bircumshaw D (1990) Making research useful to the practising nurse. *J Inst Adv Nurs* **19**: 174–179
Gibbings S (1993) Informed action: action research. Research methods. *Nurs Times* **89**(46): 28–31
Hawthorn P (1981) Supervision of dissertation of undergraduate nursing students. Occasional paper. *Nurs Times* **77**(8): 29–30
Hawthorn P (1983) Principles of research — a check list. Occasional papers. *Nurs Times* **79**(23): 41–43
Hunt J (1981) Indicators for nursing practice: the use of research findings. *J Adv Nurs* **6**(3): 189–194
Lacey E A (1994) Research utilisation in nursing practice. *J Inst Adv Nurs* **19**: 987–995
Lancaster A (1975) Reading a research report. *Nurs Times* June 12: 56
Royal College of Nursing (1977) *Ethics Related to Research*. RCN, London
Simpson A (1981) A personal view of nursing research. *Nurs Times* August 5:1393–1396.
Tireney A J (1974) Research at ward level. Nursing research. *Nurs Times* May 9: 717–718
Winter R (1989) *Learning from Experience: Principles and Practice in Action Research*. Falmer Press, London

# Assignment

The purpose of this homework is to assist you in preparing for your Workbased Assessment of Competence. As there is no pressure on you, feel free to work at your own pace, but avoid the temptation to procrastinate. After you have read your notes and suggested references, submit your work for correction. The completed work becomes part of your Personal Portfolio.

## Appendages for care: research appreciation (CU7.2, CU8.1)

1. Write a care study on a day in the life of an 85-year-old gentleman who has difficulty feeding himself (*Unit 8*).
   Length of the study: 1000 words
   Date of presentation: to be agreed with your mentor or facilitator.
2. Carry out and present a project work to members of the care team in your area of work on how you would enable clients to maintain and improve their mobility (Unit Z5.1).
   Length of study: 1500 words
   Date of presentation: to be negotiated with members of the care team.

## Advocacy for clients (Z2: 1–4)

The word 'advocacy' has been linked with the legal profession for many years, ie. a barrister or an attorney represents and pleads on behalf of his or her client in a court of law and is known as an advocate. This is because the person may not have the necessary knowledge or skill to be able to make his or her wishes known. In recent years the advocacy scheme has become a familiar idea in the care of children with special needs, in which someone who is qualified would represent their wishes and rights. The scheme has now been extended to the care of the elderly and people with mental health problems. It was reported that in 1992, five charities including MIND and the Spastics' Society joined together to form the Advocacy Alliance. Since then, there has been a rapid growth of advocacy groups, including provision of courses by Citizen Advocacy Information and Training, in the United Kingdom.

## Definition

Williams and Schoultz (1982) define advocacy as the process of 'acting for, or on behalf of another person who is unable to do so himself or herself'. They believe that it involves 'speaking or acting on behalf of oneself, or another, or issue, with self-sacrificing vigour and vehemence'. Advocacy actually takes place when a person enters into a relationship with, and represents the interests of, another person. It requires complete loyalty on the part of the advocate, by representing the wishes, needs and interests of the partner or other person as if they were their own.

## Forms

There are various forms, but the current ones in use are:

### *Self-advocacy*

Self-advocacy or speaking up for oneself, is something which some older people already do. It has become a key tool for encouraging people with learning difficulties or mental-health problems to express their own needs and promote their own interests.

### *Legal advocacy*

This involves lawyers or those with legal knowledge protecting their clients' rights and interests under the law. It requires the preparing of 'briefs' or casework as may be necessary to represent their clients in the courts of law, or tribunal, eg. in the case of compulsory treatment or discharge from compulsory order. There is also a public advocacy where a group or organisation campaigns for a particular change, eg. MIND or MENCAP.

### *Citizen advocacy*

This may be especially relevant to the needs of those older people who cannot achieve what they want on their own, but does not necessarily involve the legal system. They may be represented by people who are not health care professionals.

## Advocacy scheme in care

The process usually begins with carers and clients accepting that their relationship is based on equality, trust and mutual respect. The idea is to empower people, help them defend their rights, speak up for themselves and make their views and wishes known. In so doing, carers should avoid patronising their clients and focus only on personal or professional issues. Generally, the needs of elderly people change constantly as they get older, to the extent that they are often faced with considerable worry when dealing with a complex system like the social security. Research shows that some elderly people are not aware of their entitlements and, accordingly, may not be claiming their full benefits. On the other hand, those who are aware of their allowances do not claim because they do not 'want hand outs', or to 'bother anyone'. Therefore, they need a trusted friend to act as an advocate and look after their interests by giving them good advice. A number of elderly people, especially in the community, fall into one of these two categories.

## Residential care setting

In hospitals, social workers act as advocates in the interests of their patients. Nurses and care assistants, especially in privately owned health care homes, have always acted on behalf of some of their residents. However, it is believed that some clients do not see carers as truly representing their interest, especially if they have been subjected to institutional abuse. On the other hand, some carers regard the role of advocacy as an optional extra which is 'not in my job description'. It follows that a progressive care plan cannot be delivered if this is the prevailing attitude. There is an increasing awareness of the need for an advocacy scheme in the care of clients with dementia, mental health problems and learning difficulties, who cannot speak out for themselves. The objective is to enable them to improve their quality of life and obtain their full rights and entitlements.

The elderly usually appreciate and value emotional support through friendship. They need someone to speak on their behalf, the opportunities to learn new skills and to obtain the services they need. There are a number of practical considerations, such as estimation of risk, and approval of the action chosen by the clients themselves, which may not always be approved by trained staff. The process involves power shared equally between clients and carers.

## Skills needed

The care of elderly people and a significant number of people with mental health problems requires carers to focus on developing essential skills that are necessary to support the scheme, for example:
- good interpersonal relationship skills based on trust and mutual respect
- assertiveness, negotiating and communication skills
- counselling is a prerequisite, and ability to share information
- paraphrasing follow-up interviews, confirming the extent to which clients have understood the explanation given for diagnosis and treatment. Clients appreciate a simple explanation in a relaxed atmosphere after the initial interview, eg. with a consultant
- maintaining confidentiality. This includes responsibility to clients and employers, who protect clients' records within an agreed policy and philosophy of care.

## The role of carers

In recent years the carer's role has seen remarkable changes, with emphasis on an individualised care plan based on good interpersonal relationships. Those involved in the care of people with mental health problems and the elderly are usually involved in admission and discharge procedures and more so in medical treatment. These are 'at-risk' areas in which carers should be adequately prepared in order to advocate effectively. Murphy and Hunter (1984) believe that the role of carers should be to help their clients obtain the best care even if this means going against hospital administration and other health care professionals' wishes. The role of carers, therefore, focuses on the ability to:
- act always in the person's best interests by declining duties or responsibility for which you have not been trained adequately
- provide friendship and warm emotional support to your clients
- act as middle person between your client and those providing or seeking to provide services for him or her
- act as a guardian of your client's rights and protect the person from abuse, eg. verbal, financial, physical
- preserve your client's values, dignity and self-respect and speak out on his or her behalf, ie. if the person is woken up and given a bath at 5 o'clock in the morning in order to help the day staff, or if he or she is given the wrong diet
- encourage clients to develop self-advocacy skills that enhance their ability to speak out and act on their own behalf
- assist in transforming a custodial or protective care system to a dynamic one in order to prevent the onset of institutionalisation for your clients and colleagues

- observe local policy on maintenance of records, but seek and provide your client with information to enable him/her to make informed choices. Maintain complete loyalty
- ensure that your clients have information about the local 'Patient's Charter'. This includes complaints procedures and tells clients how to contact the District Health Authority.

## Evaluation by client

A major part of an advocacy role is the extent to which the carer succeeds in empowering clients so that they can actively identify their own needs and determine their own future. This will include decisions about their health welfare and the provision of care. Due to extenuating circumstances, eg. confusion, the process may take some time, but the intention is to promote benefits for the clients, especially the elderly person.

## Problems of advocacy

The main issue is how should carers report abuses which they observe? Should they do it through their trade unions and professional bodies or 'blow the whistle', and risk their jobs? This is a dilemma facing the scheme. It is believed that advocating for clients always involves some form of confrontation or antagonism with a conflict of interests. The outcome may be victimisation by colleagues and management. There can be no doubt that many carers would not become advocates for these reasons. Wertheimer (1993) says that a conflict of interest will often prevent carers from representing the interests of their clients. The UKCC (1989) guidelines on 'Exercising Accountability' note that advocacy is concerned with promoting and safeguarding the well-being and interests of clients. It is not concerned with conflict for its own sake. These guidelines, therefore, apply equally to everyone involved in care in the clinical setting, including care assistants.

Beardshaw (1984), found that nurses who wish to represent their clients can experience conflicts of loyalty with their peers and their employers, which may lead to formal sanctions being placed on their activities. But the staff concerned developed other ways of gaining job satisfaction. However, there is now a movement within the profession towards the protection of 'whistle blowers', as demonstrated by the case of Graham Pink. Basically, conflict cannot be avoided if carers are to represent their client's best interests, especially when these are clearly being ignored. The standards and quality of care are too often reduced to an unacceptable level by:

- poor staff/client ratio
- lack of resources
- care and treatment prescribed for people who are unable to give informed consent
- clients discharged early without appropriate arrangements being made for their subsequent care.

Under the topic of confidentiality of information in care, reference is made to the act of truth-telling. However, disclosing unacceptable standards of care can be threatening. The carer may face rebuke from management or even lose his/her job. This is a matter of conscience and a moral dilemma, highlighting the extent to which carers can be true advocates for their clients. Carers who have 'blown the whistle' may be singled out for criticism or labelled as 'mischief' or 'troublemakers'. Breadshaw observed that nurses have good reasons for keeping quiet about abuses, as silence is a normal, human response to intimidation and fear. Moreover, this enforced silence causes suffering to clients and 'caring nurses are deprived of free speech and are effectively prevented from following their profession's basic tenets' (Breadshaw, 1984).

It could also be argued that, far from empowering people, these initiatives have actually reduced people's rights. Whatever view is taken, the net result has been to make a large part of the population start thinking about what is and is not a 'right'. The scheme presents important issues and principles, which encourage carers to make their own decisions and judgments in their work area.

## References

Breadshaw V (1984) *Conscientious Objectors at Work. Mental Hospital Nurses. A Case Study*. Social Audit, London

Booth B (1994) A guiding act? Advocacy. *Nurs Times* **90**(8): 30–31

CAIT (1996) *Citizen Advocacy — A Powerful Partnership*. Citizen Advocacy Information and Training, London

Cohen P (1994) Advocates of independence: advocacy, older people. *Nurs Times* **90**(9): 67–69

Murphy C, Hunter H (1984) *Ethical Problems in the Nurse-Patient Relationship*. Allwin and Bacon, Boston

Nash A (1993) Point of contact. Advocacy, community care. *Nurs Times* **89**(26): 52–54

Redefern SJ (1991) *The Elderly Patient. Nursing Elderly People*. Churchill Livingstone, Edinburgh.

Sines D (1993) Balance of power: mental health. *Nurs Times* **89**(46):52–55

United Kingdom Central Council for Nursing, Midwifery and Health Visiting (1989) *Exercising Accountability*. UKCC, London

Werthemier A (1993) *Speaking Out: Citizen Advocacy and Older People*. Centre for Policy on Ageing, London

Williams P, Schouldz B (1982) *We Can Speak for Ourselves*. Condor Books, London

### Audio visual aids

*Format: VHS video*
Ref: *Powerful Partnerships*
Ref: *Taking Sides*. Citizen Advocacy Information and Training, London

## Effectiveness of Teamwork (CU9: 1–3, CU10: 1–2)

A team can be defined as a group of people who willingly work together for the benefit of the group rather the individual. The concept of people working as a team is not new to the caring profession, but has received prominence following recent developments in models of care. Modern management of care requires effective teamwork, which starts immediately a client is diagnosed as in need of care, and continues until he or she is discharged. This may be into the care environment or to the client's home in the community. Consequently, every member of the team should be aware of their individual management skills and practise them in a disciplined way until they can work effectively in their roles, and with others in teams.

### Team building

Team building is not easy and requires the right mix of people and their commitment to the job. A number of people are employed in care settings, ie. the doctor, manager, matron, nurses, cooks, domestic staff and general handyman. However, in some care environments, the medical model of care is still being used. This model implies 'ownership of the patient' by the doctor or consultant. This means that it is the doctor who has both responsibility and accountability for client care, and it suggests that the nurse does not have a decision-making role. This is not the case as the decision-making process uses a multidisciplinary team approach, and the team is jointly responsible for providing the benefits of the service.

The process of building a team is not simple. It requires careful planning by those in authority if it is to work effectively and improve the way things are done. Much thought goes into planning, organising and developing a team into a high performance unit capable of providing the service needed. Also, effective team building calls for considerable confidence and a willingness on the part of everyone involved to pull together.

## Manager

The starting point of a team building exercise is the selection of a team leader. This may be the matron, manager or the person-in-charge. He or she assumes responsibility for day-to-day care of clients, supervises the work of other team members, and knows that successful outcome depends upon his or her management style. The role is managerial and entails allocating tasks to team members, consultation, successfully selling ideas. The leader should be capable of assessing the nature of the work and the needs of the service. He or she should be able to identify the differing skills, knowledge and experience of employees, and use and develop them to bring about the best practice in the team.

It is important that the leader develops an effective communication system and good interpersonal relationship skills. The most important aspect of this role is to treat all employees as adults, respecting and consulting them when making changes. He or she should help their team to develop team management skills, and practise these skills in a disciplined fashion until they work easily and well together. The person-in-charge must rely on good teamwork and **delegation**, deciding what should be done and then allocating these tasks to other people. The manager should:

- be aware of and develop existing working procedures to suit the culture of the care establishment
- be aware of opportunities available for staff development
- seek and identify key activities or work functions that need to be present if the team is to function at its optimum level, eg. opportunity to network, experiment on new ideas
- appraise, motivate and check regularly on staff performance
- encourage team members to think about and identify their strengths and weaknesses.

## Team members

Care assistants as members of the team can contribute to the decision-making process, which requires a high level of participation. Everyone is expected to function to the best of his or her ability by continuously evaluating what they are doing in terms of quality assurance. It is known that, for various reasons, eg. personality clashes, people fail to work together. This can result in a lowering of morale, loss of self-esteem and poor job performance. Some people may respond in a rather sensitive and touchy way to a situation which is anathema to effective teamwork. The problem should be investigated. Tolerance and sensitivity to other people's feelings are the hallmark of adult behaviour. Employees should be encouraged to identify their own individual strengths and weaknesses and areas to be developed, to set goals and work towards achieving them. A record of a personal goal and action plan should be kept in the staff's personal portfolios, and discussed from time to time with the person-in-charge or matron .

## Teamwork

The topic of team nursing has been dealt with under models of care. It follows that in order to function effectively, every member should be responsible for achieving results with other members of the team. The process is that the person-in-charge assigns specific clients to each caring team. Alternatively, the team leaders develop care plans for all clients assigned to their teams. Rather than allocating specific tasks to themselves, leaders should circulate between teams, supervising the work of the other staff who are helping to care for clients. This practice creates a learning opportunity for everyone, and good habits are developed and maintained.

### *Guidance*

Members of the team should be able to:
- assist the team leader in ensuring that care plans are properly implemented and evaluated
- observe and report on the response of each client to care, procedures, practice and suggest ways of improving these.
- observe and report on the behaviour and attitude of colleagues to the team leader
- show alertness to opportunities for improvement and change. Encourage others to do the same
- continually examine their own role and suggest or 'sell' new ideas to the person-in-charge
- manage different clients' needs as assigned, maintain accurate records and report any problem
- detect and report on defects of equipment and see that the equipment is serviced regularly
- network and help others to learn by sharing ideas and information with them. Seek permission to discuss or report any matter of personal concern to the person-in-charge
- maintain an open communication channel with everyone, including clients, their relatives and visitors and report any untoward incidents, no matter how trivial to the person-in-charge
- attend lectures and staff development programmes
- evaluate and monitor work continuously in terms of quality assurance
- support and use time effectively so that resources can be made available at the right time
- ensure that there is a minimum overlap of tasks and provide positive feedback to the person-in-charge or the team leader
- seek opportunities to develop by enrolling on a vocational training programme and encourage others to do the same.

## Influencing factors

There are many factors which may impede the work of the team, including:
- staff attitude, lack of co-operation and friction, 'in fighting' and poor morale
- poor staff ratio or inconsistency in the deployment of staff leading to lack of continuity of care
- inadequate resources and ineffective use of time and skills
- poor working environment, dictatorial style of the manager and lack of co-ordination
- poor sickness and absence record among members of the team
- inadequate training and poor or inaccurate maintenance of records.

## Time management

Teamwork is linked with time and ways of carrying out procedures, but often time seems the more important of the two. Generally, it is a scarce resource and staff have been reprimanded for 'wasting valuable time'. Some managers mistakenly regard talking to a resident as a waste of time. This approach tends to be very rewarding and fulfils the social needs of clients'. It also offers the opportunity to get to know clients and for clients to get to know their carers. Time cannot be wasted, but only used effectively.

## Use of time

This concerns those matters relating specifically to your work as well as the time spent in personnel relations' activities, eg. dealing with a new or junior colleague.

Time can be used creatively if you spend it thinking about the task; how you are going to tackle the job and get it done in the shortest time with the minimum of effort. Time taken to think sensibly about the task is time well spent and pays dividends.

*Guidelines*
- analyse and assign priority to your tasks
- plan procedures by ensuring that all equipment is on hand when you carry out the task. It is disheartening to run backwards and forwards and wastes precious time
- break the task into simply managed elements and into the sequence in which you are going to tackle it
- allocate a realistic estimate of how much time each task will take and stick to it
- delegate or get someone else to handle the problems
- embark upon the task and try to keep unplanned jobs to a minimum
- monitor yourself against your own time standards.

## References and further reading

Belbin RM (1993) *Team Roles at Work*. Butterworth-Heinemann, Oxford

Humphries J (1992) *How to Manage People at Work*. How to Books Ltd, Plymouth

Lemin B (1981) *First Line Nursing Management*. Pitman Books Ltd, London

Masrgerison C, McCann Dick (1991) *Team Management. Practical New Approaches*. Mercury Books, Oxford

Rowden R (1984) *Managing nursing. A practical introduction to management for nurses*. Bailliere Tindall, London

Stewart R (1997) *The Reality of Management*, 3rd edn. Butterworth-Heinemann, Oxford: ch 11

Wagner G (1988) *Residential Care. A Positive Choice. Report of the Independent Review of Residential Care*. HMSO, London

## Management of change (NC2: 1–2)

Everyone is faced daily with the problem of change, not only in our work but in our everyday life, what we read in newspapers, new technology, new ideas. Changes in the workplace make demands on everyone including clients, their relatives and people significant to them. A change is a deliberate intention to alter something, such as the behaviour of other individuals or a group of people. Whenever change occurs, adjustments on a large or small scale need to be made. Changes may be desirable or undesirable, destructive or constructive in nature, but people concerned should be helped and supported to enable them to make the necessary readjustment. A change can be described as 'trial by ordeal', while others say it is as good as a rest. Change, however necessary, should not take place just for its own sake.

### Sources of change

Change may be the resiult of a general dissatisfaction. In the care setting, the need for change may be necessary in order to respond to clients' differing physical, social, psychological, economical and environmental care needs. For example, preparing a client and his or her family for home care, or care of the elderly in their own homes. From the carer's point of view, the need for change may follow from how care is managed and delivered to clients.

Other sources may include structural alteration of the care environment, the introduction of a computerised service or changing suppliers for economic reasons. Demands for high standards and quality of care, including value for money service are changes which face both managers and employees. The most traumatic adjustment people have to make relates to bereavement. Management of bereavement requires the use of special skills, such as counselling, to help clients, their partners, relatives and friends to explore and manage the situation themselves. This is no easy task. In all cases of change, people should be properly prepared and supported if change is to be successful.

## Management

Changes that concern clients, their partners, relatives and friends are the responsibility of a team and should be introduced with great sensitivity and constructive support. The general principles are:
- effective communication and consultation to seek views, attitudes, wishes and needs of clients and their families if the change is to be successfully implemented
- education and preparation of all those who may be connected with the change including members of the health care team and any responsible social workers
- designing an action plan and checking the effect of change on resources
- provision of specialist staff, eg. counsellors, speech therapists, physiotherapists
- induction of clients and their families on the use of any new equipment or machinery required for the successful implementation of the change.

## Framework for preparation

The aim of the plan is to seek accurate information in order to identify any pre-existing needs which may interfere with the ability of clients and their family to adjust to the change without causing one another stress, conflict and anxiety.

Changes relating to the needs of specific clients and relatives require staff to be familiar with, and plan care to meet those circumstances. For example, a change from residential to home care will require the use of procedures similar to those for transfer and discharge of clients (see *Unit 5*). The following factors will be considered and preparation carried out as follows by:
- the matron or a senior member of the multidisciplinary care team from the nursing home
- members of the community primary health care team, eg. family doctor, district nurses
- staff from the social services department with interests in older people
- clients and relatives based on their assessment and evaluation.

## Support for partners and relatives

The most important aspect of implementation relates to monitoring and evaluating the work carried out, allowing clients, their partners and relatives to adjust and to assume control of their lives. It is also important to ensure that, regardless of the team's enthusiasm for change, the family will share the responsibility for change, and will be able to cope and support one another. Initially clients may require moral support and counselling to manage at home, especially if they encounter feelings of guilt and hostility. In some cases clients and their partners will be introduced to services and schemes provided by local social services in support of elderly people in the community, eg. home care, crossroads scheme (see 'Services and facilities in the community for the elderly', *Unit 17*).

Clients and their families may decline an option offered, but they should be supported in their decision. In some cases clients may be going home to face terminal illness and, while at home, may deteriorate. It will then be the responsibility of carers and other health care professionals to offer support to the client enabling him/her to die with dignity, and to offer care to the whole family. The support for relatives following bereavement is discussed in 'Care of the dying' (*Unit 18*).

## Resistance to change

Clients and their families may resist change for any of the following reasons:
- insufficient knowledge or understanding of the reasons for the change
- lack of consultation and involvement in the arrangements
- habits and fixed patterns of living with particular reference to the cultural needs of clients, their partners and relatives
- poor communication and lack of understanding, possibly due to language barriers
- inflexibility: people being unwilling to make the necessary adjustments
- speed of proposed implementation of change causing anxiety and fear of failure
- lack of careful planning and failure to identify any pre-existing needs may hinder the exercise
- poor accommodation and overdependence on staff
- excessive pressure on the people involved
- cost, inadequate resources and preparation
- prejudice, due to lack of trust
- satisfaction with the status quo
- domineering and other cultural influences which may reduce the self-esteem of those involved.

Resistance may be lessened by:
- building up good interpersonal relationships, being flexible in approach and a good listener
- careful and intelligent planning, together with effective communication
- reasoning with clients and encouraging their involvement
- identifying and discussing possible obstacles which may be encountered during the process, and devising ways of eliminating them
- using suitable supporting skills, eg. counselling, advocacy
- encouraging clients to participate by asking questions
- networking and adequate preparation of members of the care team involved in the exercise.

## Role of care assistants

As members of the multidisciplinary team, care assistants may help by demonstrating an ability to:
- maintain good interpersonal relationships with clients, their partners and relatives
- develop and use counselling and communication skills
- act as advocates and give explanations which ensure that clients, their partners, relatives and friends understand what is required of them
- give any available written information, make time to go through it with clients and make an accurate record of information given
- be approachable and encourage clients to ask questions, which must then be answered as truthfully as possible. Refer difficult questions to the person-in-charge.

The successful implementation of change depends on many factors, especially how the individual and the organisation manage the situation. In the majority of cases, very little supervision and monitoring may be necessary.

## References

Baly M (1973) *Nursing and Social Change*. Heinemann Medical Books Ltd, London
Lemon B (1978) *First Line Nursing Management*. Pitman Books Ltd, London
Schuss MC (1975) *Nursing and Management*. English Universities Press Ltd, London

Steward R (1991) *Managing Today and Tomorrow*. Macmillan, London

**Audio visual aids**

*Format: VHS video*

Ref: CEM 6534: *Effective Interpersonal Communication*
Ref: CEM 6622: *Planning and Preparing for Negotiation*
Oxford Educational Resources Ltd

# Section III: The delivery of care: mandatory units

At the end of this section, candidates should be able to demonstrate an understanding of the basic principles of delivering care defined by the following units.

| | Units and elements of learning | |
|---|---|---|
| **Unit 1: Foster people's rights, beliefs and equality** | O1, O2, O3, CL1, CU5, NC10, W1 | 63 |
| o Rights of individuals in care | O1.1 | 63 |
| o Personal beliefs and identity | CL1.1, NC10: 1–2, W1 | 65 |
| o Promote equal opportunity for all individuals | O1: 1–2, O2: 1–2, O3: 1–2 | 69 |
| o Information in care | CU5.1, O1.3, O2.3, O3.3 | 73 |
| o Confidentiality of information in care | O1.3, O2.3, O3.3 | 76 |
| **Unit 2: Promote effective communication and relationships** | CL1, CL2 | 80 |
| o Effective communication | CL1: 1–2 | 80 |
| o Interpersonal relationship skills | CL1.1 | 84 |
| **Unit 3(a): Health, safety and security in the workplace** | CU1 | 89 |
| o Health and Safety at Work Act 1974 | CU1.1 | 89 |
| o Fire precautions | CU1.1 | 93 |
| o Health emergencies (first aid) | CU1.2 | 96 |
| o Other health emergencies | CU1.3 | 99 |
| o Falls and accidents | CU1.3 | 105 |
| o Care during epileptic seizures | CU1.3 | 111 |
| **Unit 3(b): Assist in the control of infection** | CU1, CU2, OD1, X1, X13, Y4 | 113 |
| o Sources and mode of spread of infection | CU1.1, OD1 | 113 |
| o Management and control of infection | CU2.1, OD1 | 117 |
| o Infestations | | 121 |
| o HIV/AIDS and hepatitis B | | 124 |
| o Wound care — aseptic technique | CU1.3, X13.1, Y4.1 | 127 |
| o Isolation nursing | CU1: 2–3, X1: 1–3 | 131 |
| **Unit 4: Contribute to the protection of individuals from abuse** | Z1, Z18 | 136 |

# Unit 1
# Foster people's rights, beliefs and equality (O1, O2, O3, CL1, CU5, NC10, W1)

## Rights of individuals in care (O1.1)

Rights are something that we cherish dearly and relate to what is just, equitable, morally good and fitting. They are our legal and basic human rights which we will do everything possible to retain. They are an absolute entitlement which is non-negotiable and cannot be taken away, given away or swapped. The rights of justice, privacy, choice, personal identity and fulfilment are individual entitlements, essential to maintain self-respect, dignity, lifestyle and independence. The principles of care demand that the rights of clients, including cultural and personal beliefs, must be recognised, respected and fulfilled at all times. This means that clients have the right to choose their own doctors, and admission to hospital or health care homes does not interfere with this right.

Therefore, on admission, clients should be taken into partnership and consulted during the assessment and planning stages of their total care needs, with regards to their individual choice and preferences. The whole concept of rights and choice reflects the quality of interpersonal relationships between staff and their clients and this, in turn, determines the standard and quality of care, and clients' satisfaction. At times and unwittingly, staff can forget these basic rights in an attempt to provide care in an emergency situation. During procedures, such as bed-baths or bed-making, privacy may be infringed and the patient or client may be exposed unnecessarily.

In general, residents have the right to privacy without unnecessary intrusion, the right to express their sexuality and to be involved in sexual activity and relationships. They have the right to cry or laugh if they want to, to take risks and to worship according to their faith, wishes and custom. It is important to remember that people from different ethnic minority groups have different lifestyles, dietary needs, attitudes and viewpoints with respect to their health and welfare. These must be taken into account when planning and providing care. All clients have the right to maintain contacts and links with their family and they should be consulted and given the opportunity to choose and contribute to their own care.

### Legal rights

Over the years, there have been changes in the law which have given people increased rights to know what is said or written about them in their personal records. So, subject to adequate safeguard and counselling, individuals should be able to see the records about themselves that are kept by the care establishments. In addition, various legislation has been introduced to ensure that clients have more efficient and better standards of service that put the 'patient first', no matter where they live.

The Patient's Charter (1990) and the National Health Service Community Care Act 1993 set out various rights that patients are entitled to. Also, the Data Protection Act 1984 offers people the right to access their personal records, especially those maintained by the use of automatic processes such as computers, card indexes but excluding those maintained manually. Clients rights and conditions of access to certain records have been dealt with under Confidentiality of

Information. There are certain legislation and procedures which are designed to support the rights of individuals such as the Children's Act 1989, the Sex Discrimination Act 1976 and the Mental Health Act 1983. However, there are certain exceptions whereby an individual's right may be temporarily affected if he or she is detained under specific sections of the Mental Health Act 1983.

**Choice**

Choice means giving a person two or three alternatives to choose from and depends largely upon the ability of the individual to communicate and express his or her wishes. Those who are confused, very sick, unconscious, mentally infirm and some of those who are visually handicapped may be helped in making their choice. In some cases, carers or relatives could be invited to help in making a choice for their relations. However, the majority of clients should be encouraged to choose their clothes according to the weather, food from a menu, when to go to bed at night and when to get up in the morning.

**Promotion of clients' rights**

There are many ways in which the right of individual clients can be promoted. In providing care, the rights of the person to individualised care based on a holistic approach should be accepted. Therefore, an attempt should be made to assess and identify his or her needs, ie. cultural needs, functional capability and disabilities, and then plan service to compensate for each disability. Care should be taken to ensure that such rights are not breached through the use of restraint, medication or withholding information. Clients have the right to know how and where to contact the registration authority if they wish to make a complaint or discuss some matter which has not been resolved between themselves and the management. Information on whom to contact should be clearly displayed, preferably near to the registration certificate.

> *Guidance*
> Every resident or client should be provided with:
> - a contract of care. This should reflect the aims and philosophy of the home, rights and obligations including complaints and appeal procedures. It should include information on fees and retainer fees and periods of notice
> - the opportunity for privacy and the practice of their beliefs
> - information on ways and methods of appeal against inadequate or enforced services
> - privacy without unnecessary intrusion
> - the opportunity to retain and use personal property and private space
> - a review of the service being provided at appropriate intervals
> - an opportunity to participate in the social, political and economic activities of society in accordance with their ability and social standing, eg. voting in elections.

Residents should always be offered the choice of being addressed according to their individual wishes and preferred title but never as 'pop', 'gran' or other nick names. When talking to them, especially in a group, make sure you listen to what individual clients say; support and encourage the person to express his or her needs, for example, sexuality and lifestyle. Also, take note of what is said and the way it is said (eg. the person may express intentions of self-harm) and report your observation to the person-in-charge. It is important to be aware of your local policy on equal opportunities and anti-discriminatory practice.

Carers should be aware that denial of rights or needs can bring about lack of progress in a client's treatment and may result in temper tantrums, crying, frustration, depression, aggression, violence, isolation, refusal of food, regression, depersonalisation or other psychological problems.

It is important to have in-depth knowledge of all clients, show sensitivity to each person's needs, treat everyone with respect and act as an advocate on their behalf.

# References

National Consumer Council (1983) *Patients' Rights. A Guide for NHS Patients and Doctors.* NCC, HMSO, London

Booth B (1994) A guiding act? *Nurs Times* **90**(23): 30–31

Tyler J (1992) Travesties of care. Nursing the elderly. *Nurs Standard* **4**(3): 24–5

Wager G (1988) *A Positive Choice. Report of the Independent Review of Residential Care.* HMSO, London

## Audio visual aid

*Format: VHS video*
Ref: *Life in a Nursing Home*
BBC, London

# Personal beliefs and identity (CL1.1, NC10: 1–2, W1)

Everyone has certain inborn traits inherited through their parents who are themselves the products of their ancestors. The person the individual becomes, and all that he or she does, is determined by the complex interaction of these inherited characteristics and the environment. These personal attributes may be tastes, habits, intelligence, even finger prints, which can help in determining the person's ability to adjust to his or her social surroundings.

## Belief

During our lives we are faced with a choice of things to do and, without some guidance, we may end up doing nothing at all. Belief is the act of accepting as true what is said, providing us with the guidance we need to select a particular course of action. It is a trust which is based on faith rather than fact, and it encourages a sense of purpose necessary to carry out our goals. Therefore, belief is an essential motivating factor.

## The belief system

The system comprises a variety of beliefs, such as opinion, religion, magic, political ideologies or science, which motivate us to hold a particular conviction. It means that the actions we take to deal with a situation will be based on our convictions. Beliefs do not exist in isolation, but are associated with the complex systems which are taught by society. They are absorbed in the same way that people absorb other aspects of their culture.

## Identity

Identity is the sum total of the individual's persona which constitutes his or her personality and includes feelings, attitudes, beliefs and memories. There are many factors which may influence identity. These include personal beliefs and preferences, legal constraints, organisational policies, other peoples' tastes, ignorance and discriminatory practices.

In providing care, it is important that attempts should be made to protect and foster identity and beliefs. The following approaches aim to fulfil these objectives:

## Legislation

Certain acts of parliament were passed to protect the rights of individuals. These include the right to make personal choices and the right to our own beliefs. Some of these acts are: the Children's Act 1989, the Sex Discrimination Act 1975, the Race Relations Act 1976, the Disabled Person's Act 1974, the Fair Employment Act 1989 and the Equal Opportunities Commission Code 1985. Other acts relate to specific care settings or client groups, such as the Mental Health Act 1983, The National Health Service and Community Act 1993 and The Patient's Charter 1990. Implications and penalties are incurred for any infringement of these regulations (see *Chapter 2*, page 9–10).

## The care environment

Managers of care environments are obliged to provide their residents with a contract of care. This is an agreement which reflects the aims and objectives of the home, rights of individuals, information on fees, period of notice and an opportunity to make complaints. Residents should be offered an opportunity to make and test initial choice, and to maintain contact with their previous life as far as possible. They should be encouraged to retain and use their personal property and private space. Their relatives and advocates should be given an opportunity to participate in certain aspects of care, which should be consistent, and reviewed at appropriate intervals.

## Care plan

This forms the basis on which care is given and involves identification of a range of clients' interests, hobbies, beliefs, and specific needs. It is formulated by members of the care team, residents and their relatives. The idea is to help residents to pursue and achieve these goals, according to individual abilities and capabilities. It should explore ways in which individual clients' abilities could be used in their care. Emphasis should be focused on helping them to maintain their individual lifestyle, privacy and live as independently as possible, using their remaining life skills. The care plan should help them to:

- express their preferences, needs, feelings, rights for self-respect, dignity, privacy, make choices and take risks
- use opportunities offered to show their interest, participate and share their life experience with others in leisure and social activities
- express their sexuality in private without unnecessary intrusion and offence to others.

The implementation of the care plan is based on encouraging them to assume responsibilty for their lifestyle, and make known their wishes and choices. Within this framework, care is provided irrespective of race, ethnic group, colour, creed, gender, social status, religious or political persuasions, so that they can live as full a life as possible. It follows that, on admission, a care plan should be designed to reflect their physical, social and psychological well-being. An attempt should be made to assist the individuals in maintaining their values, culture, personality and belief.

## Values

These are the measures, worth and qualities which we place on ourselves and on others. They are shaped by our dreams, memories and associations. Society, background, upbringing, temperament and training are also responsible for forming our values.

## Culture

Culture is a social inheritance made up of techniques, ideas and habits that are passed from one generation to another. Collectively they are responsible for providing knowledge that, over time, people from the same ethnic groups may use to solve problems. Culture is regarded as a social inheritance and a learned behaviour.

## Personality

Personality is complex and diverse. It is the sum total of a person's behaviour, the way he or she feels, thinks or acts and differentiates him/her from others. Personality is formed by appearance, attitude, values, culture, beliefs and inherited characteristics. These will define the way in which the individual socialises with others in his or her community. It is important to respect other people's qualities and their role in life. In this way, carers will help their clients to adapt, co-operate and live as independently and harmoniously as possible.

When a client is admitted into care, especially for the first time, note should be taken of his or her distinguishing features, such as height, facial expression, posture, clothes, colour of the eyes, skin or race. These features give an overall impression of the person, setting him or her apart from other people. The impression may affect the way we perceive the person and any prior contact with him or her may also influence this image. It can be reinforced by observing, talking and developing a good interpersonal relationship.

### *Factors which influence personality*

In a care environment, there are many factors that can influence and perhaps impose restraint on a personality. These include:

#### *Social isolation and loneliness*
- These factors can make it difficult for clients to join in activities involving effort, because of a gradual decline in the quality of their sense organs. This decline may result in deafness and failing eyesight. These disabilities may isolate the client.

#### *Lack of interest*
- As one gets older, interest changes. More importantly, interest in physical activities usually decreases with age. The elderly may prefer to do odd jobs in the home where they can take a less active role, or going to the theatre, watching television, playing board games or reading.

#### *Restraint*
- The rights, dignity and self-respect of individuals are infringed by the use of physical restraint. Any form of restraint should be barred and residents should be treated with courtesy and respect. Risk assessment should be carried out on all residents to identify those at risk and care plans should be introduced to meet their individual needs.

#### *Clothing*
- The use of a 'pool' of clothing is an insult and slur on the individual client's personality. Such clothing never fits properly and only personal clothing and objects should be used.

#### *Consent for treatment*
- Medical treatment cannot be given without valid consent. If a client refuses to take medicine or nourishment, this should be reported to the person-in-charge. Never use coercion to force treatment on the individual. Only those patients or clients who are detained under the provisions of the Mental Health Act 1983, or have a notifiable disease such as typhoid can be treated without consent.

#### *Other factors may include:*
- breakdown of personality — may be due to the effects of the care environment which are known as 'institutionalisation'
- anti-social behaviour, mood changes and irrational behaviour
- low self-esteem leading to mental health problems in the elderly.

### Promoting clients' personal beliefs and identity

This is a very important role which requires knowledge of individual clients' personality, culture, values, beliefs and above all, encouraging their rights to express their lifestyles and sexuality.

Clients must always be treated with empathy, respect and dignity and encouraged to use their remaining life-skills to maintain their self-esteem and worth.

## Guidance

- identify the range of clients' interests, needs and hobbies and encourage them to pursue these based on their ability and capability
- address clients according to individual wishes and preferred title. Never use 'pop', 'gran'
- promote effective communication and treat clients with respect and dignity; allow them sufficient time and space to express personal views and make suggestions
- encourage clients to maintain contact with their family and others significant to them
- encourage clients to exercise their civil rights by participating in social and political activities, such as voting during local and general elections
- encourage visits from spouses, friends, relatives, and pets in accordance with local policy
- encourage clients to worship according to their faith. It is not necessary to be a member of an organised religion to have spiritual needs, as these can be expressed by a way of living
- encourage clients to continue their religious practices and in some cases transport could be arranged to take them to church services
- be aware of special religious customs and needs, as some religions forbid certain food, and require believers to have certain articles, eg. Orthodox Jews; the last offices are carried out by a Rabbi after death. Also, be aware of days celebrated as holidays with special ritual, eg. Ramadan
- provide adequate facilities and privacy when clergy visit to minister to clients
- be aware of medical treatments that are not allowed, eg. blood transfusion for Jehovah's Witnesses
- act as an advocate for the person.

## References

McMahon C, Harding J (1994) *Knowledge to Care: A Handbook for Care Assistants*. Blackwell Scientific Publications, London

Robertson B (1992) *Study Guide for Health and Social Care Support Workers*, NVQ level 2. First Class Books Inc, USA

Tyler J (1992) Travesties of care: nursing the elderly. *Nurs Standard* 4(3): 24–25

Wager G (1988) *A Positive Choice. Report of the Independence Review of Residential Care*. HMSO, London

## Assignment

The purpose of this homework is to assist you in preparing for your Workbased Assessment of Competence. As there is no pressure on you, feel free to work at your own pace, but avoid the temptation to procrastinate. After you have read your notes and suggested references, submit your work for correction. The completed work becomes part of your Personal Portfolio.

## Rights of individuals (O1.1) and personal beliefs and identity (CL1.1, NC10, W1)

1. Define the terms 'rights', 'beliefs' and 'personality'.
2. List various approaches which can be used to protect clients' rights, identity and beliefs.
3. Discuss how you will protect the rights and identity of clients in your care.
4. Discuss how the knowledge of a client's personality could be used in his or her care.

5. Describe in what circumstances you would offer choices to your clients.
6. A restriction has been placed on one of your clients. Discuss how you would explain to him, the reasons for this restriction.
7. Discuss how you would support and encourage the rights and choice of your residents at risk in relation to their health and safety, for example if your client is confused.
8. Discuss how you would help a client to overcome the effects of prejudice and institutionalisation.

## Promote equal opportunity for all individuals (O1, O2, O3)

### Anti-discriminatory practice (O3.1)

One of the fundamental qualities of carers is an ability to maintain at all times the highest standards of care, within the principles of good professional etiquette. Basically these are unwritten rules of professional conduct, which guarantee that everyone is treated fairly, justly and without any form of discrimination. This is to enable the person to meet his or her own essential and basic rights for recognition, self-respect, privacy and dignity. Generally, it involves the delivery of service within a prescribed code of professional conduct.

### Codes of professional conduct

Each profession has a set of rules and regulations regarding behaviour which its members have to obey, and the caring profession is no exception. Quite often, carers are faced with issues requiring personal judgment. For example, you have been asked to attend to two residents who both need urgent personal attention. Which one would you attend to first and why? Obviously, whatever your decision, you will be influenced by some ethical issues, which may result in conflict with your responsibility in patient or client care. These codes deal with human moral conduct as rational, good or bad, fair and just. To ensure that the profession is not brought into disrepute, sound personal judgment should be exercised.

Care assistants are not within the jurisdiction of the UKCC (United Kingdom Central Council for Nursing, Midwifery and Health Visiting). They are obliged by legal, ethical, moral and personal responsibilities to carry out their duties under the direction of qualified nurses. Although not bound by the UKCC Code of Professional Conduct, they are indirectly affected. It is, therefore, right and proper for them to understand the correctness of their action and the level of responsibilities within the care setting, as a breach of this Code of Conduct could lead to a severe reprimand, as well as the possibility of disciplinary action by employers. More importantly, a client or patient could bring legal action against the employee. Everyone should be able to show honesty and loyalty, with the right to refuse delegated duties which they are not competent to perform. They should also show a caring attitude and seek to promote actions aimed at helping clients to maintain their individual lifestyle, beliefs and self-respect without prejudice.

### Discrimination

This means treating people less favourably than others in the same position. It is deemed to occur when, for instance, a woman is treated less favourably than a man or if a person is treated less favourably because he or she is black. Discrimination signifies the way we feel about certain members of the society, ie. if we treat a person with disdain solely on the grounds of nationality, citizenship, ethnicity or origin. But discrimination could occur in other settings, for example, if people who are confined to wheelchairs have no access to public places because of a lack of ramps.

Prejudice is widely experienced in employment, housing, education and training. Within the profession, intolerance raises many issues about our attitudes towards clients, colleagues, black and ethnic minority groups, and other people who we meet from day to day. Since the primary duty of a carer is to provide a service to people, it follows that care must be provided in an atmosphere of trust, justice and equality for all individuals.

## Forms of discrimination

1. **Direct**: That which is obvious. It may include open harassment, abuse, physical attacks, denial of needs and opportunities, degrading or demeaning behaviour.
2. **Indirect indiscrimination**: This occurs when a specific requirement or condition is unfair or unjust. It is hidden, subtle and difficult to prove. In most instances, it is practised unintentionally and is therefore difficult to deal with or detect.
3. **Institutional discimination**: This takes place when particular policies, practices or procedures have a discriminatory effect on someone, eg. nursing homes may not have facilities for providing vegetarian food and so discriminate against those individuals who do not eat meat by limiting their choice of food.
   The condition known as institutionalisation could arise as a result of a rigid routine and institutional practices which put a barrier between residents and the outside world. Clients are made to conform to the strict regime with a loss of rights, self-respect, dignity and independence.

## Areas of discrimination

Research shows that prejudice has no boundary, and can be aimed at anyone irrespective of age, including children and babies. There are a number of ways in which people could be targeted by prejudicial remarks, such as physical attractiveness in which some are described as beautiful and others as ugly, some as thin or others as fat. However, the most common areas recognised by law are discrimination by age, sex and sexual harassment, creed, race, culture, colour, ethnic origin, marital status, disability or personal attributes, mental health problems, health status, people with HIV, political and religious persuasions, sexuality, sensory ability and learning difficulties.

## Effects of discrimination

The effect of discrimination is a fluid and changing experience, and reactions depend on a number of factors, such as the frame of mind of the person who discriminates, position of authority, the situation and circumstances. Different people react in a variety of ways to discriminating situations, and quite often less attractive people are more likely to experience lower self-esteem, marginalisation, rejection and isolation. In the care situation, there may be a noticeable change in a client's behaviour which may indicate a feeling of alienation, depression, withdrawal, shame, anger, rejection, frustration or displays of aggression and violence.

## Approaches to combat discrimination

Parliament has passed certain acts which require organisations to formulate their policies and guidelines for good practice. These acts are the Sex Discrimination Acts 1975 and 1986, the Race Relations Act Act 1976, the Children's Act 1989, the Disabled Persons Act 1974, the Equal Pay Act 1970, (amended 1983), the Health and Safety at Work Act 1974. In order to see that these acts are implemented, various commissions were set up to try to combat discrimination. These include the following:

## Equal Opportunities Commission
This is a public body which was created by Parliament in 1975 to work towards removing unlawful discrimination on grounds of sex, and to promote equal opportunities for women and men. It has the power to investigatge discriminatory practices and take direct action to make people change and comply with the law. If the employers persistently discriminate, especially through unlawful advertisement, the Commission can take legal action against both the employer and publisher. If anyone experiences any problem relating to sex discrimination, especially at work, the Commission can help in various ways, eg. by giving advice, putting one in touch with other agencies who may be able to assist, such as the Arbitration, Conciliation and Advisory Service (ACAS) or take the offender to an industrial tribunal.

## Commission for Racial Equality
Under the Race Relations Act 1976, it is unlawful to publish advertisements that discriminate on racial grounds. The law relates to discrimination of a person in housing, recruitment, jobs, goods, facilities and services, education and training. Individuals who believe that they have been the victims of discriminatory practices, especially at work, have a right to take legal action or go to a tribunal. But there are general exceptions, eg. in sports or games where discrimination is allowed in selecting a person or a team to represent a country or place of birth.

## Religious organisations
Religious bodies recognise the problems of racism which involve marginalisation and isolation of people from ethnic minority groups. The Church of England recognises this through its report on the *Seeds of Hope* (1991), which it sends out in Parish Study Packs to combat racism in all the dioceses throughout England, Northern Ireland and Wales.

## Statutory bodies
The United Kingdom Central Council for Nursing, Midwifery and Health Visiting (UKCC) (1992) *Code of Professional Conduct* No 7 requires registered nurses to 'recognise and respect the uniqueness and dignity of each patient and client and respond to their needs for care irrespective of their ethnic origin, religious beliefs, pesonal atributes, the nature of their health problems or any other factor'.

## Responsibilities under the acts

### 1. Employers
They are required by law to accept and promote the principles of equal opportunities as being an essential part of good employment practice. The Patient's Charter requires them to have policies that reflect the rights and standards set out in the Charter. Also to develop and establish:
- A complaints procedure so that everyone including clients, staff and visitors have the right to make complaints, and should be aware of the organisation's procedure should they wish to lodge a complaint. Complaints may be verbal or written and should be attended to swiftly and thoroughly, in order to maintain standards and quality of care
- A local policy on equal opportunities and anti-discriminatory practices — the policy should reflect a positive outlook and value for people, in order for them to maintain their self-respect and individuality. All cultural groups should be catered for in order to ensure equal access to treatment and care, education and training. They are required to:
  - provide a system for monitoring local implementation of the policy
  - provide an ongoing in-service training programme on equal opportunities for all grades of staff and ensure that they attend

- carry out an investigation on all reported cases of sexual, racial or other harassment, and actively discourage discrimination by victimisation
- review local policies in the light of national developments.

## 2. Employees

Employees (eg. care assistants) are required to:
- assist in monitoring the implementation of equal opportunities policies and provide ways of challenging discriminatory behaviour and attitudes
- address the issue in a sensitive way and accept responsibility for their own individual attitudes and thoughts
- be familiar with organisational policies concerning equal opportunities, health and safety policies and the Mental Health Act 1983 for those who work in the mental health fields
- be aware of local policies and procedures for making complaints
- be aware that individual rights may be affected by other people's behaviour
- avoid using a uniform, appearance, personality, beliefs and behaviour in a way that may be regarded as confusing or threatening to individuals
- be aware of the effects of stigma, institutionalisation and prejudice on the delivery of care
- act as an advocate to clients and be aware of methods of challenging discriminatory practices, for example in face-to-face interactions
- report to the person-in-charge any form of discriminatory practices and give support to individuals who may be at risk
- answer to employers on the level of responsibilities under the freedom to act.

## Other responsibilities

These should include the willingness to:
- learn about health and sickness in different cultures
- provide a variety of food on the menus
- ensure that, where requested, patients have access to female medical staff
- provide clients with information on specific topics, for example, the organisation's Charter of Care.

## References

CMAC (1996) *Seeds of Hope in the Parish* (study pack). Committee for Minority Anglican Concerns. The Ludo Press, London

Equal Opportunities Commission(1986) *A Guide to Employers to the Sex Discrimination Acts 1975 and 1986.* EOC, London

Equal Opportunities Commission(1995) *A Short Guide to the Equal Opportunities Commission.* EOC, London

Home Office (1976) *Racial Discrimination: A Guide to the Race Relations Act 1976.* HMSO, London

National Health Service (1990) *The Patient's Charter.* HMSO, London

Stevens MK (1965) *Personal and Vocational Relationships of Practical Nursing.* WB Saunders Company, London

The General Synod (1991) *The Seeds of Hope Report: A Report on the Study of Combating Racism in the Dioceses of the Church of England.* General Synod of England, London

Tingle J (1990) Ethical way. *Nurs Times* **86**(43): 60–61

United Kingdom Central Council for Nursing, Midwifery and Health Visiting (1992) *Code of Professional Conduct.* UKCC, London

Whitehead E (1995) Prejudice in practice. *Nurs Times* **91**(21): 40–41

## Assignment

The purpose of this homework is to assist you in preparing for your Workbased Assessment of Competence. As there is no pressure on you, feel free to work at your own pace, but avoid the temptation to procrastinate. After you have read your notes and suggested references, submit your work for correction. The completed work becomes part of your Personal Portfolio.

## Anti-discriminatory practice (O1.2)

1. State your understanding of the concept of the Code of Professional Conduct.
2. Define the term 'discrimination', and give examples of various forms of discrimination.
3. What do you understand by the term 'anti-discriminatory practice'?
4. Identify six ways in which a person may experience discrimination.
5. Give an example of discrimination that you have witnessed or experienced.
6. State briefly what you would do to protect a client who complains to you that he or she is being discriminated against by a senior member of the staff.
7. List various legislation and policies aimed at protecting and supporting the rights of individuals against discrimination.

## Information in care (CU5.1, O1.3, O2.3, O3.3)

The background to providing care involves the use of information science which is the study of the process for collecting, storing and retrieving information. This is needed by members of the health care team to decide on the diagnosis, treatment and subsequent rehabilitation of clients. *The Pocket Oxford Dictionary* (1987) defines information as 'what is told, knowledge, items of knowledge'. In the care setting, this relates to facts, inside stories, news and reports, including information about the person's social life that is relevant to care. Knowledge of individual residents' financial standing is essential, because they may need financial help to contribute to their care in nursing and residential homes.

### Sources of information

Initial sources of information may include clients themselves, relatives, next of kin, spouses, friends, colleagues and anyone with whom clients may have had close contact, such as solicitors, family general practitioners, community nurses and clergy. Clients' previous records can provide useful information, but it is important to understand the background from which this information comes if its accuracy, validity, credibility and relevance in care is to be considered reliable.

### Methods of obtaining information

Face-to-face interviews are the most common way of obtaining information from clients, their families, friends and other people who may be significant to them. Data may also be obtained through electronic means, the telephone, written or orally (face-to-face). Any member of the care team may obtain information according to his/her professional role. But it is vital that those who are taking information adopt non-threatening sympathetic attitudes during these interviews. Even the way we stand or move, the uniform we wear, our personal appearance, facial expression, gestures and tone of voice may influence the way clients react to staff and the quality of information given. It goes without saying that good interpersonal relationships are important, and that clients should be treated with respect, dignity, and without intimidation. Information about residents is highly confidential and access should never be given to unauthorised persons.

**Methods of sharing information**

It is considered good practice for staff to share information with residents, in an attempt to maintain an open professional relationship. Information is usually disseminated at staff and resident meetings, which are held regularly in the home or where care is given. The Data Protection Act 1984 encourages openness and gives individuals the right of access to personal information maintained on computer. Staff and client notice boards can be installed on which information can be posted, but an attempt should be made to ensure that the information displayed is current. Information given in handbooks and leaflets should also be regularly updated.

**Forms of information**

It is a requirement of the Nursing Homes Act 1984 that health care establishments should maintain the following records:

*Register of patient*
A register must be accurately maintained giving detailed information of name, date of birth, address prior to admission and marital status.

*Records*
A written account must be made of all aspects of care required by each individual client. It should contain entries recording facts and observations on the clients' needs and actions taken by members of the health care team to meet these needs, for example X-rays, laboratory reports and charts. All records should be completed in such a way as to assist in monitoring the standards and quality of care, including investigations of complaints.

*Medical and nursing records*
Individual clients' records should contain entries relating to:
- the administration of all medicines, with notes of particular interest
- personal belongings and valuables held
- financial affairs relating, for example, to a Court of Protection Order
- daily and periodical statements on health and well-being.

*Staff records*
- records of professional staff employed should include employment details, educational and professional qualifications, skills and any other relevant information
- register of all staff employed.

*General and administrative records*
- management of drugs — a central record for ordering, storing and administration of medicines
- complaints and procedures for making complaints
- fire drills
- notification of accidents, illnesses or death
- various records, such as relatives, seclusion of clients, visits by authorised person to inspect the home, nutrition of clients, scale of charges, accounts held in respect of individual clients, all maintenance for medical, surgical and nursing equipment.

## Methods of storing and retrieving information

There are a number of methods for storing and retrieving information. Records maintained must be appropriately secured under lock and key at all times.

### Written reports
These are usually in files and folders and stored in filing cabinets. Written records must be legibly written. In accordance with local policy, each entry must accurately chronicle the date and time of the report and the signature or initials of the person making the entry should be included.

### Electronic devices
Electronic devices can include computers, audio tapes, telephone, micro film and compact disks.

## How to deal with information

A local policy should be in place which identifies a designated person or the grade of staff who can disclose information to approved relatives and friends. The purpose of the policy should be to:
- discourage disclosure of information over the telephone except by an authorised person, as agreed by members of the health care team
- maintain and conform with the requirements of the Data Protection Act 1984, if personal information is held on a computer
- adopt appropriate methods to ensure that confidentiality is not contravened in public places, especially that relating to specific client groups, for example those protected by the Mental Health Act 1983
- secure client and staff records in appropriate locations when not in use, and instruct staff on how to obtain proof of identity from callers
- mark records and other information with confidentiality ratings, such as very/highly confidential.

## Care assistants

Carers should be able to demonstrate skills in the use of electronic devices.

### Receiving telephone information:
- be aware of local policy for dealing with information over the telephone
- identify yourself and place of work to the caller
- demonstrate tact in answering questions put to you over the telephone
- make a brief note of date, time, matters discussed and any other action required
- refer any 'difficult' enquiries to the person-in-charge
- pass any relevant information immediately to the individual concerned
- seek proof of caller and never disclose any personal information on staff and clients to anyone. If pressed, ask for the caller's name and telephone number or any messages for passing onto the person concerned.

### Making a telephone call:
- think and be clear in your mind about the message that you want to transmit
- check that you have the correct telephone number and make the call
- confirm that the location is correct, note the time and identify the name of the person to whom you are speaking
- state briefly the nature of your message and the action needed
- ascertain that the message is understood by asking the recipient tactfully to confirm details of the message
- listen attentively to the reply, correct any misunderstanding and make a brief note of the sequence of events
- if appropriate, provide a brief summary in the right sequence to the person-in-charge or the person concerned, eg. the client.

## Computer information

Some care establishments maintain a computer information system which can be accessed by members of the health care team. In general, detailed information on clients is computerised at the time of admission or registration, but professionally qualified staff involved in their care may update the data at any time, for example changing the name of the next of kin or an address. The use of computer information in care requires a knowledge of the 'menu' and operating instructions of the computer and, more importantly, the requirements of the Data Protection Act 1984.

## References

Lelean SR (1973) *Ready for Report Nurse?* Royal College of Nursing research series. RCN, London

National Association of Health Authorities in England and Wales (1985) *Registration and Inspection of Nursing Homes. A Handbook for Health Authorities*. NAHA, Birmingham

Oxford University Press (1987) *The Pocket Oxford Dictionary*. OUP, Oxford

Vousden M (1987) Do you really need to know? *Nurs Times* **83**(49): 28–30

## Assignment

The purpose of this homework is to assist you in preparing for your Workbased Assessment of Competence. As there is no pressure on you, feel free to work at your own pace, but avoid the temptation to procrastinate. After you have read your notes and suggested references, submit your work for correction. The completed work becomes part of your Personal Portfolio.

## Information in care (CU5.1, 01.3, 02.3, 03.3)

1. What is meant by the term 'information in care'?
   a) Discuss the importance of this information
   b) List various forms of information that may be required
   c) State in what circumstances could this information be shared with clients.
2. Discuss sources and methods which may be used to obtain information, touching on how the quality and validity of information may be affected.
3. Describe methods of storing and retrieving information for care in your area of work.
4. Discuss your role in giving and receiving telephone information and the precautions you would observe in carrying out these processes.

## Confidentiality of information in care (01.3, 02.3, 03.3)

Confidential information means classified records which include spoken or written information. The purpose of seeking information in care is to enable members of the health care team (doctors, nurses and paramedical staff) to make informed decisions concerning diagnosis, treatment and the well-being of their clients. This means sharing information, but effective communication can be hampered by the need to maintain the confidentiality of the information entrusted to members of the team. This confidentiality covers facts and data of a sensitive nature, intimate and private to the individual client concerned. Consequently, such information must always be protected in order to safeguard the interests and welfare of the clients involved, and to preserve their self-respect and dignity. A breach of this confidentiality may result in litigation.

## Complexity of confidentiality

The issue of confidentiality is a complex and cruical one, as it is based on the principles of telling the truth. Moreover, the profession is moving towards a position where clients receiving care should have full and open access, at any time, to all the information about them. It follows that, within this context, confidentiality does not indicate secrecy or exclusive possession of information, rather it involves the disclosure of certain information to specifically authorised persons under trust.

This means that information about the client will be shared with people who are directly involved in his or her care in the form of verbal reports and written notes. This is essential with the proviso that everyone will work together as a team under a code of professional ethics of mutual trust, respect, honesty and dignity to protect the dignity, self-respect and freedom of all individuals concerned. Such information should remain confidential to members of the health care team, and this should be clearly explained to individual clients.

In this respect, managers of care establishments should be able to provide local guidelines on the control of information, and ensure that such information remains confidential between clients and members of the care team. In all care establishments, information maintained in manual records is entrusted to authorised personnel, such as matrons, care managers, sisters and charge nurses, with reasonable access to designated members of the health care team.

## Legal aspects of confidentiality

The legal aspects of confidentiality are particularly related to the clients' records and the forms signed before administration of anaesthetics and performance of operations.

## Consent for treatment

It is important that clients give written or verbal consent for their treatment, especially if they are undergoing medical procedures or operations. Consent may be given by a parent or guardian if the client is under the age of 16. Failure to obtain consent may be regarded as an assault on the person.

There are certain circumstances in which clients admitted under Section 3 of the Mental Health Act 1983, can receive treatment without consent. The Act states that 'if it is necessary for the health or safety of the patient or for the protection of other persons that he should receive treatment, and it cannot be provided unless the patient is detained under this section'. But Section 57 requires that a patient who may need psycho-surgery or any other more serious treatment should give consent in the normal way. If the patient is not capable or does not give informed consent, he/she cannot be given treatment.

## Disclosure of information

The following is the main legislation which provides guidance on the release of information on request:

### *Data Protection Act 1984*
The Act gives the client access to all handwritten health care records written after November 1991. The importance of this is not so much that it extends individual rights and freedom, but that it lays new responsibility on members of the health care team to share their working methods and conclusions with clients as partners in care.

### Access to Health Records Act 1990

Clients have the right of access to recorded health information about themselves as from 1 November 1991. The requests must be made in writing directly to the doctor or consultant. An administrative charge may be made.

### Access to Medical Record Act 1988

The Act covers requests from employers or insurance companies seeking medical reports on clients. But information cannot be given without the person's knowledge or consent and he/she has the right to refuse permission. The individual also has the right to see the report and request that corrections be made before it is passed to the employers or insurers.

### The role of qualified nurses

Although the UKCC *Confidentiality of Information* (1987) holds registered nurses, midwives and health visitors accountable for confidential information obtained in the course of their work, it lists four categories under which information may be disclosed:
- with consent of the patient or client
- without the consent of the client when disclosure is required by law or order of a court of law
- by accident
- without the consent of the client or patient when disclosure is considered necessary in the public interest.

The last category presents most difficulty as it covers issues such as child abuse, drug use, drug trafficking or other illegal acts. Recently, confidential information and practices have been disclosed by 'accident' through rumours.

### Role of health care assistants

As members of the health care team, care assistants have a moral and legal liability to maintain confidentiality of the information obtained during the course of their duty in accordance with local policy, especially in relation to clients at risk of abuse, drugs and effects of drugs.

> ### *Guidance*
> - seek and obtain a copy of an employer's policy on confidentiality of information
> - be aware of information which may indicate that the client or others are 'at risk', ie. taking drugs or they intend to commit suicide, and of local policy on handling the confidentiality of such information. Listen attentively to what is being said and report immediately to the person-in-charge
> - assist in ensuring that records are kept securely locked at all times
> - respect individual choice regarding the confidentiality of information as far as possible
> - be aware of circumstances which may override individual choice, eg. legal affidavits
> - do not give information concerning clients to any unauthorised person either orally or in writing. At times clients and their relatives may seek information. Offer help of a practical nature, eg. 'I will ask the matron to speak with you'
> - never disclose information about staff and clients. Refer 'difficult' queries to the person-in-charge or ask the caller to leave a contact number for a return call
> - be discrete and demonstrate tactfulness in answering telephone enquiries
> - do not engage in conversation relating to confidential matters where this may be overheard by a passer-by, eg. in corridors, lifts or reception areas
> - do not discuss with third parties any matters of a confidential nature about clients, outside the place of work
> - maintain confidentiality relating to your care environment at all times.

## Breach of confidentiality

A breach of confidentiality is deemed to have occurred when there is:
- a disregard of local policy on release of information
- a removal, falsifying or altering of any records, or reports or important notes are left unattended
- tactlessness, flippancy leading to disclosure of information to any unauthorised person(s)
- a failure to report and refusal to disclose information which may be of importance in the care plan, following a reasonable request to do so
- leaving information on visual display units visible to the general public.

Confidentiality of information is a complex issue in which every member of the health care team is held accountable within the organisation, and any of the above indiscretions, may lead to serious consequences and disciplinary action.

## References

Barber B (1992) Security screening. Confidentiality of patients' records. *Nurs Times* **88**(49): 50–52

Davies Report (1974) *Report of Committee on Hospital Complaints Procedure*. HMSO, London

Department of Health and Social Security (1981) *Access to Health Records Act 1991*. HMSO, London

Department of Health and Social Security (1984) *Data Protection Act 1984*. HMSO, London

Hyland M, Frapwell C (1986) Rough justice. *Nurs Times* **82**(41): 32

Inglesby E (1988) Moral matters. *Nurs Times* **84**(19): 49

Marsh G (1984) Complaining to effect. *Nurs Times* **80**(9): 36–37

Robertson B (1992) *Study Guide for Health and Social Care Workers: NVQ in Care Level 2*. First Class Books Inc, USA

United Kingdom Central Council for Nursing, Midwifery and Health Visiting (1987) *Confidentiality*. UKCC, London

## Assignment

The purpose of this homework is to assist you in preparing for your Workbased Assessment of Competence. As there is no pressure on you, feel free to work at your own pace, but avoid the temptation to procrastinate. After you have read your notes and suggested references, submit your work for correction. The completed work becomes part of your Personal Portfolio.

## Confidentiality of information in care (01.3, 02.3, 03.3)

1. Maintaining confidentiality of information is an important aspect of care.
    a) Define the term 'confidentiality of information'
    b) How would you help to maintain confidentiality of clients' information?
2. Discuss circumstances in which clients may exercise their rights to access of information.
3. A caller rings up to seek information about a client, and he or she is not known to you.
    a) Discuss how you would check the caller's right to this information.
    b) How would you deal with the situation and what information would you divulge?
4. Discuss what you understand by the term 'breach of confidentiality'?
    a) How would you help to maintain confidentiality of information in your area of work?
    b) In what circumstances would you disclose information?

# Unit 2
# Promote effective communication and relationships (CL1, CL2)

## Effective communication (CL1, CL2)

One of the essential attributes for delivering any service, is our ability to develop and maintain a dynamic *interpersonal relationship skill* which is, perhaps, the most difficult aspect of care to satisfy. It has three main parts comprising communication, social and assertiveness skills. It is, therefore, important that there should be a dynamic and intimate relationship between members of the care team, users of the service and their relatives, in order to maintain a high standard and quality of continuity of care. We now examine aspects of this dynamic relationship, starting with communication.

### Communication

This is the process of sending and receiving messages between two or more people in order to achieve a desired action or reaction. It is a two-way process and involves talking, listening or writing and reading. Effective communication is crucial in enabling people to build good interpersonal relationships, working together as a team or living harmoniously with one another.

In the care setting, it is difficult for many elderly people to find the words to express their thoughts. This may be due to the ageing process and/or specific problems associated with physical and mental health. Being able to communicate with other people is very important and, to meet their needs, an attempt must be made to examine the effects on communication of normal ageing and specific diseases.

### *Purpose of communication in care*

The way in which knowledge of communications can be used in planning and delivering care, will depend on the relationships between the carers and the style of leadership of the person-in-charge. Generally, communication helps the staff to promote and build up good interpersonal relationships and empathy. Carers should:
- find out how patients or clients feel about the care they are receiving and exchange ideas and information with their relatives and others involved in the care
- provide high standards and quality of care by explaining procedures
- define problems, give direction to staff, clients and visitors, and reduce conflict
- allow people to express their feelings, opinions, to satisfy needs
- counsel, teach, instruct and discipline staff
- share experiences about clients' care and learn from one another.

### *Forms of communication*

*1. Verbal* (Speech) — Research shows that speech is the highest form of human communication, and an exposure to language is an essential condition of speech attainment. Children are taught to speak and should be able to do so within their first three years. In adults, speech is usually influenced by the tone of voice, accent and timing. It is used in association with facial expression, eye contact, gesture, signals and touch. Communication is more effective when simple and clear words are used together with a moderate tone of voice. Shouting should be avoided.

**2. Non-verbal** — This is known as 'body language' which is used principally to express feelings or affection, needs, sexuality and attitudes, and involves the use of:
- gesture, ie. movements of hands, feet and facial expressions
- posture, body and eye contact
- symbolic gestures, eg. shaking hands, rubbing noses, embracing according to social conventions
- touch — generally known as sensory contact.

## Methods of communication
In the clinical setting, a wide variety of methods are used depending upon the cultural background of clients. However, the most common and widely used methods are:
- listening and observing to grasp the real meaning of what is being said
- silence combined with different aspects of 'body language'
- written or recorded, eg. written reports on clients, letters.

## Process of communication
The process involves the sender who must have a thought (source) which is then put into words and sentences to convey meaning. The words are spoken using movement of the larynx, tongue and face to produce speech (encoded). At times we use hand and body movements to produce gestures, changes in voice to convey feelings together with facial expressions, eg. a smile or grimace. The listener needs to attend to both the spoken words and other information that the speaker is conveying. So listening involves using our eyes as well as our ears in order to receive and interpret (decode) the message. He or she then sends a **feedback** to confirm with the sender that the message is received and understood. The key shows areas in which **barriers** may influence the process.

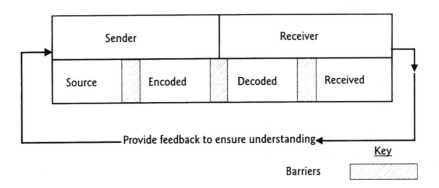

**Diagram showing the process of effective communication**

## Ageing and effective communication

The process of ageing usually causes people to react more slowly, so that talking and understanding may take longer than in younger people. Older people also have occasional difficulties in finding words that explain what they want. This is known as the 'tip of the tongue state' and happens to all of us at times. They also show differences in their style of talking. They may tend to give a great many details and perhaps 'ramble' a little. But these changes in style of communication do not affect their everyday ability to communicate. It is, therefore, important that elderly people are given every encouragement to talk and to express their opinions. A lively, interesting environment will help to stimulate conversation. It is essential that those involved should treat one another with mutual respect.

### *How to promote effective communication*

#### *Guidance*
It is important to develop and maintain good interpersonal relationships with clients based on mutual respect and trust to promote understanding. Ensure that the environment is free from distractions such as noise, and that everyone concerned is comfortable and socially approachable.

#### *Technique*
- approach the individual with a short social greeting
- to 'break the ice' and make friends, sit down and promote communication by using a 'safe' topic, such as what a lovely day etc.
- use non-verbal communication skills, eg. touch or gesture as appropriate and in accordance with established convention for both social and professional settings
- listen attentively and pick up non-verbal signals of client's needs. Tactfully confirm your observations with respect to these needs
- be aware of handicaps and show interest by occasionally posing tactful, short questions
- provide feedback to promote understanding
- do not be in a hurry and show respect for the individual's dignity and self-respect, and demonstrate honesty and undertanding by an occasional nod or 'yes'
- offer some form of refreshment. In a difficult situation with the patient or resident, conclude your conversation with a short social farewell, but do not make promises that you are unable to keep
- thank the person for his or her time.

Communication is the only way a carer can pass on information to clients about their care and maintain a good interpersonal relationship with them and their relatives. A touch coming at the right moment can convey a feeling of understanding, encouragement or compassion to a client or relative. Another means of communicating effectively, is through the sense of smell, eg. the incontinent person will be more than grateful if the carer ensures that odours are not passed on to others by the use of neutralising scent. Also, a display of empathy and humour can be considered the key to effective communication.

The measure of our ability to care depends on how we communicate and maintain good interpersonal relationships with our clients. This means finding out how individual clients usually communicate, what they know about communicating, what problems they have and ways of overcoming them.

## Barriers to effective communication

There are many circumstances which may influence effective communication. Looking at the diagram on the process of communication (see *page 81*), we can see that the *key* indicates specific areas in which communication may be impeded by factors such as:

### 1. Personal characteristics

During a normal conversation, various activities take place in a person's mind. These are attention, distraction, anger, frustration all of which could impede effective communication, and some people may claim to be too busy. Also words have different meanings to different people, for example, a 'row in the lake'. In extreme circumstances, barriers to effective communication could be due to misunderstanding and misinterpretation of what has been said because of language and cultural differences, inexperience, inadequate information or preconceived ideas.

Other factors include:
- attitude — resentment, prejudices, being submissive, patronising, threatening and speaking to someone in a 'superior or dominating' manner. Some people have a general tendency to distort what is being said
- deprivation of needs, belittling or ignoring the person may interfere with his or her ability to listen and understand. Also, irrational fears and beliefs may play an important part in impeding effective communication.

### 2. Language

Language is known as 'the psychological processes which regulate speech'. It is said that language is a man's finest asset as most human activities start with this unique process. Quite often a misunderstanding and misinterpretation of what is being said may be due to language and cultural differences because of the complexity of the English language, eg. *a row in the lake* could have more than one interpretion. However, man communicates in symbolic form and can make known his or her ideas by using these symbols. These two uses of language are very important in care because it is built around the effective communication of ideas.

### Interpreting services

The caring industry provides service for a multi-racial society with a wide variety of languages, most of which are very difficult to understand without the help of an interpreter. More importantly, some clients speak very little English or none at all, which makes it difficult for them to make their wishes known. This language problem presents a barrier to the provision of effective care and is likely to cause anxiety and stress, especially to the residents concerned. It is, therefore, essential to establish on admission the language the person speaks and arrange for someone to act as an interpreter. Some ethnic minority groups and social service departments maintain a list of approved interpreters. The British Red Cross Society and King's Fund Centre, London have picture cards with comprehensive information in many languages. It is important that each care establishment should have a means of evaluating the effectiveness of the interpreting services they use.

### 3. Environmental

The following factors may hinder a person's ability to communicate effectively. It must be said that some of these could be real or imaginary to the individual concerned:
- an atmosphere of suspicion, especially if technical jargon is used frequently
- hostility as a result of poor interpersonal relationships
- autocratic and authoritative leadership
- discomfort, eg. arising from noise and the use of 'social distance' as a barrier to personal contact.

## 4. Specific conditions:
- **physical**, eg. dysarthria and aphasia
- **mental health**: talking with clients suffering from mental health problems such as confusion, depression and Alzheimer's disease is difficult at times but becomes more so, when delusions and hallucinations are present. What we need to do is to use our own life experiences and develop some of the essential caring skills to help us communicate effectively with them.

## References

Hewitt FS (1981) The nurse and the patient, communication skills. *Nurs Times* **77**(17): 13–16

Hewitt FS (1981) Getting it across (information giving — part I). *Nurs Times* **77**(29): 25–28

Hewitt FS (1981) The geography of encounter. *Nurs Times* **77**(17): 13–16

Kershaw B (1989) *Helping to Care. A Handbook for Carers at Home and in Hospital*. Balliere Tindall, London

### Audio visual aids

***Format: VHS video***
*Interpersonal communication skills*
Career track
Ref: CEM 8289: *Exercises in Communication Skills*
Ref: CEM 6835: *Management Skills Series — Communication Skills*
Ref: CEAU 237: *Communication Problems in the Elderly 222*
Oxford Educational Resources Ltd

## Assignment

The purpose of this homework is to assist you in preparing for your Workbased Assessment of Competence. As there is no pressure on you, feel free to work at your own pace, but avoid the temptation to procrastinate. After you have read your notes and suggested references, submit your work for correction. The completed work becomes part of your Personal Portfolio.

### Effective communication (CL1, CL2)

1. State briefly what you understand by the term 'effective communication'.
2. Write down a list of methods of communication used in your area of care.
3. Discuss the factors which may hinder effective communication with clients and colleagues.
4. You seem to be having difficulty in talking with Mr James, a 75-year old resident.
   a) What do you think could be the reason for this situation?
   b) How could you bring about effective communication with him?

### Interpersonal relationship skills (CL1.1)

Belonging, being loved and being wanted are basic human needs. When these needs are fulfilled and then combined with the ability to empathise with others successfully, good human relationships develop. Relationships are the connection and warm responses that exist between people, bringing about unity, friendship and understanding. This type of relationship is an enabling one and can be compared to that which a priest might have with his congregation, a nurse with her patients or a teacher with a child. It embraces social boundaries and provides a demand service and commitment. It asks questions, has respect for others, and accepts responsibility. It is based on trust and sincerity, and must be taken seriously. This relationship means caring for people.

## Components of a relationship

There are many factors which contribute to the development of a good rapport. These include: attitudes, personal values, behaviour, custom, beliefs and culture. Within these elements, interaction goes on according to certain defined social rules. This means that a person can replace either of the two people in a particular relationship and still keep the relationship going based on an ability to demonstrate effective:

- social skills
- assertiveness skills
- communication skills — discussed in *Unit 6*.

### Social skills

These are basic social routines or greetings used to influence and interact amicably with people in various settings. They involve the use of social behaviour which allows for physical contact and non-verbal forms of communication, such as gestures, posture, facial expressions, eye contact and movements of hands and head. In western society, it is usual to offer one's hand to a stranger, followed by a verbal salutation and greetings, eg. 'good morning'. Argyle (1969) believes that this form of social contact sends out signals of liking or dominance in order to manage the immediate situation. Gestures usually replace verbal communication when noise or distance makes this impossible.

The way we approach people influences their responses and invites social responses that are translated into appropriate actions. For example, if you give a glass of water with a smile to a client, he or she may receive it and say 'thank you' with a smile in return. Awareness of an individual's beliefs, values, customs, social rules and routines avoids causing offence and maintains good interpersonal relationships. If these social conventions are observed, then communication improves even in situations where stress or illness cause social problems.

### Conversation

#### Guidelines

The approach is similar to that of communication skills with clients:
- approach the situation with a confident smile
- use social greetings or salutations, eg. 'good afternoon'
- open the conversation with safe remarks, especially if addressing a new client
- introduce the topic of conversation, eg. information-seeking or giving or social contact, such as helping a newly admitted client to settle in
- develop the topic by making a fairly general statement followed by detailed and specific information
- use non-verbal communication as well, especially a smile, eye contact or touch.

#### Termination of conversation

The end of any relationship is crucial and will govern the future behaviour or function of the individual so it is important to terminate the conversation successfully. If a carer relates closely with a client by allowing free expression and warmth of feelings to circulate between them, the client may be encouraged to seek more fulfilling relationships in the future. In this way, the carer can help the person to achieve a major life task. Always thank the person for his or her time.

## Assertiveness skills

Assertiveness is the ability to stand up for one's rights without interfering with the rights of others. It means being honest with oneself and with others. Good assertiveness skills allow you to say emphatically what you want, need or feel without offending other people.

It is a skill which carers need to acquire in order to manage their own stress, to respond to other peoples' feelings and anxieties appropriately, and to cope with situations of conflict. Being assertive is to feel comfortable with yourself. An assertive person has self-respect and is not afraid to say the right thing at the right time, and feel good about the outcome. There are times when people are assertive and do not get what they want. But you should still have confidence in yourself and behave in a positive way, negotiating and reaching a workable compromise.

## Forms of assertiveness

### 1. Passive behaviour

This means manipulating people and getting your own way at the expense of others. It also means not speaking out, being a victim and putting up with possibly antisocial behaviour in order not to 'rock the boat'.

### 2. Positive behaviour

People differ about issues that are fundamental to their view of life, and which are bound to produce a strong personal feeling and response. For instance, the matron makes a request for you to change your holiday for the second time in a year. You may say, 'oh no, not again. Why is it always me you ask to change holidays? I booked my holiday a long time ago and may lose my deposit.' Alternatively, you can be feel inwardly aggressive, but because your anger is not expressed, it will still be there hours later. The way the incident is handled should not be damaging to your self-esteem but should make you feel satisfied and positive. Therefore, compose yourself, maintain self-control and talk to the matron directly and assertively.

### *Guidance*

In an informal setting:
- first decide, what you want to say and arrange to see the matron. State your thoughts and feelings clearly and without insistence or apology. Use linking words, such as 'however', 'but', 'even so'
- listen to what is being said to you, and then show the other person that you hear and understand what they are saying. Pay attention to the other person and demonstrate empathy, even if you do not agree with the situation in which you are placed. Do not be manipulated or side-tracked
- say what you want to happen and be prepared to reach a workable compromise or 'middle way'. Give a clear and straightforward version of the action or outcome you expect without hesitating or sounding dictatorial or difficult. But aim for 'win-win'.

In a formal setting:
- sit upright and straight, relax and move your hands freely and easily
- use direct eye contact but do not stare
- use facial expressions which fit the words, and moderate the tone of your voice. Say 'no' without being frightened, maladroit or aggressive
- be positive in the dialogue, but do not try to manipulate the situation. Be honest
- help an aggressive individual to relax and listen to you by agreeing with some of what he or she says; demonstrate an ability to calm things down without losing your integrity.

## Benefits of being assertive

Carers can be advocates by standing up for the rights of their clients or patients. This will result in:
- people being happier with themselves and the way they handle difficult or tricky situations
- getting the best from people at work, including themselves
- a reduction of stress as people are more likely to manage conflict situations early and in a competent way
- the organisation having a more confident and competent workforce
- more direct talking and less 'hidden agenda'
- issues being resolved at an early stage, before they become long-term problems. So, be assertive.

## Summary

The use of interpersonal relationship skills has an important value in caring for people. Your personality can be used as a therapeutic agent, allowing healing and changes to take place. You may have noticed that at times being 'too nice' is not particularly effective, and may diminsh your self-respect. Being assertive lets you speak up confidently and people will listen to you.

## References

Argyle M (1969) *Social Interaction*. Methuen, London

Argyle M (1988) *Bodily Communication*. 2nd edn. Routledge, London

Bond M (1986) *Stress and Self-awareness: A Guide for Nurses*. Heinemann, London

Bridge W (1980) *Teaching Communication in Patient Care*. RCN, London

Burnard P, Morrison P (1991) Nurses' interpersonal skills: a study of nurses' perspectives. *Nurse Educ Today* **11**: 24–29

Dickson A (1982) *A Woman in Your Own Right: Assertiveness and You*. Quartet, London

Egan G (1990) *The Skilled Helper* (4th edn). Brookes-Cole Co, California

Hewitt FS (1981) The nurse and the patient communication skills. Part 2: getting it across. *Nurs Times* **77**(30): 29–32

Pitcher F (1986) *Business Matters*. BBC TV, London

## Audio visual aids

### Format: VHS videos

Ref: *Straight Talking: The Art of Assertiveness*. Video arts, London

Ref: *Working with Assertiveness*. BBC Enterprises Ltd, London

Ref: CEM 8187: *Decision Exercises. Dealing with Difficult Situations*

Ref: CEM 6534: *Effective Organisational and Interpersonal Communication*

Oxford Educational Resources Ltd

## Assignment

The purpose of this homework is to assist you in preparing for your Workbased Assessment of Competence. As there is no pressure on you, feel free to work at your own pace, but avoid the temptation to procrastinate. After you have read your notes and suggested references, submit your work for correction. The completed work becomes part of your Personal Portfolio.

## Interpersonal relationship skills (CL1.1)

1. Explain the term 'interpersonal relationship skills' and list its components.
2. Why is it important to develop and maintain good interpersonal relationships with people, especially those in your place of work?
3. Discuss how you would help a newly admitted client to 'get on' with other residents.
4. It is believed that social skills can be used to influence people in any setting.
    a) Discuss how you could use this skill to develop and maintain effective relationships with an elderly lady in your care.
    b) Discuss factors which may hinder this relationship, and how you would prevent this unhappy relationship from developing?
5. Explain what you would do in the following circumstances:
    a) When you returned from shopping, your next door neighbour who has not been friendly has parked his or her car in your parking space in front of your house.
    b) When you need the support of the person-in-charge to introduce a new idea at work.
6. Give three situations where it might be appropriate to encourage clients to develop and maintain good interpersonal relationships, and where it might not be appropriate.

# Unit 3(a)
# Health, safety and security in the workplace (CU1)

## Health and Safety at Work Act 1974 (HSW)

The aim of the Health and Safety at Work Act 1974, is to maintain or improve the standards of health, safety and welfare of persons at work. It also protects others against risks to health or safety arising out of or in connection with activities of persons at work. It controls the keeping and using of explosives, toxic and highly flammable substances, and the sending of harmful substances into the atmosphere. The Act replaces many regulations relating to health and safety such as the Factories Act (1961) and Offices, Shops and Railway Premises Act (1963). It identifies and places responsibilities for safety on the employer, employee and management, ie. **everyone**.

**Employers' responsibilities**

The employer has a duty under the law to ensure as far as reasonably practical, the health, safety and welfare of their employees at work. These responsibilities are an integral part of providing high standards and quality of care and include:

- taking all necessary precautions to ensure that fumes, gases, dust, noise and odours emitted are under control
- encouraging all staff to be safety conscious and to report all faults and hazards, eg. electrical wiring, loose floor tiles
- carrying out regular safety inspections within the care establishments
- displaying all health and safety information within the care establishment, and bringing new regulations to the attention of staff
- ensuring that all staff are aware of available first aid facilities and the procedures for reporting and investigating accidents
- taking precaution against fire, and providing equipment for fighting fire
- training and instructing staff in safe working practices and providing free protective clothing or equipment specifically required by law
- drawing up a health and safety policy statement if there are five or more employees, and bringing this to the attention of employees
- reporting certain injuries, diseases and dangerous occurrences to enforcing authority
- providing and maintaining equipment and systems that are safe, and without health risks in the use, handling, storage and transport of articles and substances
- facilitating and complying with all statutory monitoring processes of the Act and legislation concerning environmental health.

**Management responsibilities**

All managers have responsibility for the safety of all who come within their sphere of authority, and should be able to:

- ensure that staff adhere to orders and procedures

- provide training for safe practices and work methods
- explain hazards and safe practices to new employees in the department before they begin work
- ensure that each new employee is given an induction manual which should include the policies and procedures appropriate to their specific role and functions
- report and record all accidents
- provide written health and safety procedures for the care establishment in accordance with relevant legislation. Among other items, the procedures should cover:
    - fire-fighting equipment
    - the safe lifting and handling of residents
    - first aid procedures and location of first aid boxes
    - infection control and management
    - procedure to be followed in the event of a missing person
    - investigation of all accidents with a view to prevention.

**Employees' responsibilities**

The HSW Act requires every employee to be able to:
- take reasonable care for ensuring the health and safety of themselves and any other persons who may be affected by what they do or do not do
- co-operate in ensuring that procedures for safe working practices are observed
- make themselves familiar with the health and safety policy and any supplementary documents produced, and participate in various forms of training provided by employers
- wear the appropriate safety clothing and use appropriate safety devices where applicable, and observe safety rules at all times
- report any accidents and damage immediately to managers regardless of whether or not persons are injured
- refrain from interfering with or misusing anything provided to secure health and safety at work
- bring to the attention of the employers an act or abuse which could place patients and others in jeopardy or which militates against safe standards of practice.

Generally, all employees have a responsibility to do everything they can to prevent injury to themselves, their clients, colleagues and others. They are expected to familiarise themselves with local policy and procedures and report any incidents which may lead to injury or damage.

**The care assistants**

They should be able to take reasonable care in assisting professionally qualified practitioners in carrying out procedures, eg. security, storage and administration of medicines in accordance with the Pharmacy and Poisons Act and UKCC (1982) Guidance on Administration of Medicines. Those in residential care homes should be aware of local policy regarding administration of medicines. Knowledge of infection control is very important and includes proper disposal of syringes and needles to prevent needle-stick injuries and infection from needles and sharp objects.

*Guidance*
- report any safety hazards or accidents within local policy
- dress properly for work, wear issued uniform, comfortable fitting shoes, disposable aprons and gloves
- never try to lift heavy or awkward furniture without help or lift clients without following the correct techniques and guidelines
- carry out regular inspections, check and report on safety matters and the state of equipment, eg. beds and trolleys.

It is essential that everyone, especially qualified staff, should continually update and refresh their knowledge and skills about various aspects of the caring procedures. Care assistants should receive appropriate training and instruction on the safety aspects of client care, eg. basic lifting techniques.

### Domestic and ancillary staff
These staff should be especially careful when using cleaning fluids or gas and electrical appliances. Regular inspection and reports should be made on all equipment and faults should be repaired immediately. Domestic staff should receive instruction on the use and care of utensils, disinfectants, cleaning equipment, maintenance of floors and the importance of personal hygiene.

### Kitchen staff
The cook and other kitchen staff should be aware of special statutory regulations about Food Hygiene (General) Regulations 1990 on the preparation and handling of food. Wet floors are a common cause of falls in the kitchen. Care should be taken to dry these as much as possible. Leave a warning sign — 'WET FLOOR'.

### General maintenance staff
Most care establishments employ a general handyperson to provide regular repair and maintenance services. These employees should be familiar with the statutory regulations relating to the use and maintenance of machinery and equipment in accordance with manufacturers' recommendations. They should:
- observe the safety rules at all times and remove any equipment that is considered risky until it has been repaired or replaced
- provide safe arrangements for the handling, storage and movement of materials, equipment and substances
- inspect equipment such as lighting, passageways, fire alarms, fire escapes, fire extinguishers to ensure their efficiency and maintenance
- carry out frequent safety checks.

## New Health and Safety at Work Regulations (1992)

A set of new regulations which came into force at the beginning of 1993, apply to most kinds of work activity. Like the law on health and safety, they place duties on employers to protect their employees and others, including members of the public who may be affected by work being done. These new regulations are necessary to implement the following six European Community (EC) directives on health and safety at work.

### The new regulations cover:
1. **Health and safety management**: to assess the risks to the health and safety of employees and anyone else who may be affected by the work activity, to identify the necessary preventive and protective measures.
2. **Work equipment safety**: to ensure that equipment is suitable for its purpose.
3. **Manual handling of loads**: to assess adequately and avoid handling hazardous operations where reasonably practicable.
4. **Workplace conditions**: to make sure that the working environment, safety facilities, and housekeeping comply with new regulations.
5. **Personal protective equipment (PPE)**: to assess the risks, maintain, provide, ensure that PPE is used properly and provide training, information and instruction to employees.

6. **Display screen equipment**: to assess display screen equipment workstations and reduce risks as necessary.

## Consultation with employees

Since October 1996 it is a requirement for employers to consult their employees on health and safety matters, especially in situations where trade unions are not recognised and where there is no health and safety representatives. Areas of consultation include:
- risk and dangers likely to arise from the work and action taken to reduce or overcome these
- any changes which may affect employees health and safety at work, eg. procedures, equipment
- plans for health and safety training
- influence on health and safety of introducing new technology.

# References

Buckley N (1991) How safe is your ward? *Nurs Times* **87**(6): 31–33

Department of Social Security (1974) *Health and Safety at Work Act 1974*. HMSO, London

Finch J (1980) Who is responsible for health and safety? Law and the nurse series. *Nurs Mirror*, September: 26–27

Health and Safety Executive (1993) *New Health and Safety Regulations*. HSE, Sheffield

Health and Safety Executive (1985) *The Reporting of Injuries or Dangerous Occurrences Regulations*. HSE 11(Rev), Sheffield

Health and Safety Executive (1989) *Health and Safety Law: What you Should Know*. HSE, Sheffield

Health and Safety Executive (1992) *Essentials of Health and Safety at Work* (revised edn). HMSO, London

Health and Safety Executive (1993) *New Health and Safety at Work Regulations*. IND(G) 124 (L), Sheffield

Health and Safety Executive (1985) *Health and Safety at Work Regulations Act 1974. Advice to Employees*. HSC, Sheffield

Health and Safety Executive (1993) *Health and Safety at Work Regulations Act. Advice to Employers*. HSC, Sheffield.

## Audio visual aids

### Format: VHS Video

Ref: 331/1-2: *Health and Safety Act Part 1: Medical and Nursing*

Oxford Educational Resources Ltd

# Assignment

The purpose of this homework is to assist you in preparing for your Workbased Assessment of Competence. As there is no pressure on you, feel free to work at your own pace, but avoid the temptation to procrastinate. After you have read your notes and suggested references, submit your work for correction. The completed work becomes part of your Personal Portfolio.

# Health and Safety at Work Act 1974 (CU1)

1. Discuss your role in maintaining the health and safety of your care environment.
2. What are your responsibilities to:

    a) residents
    b) colleagues
    c) yourself?
3. Discuss how you would deal with wastage and spillage, eg. body waste, dressings, sharp implements, aerosol cans and bottles including precautions you would take.

# Fire precautions (CU1)

Fire is a possibly lethal menace in hospitals and residential care establishments. Most people consider that fire, gas escapes, water leakage and floods, bomb alerts or other emergencies will never happen to them. However, emergencies do occur and when this happens in a care establishment residents depend upon nurses and care assistants for their safety. Staff must be constantly aware of fire risks associated with flammable items such as bedclothes and mattresses. These are a source of rapidly spreading fire and toxic fumes, which can cause death.

### Legal and policies requirements

The Health and Safety at Work Act, 1974 imposes a general duty on every employer to protect the health and welfare of all employees at their place of work, and others who may be affected. Also, care establishments are required by law (Fire Precaution Act, 1971) to have their own fire prevention equipment, such as smoke detectors, fire extinguishers, and procedures in case of fire. They are required to have a secondary means of fire escape from each floor. Fire points must be clearly indicated, and all staff must be instructed in the use of fire extinguishers and other fire fighting and prevention equipment.

In practice, hospitals and residential care establishments are regularly inspected by local Fire Prevention Officers and recommendations are made to the owners of premises on what precautions must be provided. These will include:
- means of escape in case of fire
- fire alarms
- fire-fighting equipment
- any other requirements relating to building regulations.

### Preventative measures

#### 1. Training
Research has shown that all care establishments at one time or other, have small fires. But what is important is the correct use of procedures for dealing with such outbreaks. Staff training should include:
- how to raise the alarm in the event of fire
- what the alternative escape routes are from each area
- where fire extinguishers are located and their method of use.

#### 2. Fire lectures
Lectures and training should be arranged for all staff on a regular basis. It is important to pay attention to fire drills so that everyone is conversant with local recognised procedures, and are able to locate and identify different types of fire extinguishers and how they work. Staff should participate in fire drills and training programmes and maintain a record of attendance in their Personal Portfolio.

### 3. Recognising fire hazards

Awareness of fire hazards is the first step towards fire prevention and safety, followed by the precautions that should be taken by staff and residents. Remember the three elements required for a fire to start, and by removing any one of them fire can be prevented. These are:

**Heat**: a spark or flame

**Oxygen**: normal air

**Fuel**: combustible material.

*Action*
- activate the fire alarm and close all doors to contain the fire and delay its spread.

### Smoking

People whose functional abilities are reduced as a result of their physical or mental state or the effects of drugs tend to smoke but are quite often incapable of handling smoking materials safely.

*Action*
- never leave them unsupervised. Allow smoking in specially designated areas only
- provide plenty of ashtrays in that area and empty them frequently
- never allow the use of paper cups or rubbish bins as ashtrays
- never allow smoking where oxygen is in use.

### Electrical wiring

Regularly inspect electrical equipment and report any suspected fault. Do not use any equipment with frayed or worn power leads, or broken or cracked casings.

### Aerosols

Never use an aerosol spray in the presence of lighted cigarettes or naked flames. Keep in a cool place, and never on a window sill: they can easily be heated by the sun shining through the glass and may explode when the pressure, caused by the expansion of the heated gas, builds up.

### Fire extinguishers

Note the different types of extinguishers available in your place of work, how to use them and which to use on which type of fire. Also note when fire blankets should be used.

### Combustible substances

Ensure that heat-producing appliances are kept at a safe distance from bedcovers, upholstery, plastics (mugs, cups, trays) paper (charts, magazines).

### Corridors and passages

It is important to make sure that equipment and furniture do not block stairways, doors and entrances to the care establishment. Signs indicating exits must be lit at all times and failure must be reported immediately.

## Waste disposal

Refuse must always be disposed in appropriate containers which should be kept outside and well away from sources of heat. Most places now have wheeled dustbins with attached lids, but if your home still has conventional dustbins, ensure that the lids are firmly in place at all times.

### General guidance in case of fire
- be sure that you know your organisation's fire emergency procedures
- demonstrate your knowledge of the existence and position of fire points
- know how to raise the alarm in the event of fire
- ensure that fire doors are kept closed at all times, unless magnetic restraints are fitted which will be released when the fire alarm is activated
- know the designated fire escape routes
- be aware of an emergency telephone number
- ensure that everyone is accounted for, including the staff and visitors.

## Action to be taken on discovery of smoke/fire (ARCE)

1. A: *Alarm* — activate the alarm.
2. R: *Rescue* — people in the immediate danger area if safe to do so, by evacuating the premises.
3. C: *Contain* — the fire by closing doors and windows.
4. E: *Extinguish* — the fire by using the correct equipment if it is safe to do so.

## Other ways to fight fire

Smother a fat pan fire with a damp tea cloth or fire blanket if it is safe to do so, especially in the kitchen.

When the fire brigade or/and police arrive, follow the instructions of the officers responsible for fire-fighting and evacuation of the premises.

***DO NOT ALLOW YOURSELF TO BE GUILTY OF IGNORANCE IN THE CASE OF FIRE. ALWAYS ASK IF THERE ARE ANY FIRE PRECAUTION PROCEDURES YOU ARE NOT SURE ABOUT.***

# References

Dooley TP (1981) Fire! The nursing response. *Nurs Times* **77**(21):1845–1848

Department of Health and Social Security (1978) The organisation and management of fire precautions. *NHS Circular* **78**(4)

Scriptographic (1989) *Fire Safety in Health Care Premises*. Scriptographs Publications Ltd, Surrey

Home Office Public Relations Branch (1991) *Fire Safety in the Home* (FLO6). Home Office, London

Home Office Publications Branch (1991) *Fire Safety Advice for Disabled People* (FB6). Home Office, London

## Audio visual aids

### Format: VHS Video
Ref: *Firetrap*
Concord Films Council
Ref: *Fire Prevention in an Old Person's Accommodation*

Ref: 420CT: *Fire in the Home*
Oxford Educational Resources Ltd

# Assignment

The purpose of this homework is to assist you in preparing for your Workbased Assessment of Competence. As there is no pressure on you, feel free to work at your own pace, but avoid the temptation to procrastinate. After you have read your notes and suggested references, submit your work for correction. The completed work becomes part of your Personal Portfolio

## Fire precautions (CU1.1)

1. What is the first thing you should do on:
   a) hearing the fire alarm?
   b) discovering a fire?
2. Where are the fire alarm call points located in your work environment?
3. Make a list of fire-fighting equipment and their locations in your place of work.
4. Discuss your role after the fire alarm has sounded?
5. Where do the residents go to?
6. What would you do about:
   a) doors?
   b) windows?
7. How would you tell if a room is unsafe to enter?
8. If you are using a fire extinguisher, when should you stop using it?
9. Differentiate between and discuss the importance of:
   a) fire drill?
   b) fire lecture?

## Health emergencies (first aid) (CU1.2)

First aid is the skilled application of acceptable principles of treatment given to an injured person or in the case of sudden illness, using materials available, until the casualty is placed in the care of a doctor or removed to hospital. It is not a proper treatment, but a way of responding to an emergency situation as quickly as possible in order to save life.

Nurses and other carers in the health care settings are usually very knowledgeable about first aid mainly due to the fact that their time on duty is spent trying to prevent emergencies from happening. However, they rarely use their knowledge and skills in the practice of first aid except in an emergency situation.

Whoever practises first aid is accountable to the casualty, society and also to the employer if the accident happens during the course of duty. If something goes wrong, the first aider is open to civil proceedings from the casualty or his/her relatives. However, the patient should be your main concern, and as long as you act always in the interest of the casualty, providing you know what you are doing, and are prepared to justify it later to uphold professional standards, the threat of legal proceedings should not inform your practice. Many people feel apprehensive when faced with an emergency. People who offer first aid must accept that, however hard they try, casualties may not respond as expected.

### Aims of first aid:

1. To sustain life by:
   - performing emergency resuscitation, stopping bleeding, sending for help.
2. To prevent the condition from becoming worse by:
   - covering all wounds and immobilising any fractures
   - placing the casualty in the correct or comfortable position.
3. To promote recovery by:
   - reassuring the casualty and friends
   - relieving any pain through careful moving and handling of the casualty
   - protecting the casualty from extreme temperature or adverse weather conditions.

### First aid needs in workplace

Under the Health and Safety at Work Regulations 1981, workplaces must have provision for first aid. The form it takes depends on various factors, especially, the nature and degree of hazards at work, whether there is shift working, what medical services are available and the number of employees.

### First aider

This is a person trained to provide first aid at work. He or she is authorised to take charge of the situations, eg. call an ambulance if there is a serious injury or illness, identify and deal with hazards and advice on the necessary training.

### Accountability

A nurse is legally accountable for his/her practice when administering first aid. The nurse as a professional has no formal role to play in first aid, but should be aware of the legal position of a nurse carrying out first aid in an emergency situation. If something goes wrong at an accident, the first aider is open to civil actions from the casualty or his/her relatives. What the casualty seeks is compensation or, 'damages'. It is not about punishment, but an attempt to put the injured party back, in financial terms, in the position he or she would have been in if he or she had not been wronged. A direct claim will not be made against the nurse, but against his or her employer.

### First-aid boxes

It is the responsibility of employers to provide first-aid boxes containing items that a first aider has been trained to use. The boxes should always be checked to ensure that they are adequately stocked and do not contain medication of any kind.

#### *Content*
- guidance leaflet *First Aid at Work*
- individually wrapped sterile adhesive dressings of assorted sizes
- sterile eye pads, with attachment
- individually wrapped triangular bandages
- safety pins
- individually wrapped sterile undedicated wound dressings of various sizes

- individually wrapped moist cleaning wipes.

## Action at emergency situations

In an emergency situation, many different things may happen at once, and this may affect your concentration, but remember that someone's life may depend upon what you do and how you do it. Remain calm and in control. Observe the following principles:

### 1. Assess the situation
- identify any danger to yourself, the casualty and bystanders
- find out what resources are available and what may be needed
- ask the casualty or a bystander what happened, and obtain a history of the accident
- examine the casualty if possible to determine signs and symptoms
- note the time of accident on your arrival at the scene and if there are any witnesses
- check to see whether there is anyone else with first aid training available.

### 2. Make the area safe
- ensure that there is no further danger to yourself, the casualty or to bystanders
- remove the casualty from the cause or the cause from the casualty, eg. cut the electric current
- seek specialist help and equipment if you cannot remove a life-threatening danger
- do not move the casualty unnecessarily. If you must, immobilise any fractures and dress large wounds.

### 3. Give emergency aid
- check that the casualty is breathing, conscious and not bleeding
- give priority to the most urgent conditions in the following order
  - those who are unconscious
  - those who are bleeding
  - those who you know or suspect to have fractures, and other casualties
- position the casualty correctly and protect him/her from inquisitive bystanders who have not seen the actual incident
- observe carefully for any changes in his/her condition
- maintain the casualty's right for privacy, self-respect and dignity
- never give a casualty anything to eat, drink or smoke.

### 4. Get help
- invite bystanders to dial 999 or to carry out other tasks, eg. maintaining safety
- send for the person-in-charge in the care setting
- make use of all the resources available
- reassure the casualty constantly
- do not attempt to do too much.

## Recovery position

This position may be necessary to prevent the casualty from choking on his/her tongue or vomit, especially if the person is unconscious and lying on his or her back.
1. Kneel beside the casualty and place both his/her arms close to the body.
2. Turn the casualty gently onto his/her side (left or right lateral position).
3. Tilt his/her head with his/her jaw forward to maintain the open airway.

4. Draw the upper arm and leg upwards and outwards to form right angles with the body, and prevent the casualty from rolling forwards or backwards.
5. Check that he or she is breathing and take the pulse frequently. If there is a pulse but no breathing start artificial ventilation or resuscitation immediately.

**Cessation of breathing**

In all cases of cessation of breathing and heartbeat, artificial respiration must be started at once to supply oxygen to the blood which must reach the brain within three minutes otherwise irreparable damage will be done.

**The DRABC of resuscitation**

Techniques aim to preserve life by maintaining an adequate supply of oxygen to the brain. If breathing and pulse are present, put the casualty into the recovery position and monitor his/her condition. But if there is pulse but no breathing, start artificial ventilation.

D — remove danger
R — check for response
— talk to the casualty
— shake gently
A — open the airway
— remove any obvious obstruction in the mouth
— lift the casualty's jaw and tilt the head backwards
B — check breathing
— look to see if the chest is rising
— listen and feel for the casualty's breath against your check for at least five seconds
C — check circulation
— check for a pulse by palpating the carotid artery for at least five seconds
— get help immediately if there is no pulse or breathing.

**Looking after yourself**

*Guidance*
When rendering first aid, you should be aware of the risks of HIV/Hepatitis B, and always take steps to protect yourself. Always wear disposable gloves if available and use face shield or mask when giving artificial ventilation if you have been trained to use one.

# Other health emergencies (CU1.3)

An emergency is a crisis situation which is usually unplanned and happens suddenly. Someone's life is in danger and you must act quickly. Although it is important to summon help, you must also act quickly. Assess the situation and make sure that there is no further injury to the casualty, everybody is relatively safe and you are not exposed to danger. It is important to be alert and be aware of simple remedies that can prevent serious injuries if action is taken promptly in emergency situations, such as:

**Shock**

This is a condition in which there is a sudden fall in blood pressure as a result of major injuries.

### Signs and symptoms
The following symptoms may occur:
- the casualty may feel sick, vomit or complain of thirst
- the skin will be cold, moist and clammy to touch
- breathing will be shallow and rapid, and at times the casualty will yawn and sigh
- the pulse is fast and feeble with low blood pressure
- the casualty will be restless, and if untreated may become unconscious and die.

### Management
The aim is to ensure an adequate blood supply to vital organs of the body.

#### Guidance
- summon help immediately
- reassure the casualty and lay him or her down with head lowered and feet raised
- loosen any tight clothing to help breathing and blood circulation
- keep the casualty warm with space blanket if available or a thick coat, but *never* with added heat such as a hot water bottle as this will prevent blood from reaching the vital organs
- place the casualty in a recovery position if he or she is unconscious, and move him/her as little as possible
- give nothing by mouth as this may cause vomiting, but moisten lips with water or soak a piece of cloth with water and allow casualty to suck if he or she complains of thirst
- carry out artificial respiration if breathing or heartbeat stops
- complete the accident and emergency book in accordance with local procedures and practise.

## Obstruction of airway

A person may choke if a foreign body, such as a piece of food completely blocks the airway. The person tries to clutch his/her throat and coughs in a self-rescue attempt to clear the obstruction. If this is the case, do not interfere but observe and support the person by placing your hand on his or her back.

### Management
If the victim cannot cough or speak, stand behind and bend him forward with his head low. Give two or three hard slaps between the shoulder, repeating if necessary.

If the casualty is a child, hold the head down, place him/her over your knees, and give a few taps on the back of the chest as this action may dislodge the object. Carry out Heimlich manoeuvre if the victim is still choking.

### Heimlich manoeuvre
- stand behind the victim, slide your arms under his arms and encircle him around the waist
- clench a fist with one hand and place it firmly in the soft space between the lower end of the breast bone and the abdomen at the level of the navel where the rib cage meets. Be careful not to touch the sternum (breast bone)
- hold the fist tightly with your other hand and give a hard sharp thrust with an inward and upward movement, pushing the upper abdomen against the lungs to force the air violently upwards. Give four rapid thrusts and repeat the procedure if necessary.

These thrusts should dislodge the obstruction, forcing it upward and out through the throat. But if the person loses consciousness from choking, the muscles of the neck may be sufficiently relaxed so that the airway is not completely blocked, thereby allowing removal of the obstruction. If the victim has fallen to the ground, send for help and commence artificial respiration immediately.

## Burns and scalds

These are injuries to the tissues of the body caused by dry heat such as electricity, nuclear radiation, corrosive chemical agents, eg. acids, sulphuric or caustic alkalis, or extreme cold, ultraviolet sunlight, friction and lightning.

### *Signs and symptoms*
The casualty usually complains of severe pain and there is redness of the skin. Blister formation may follow and if burst, may result in fluid (plasma) loss. Acute shock is usually present.

### *Management of burns and scalds*
If clothes are on fire, put out the fire with water or smother the area of the body with the nearest available thick cloth, rug, towel or a jacket or coat. Remove anything that may be constricting immediately, eg. rings, bangles, before swelling starts.
- wrap clean material such as a handkerchief over the burn area to exclude air
- do not tear off burnt material which may be stuck to the skin.

### *Management of burns*
The immediate first aid treatment is to put the affected part into cold water as quickly as possible. A cold compress will reduce the amount of tissue damage produced by the heat.
- seek immediate help
- immerse the injured area in cold water or place it under slow running cold water
- apply a large thick pad soaked in cold water to other parts of the body such as the face or abdomen and repeat as necessary
- keep the area cool and renew the cold pad every 10 minutes
- elevate and cover the area with the cleanest material available
- do not use ice water as ordinary tepid water from the tap is sufficient
- treat for shock by keeping the casualty warm
- give small amounts of cold drinks at frequent intervals to maintain body fluid if the casualty is conscious
- do not apply any lotions or ointments to the area
- do not prick or burst the blister, breathe, touch or cough over the burned area.

## Chemical burns

- wash the area very quickly with plenty of running water
- remove any contaminated clothes
- summon help immediately.

## Scalds of the mouth

These are injuries to tissues caused by hot or moist liquid, eg. boiling water or steam.

### *Management*
If casualty is conscious, give ice to suck or repeat sips of cold water as often as possible.

## Bleeding — haemorrhage

This is defined as an escape of blood from an injured or ruptured blood vessel.

### *Classification*
There are three main groupings:

**Arterial:** an escape of bright red blood in which the pumping action corresponds with the beating of the heart. Bleeding will be profuse if an injury has severed an artery.

**Treatment:** local pressure over the artery supplying the wound area, follow by raising the injured part of the body.

**Venous:** this is dark red blood slower flowing and not pumping out.

**Treatment:** put a pad on the wound, raise the limb and wait for bleeding to stop

**Capillary:** bright red blood oozes from the capillary blood vessel. Treatment is application of a local pad over the wound area.

## Types of bleeding

There are two main types.

### Internal Bleeding

As its name implies this is bleeding that occurs inside and cannot be seen from outside the body.

### Signs and symptoms

- deep sigh breathing with a feeling of faintness leading gradually to loss of consciousness
- thirst with blurred vision and increased restlessness
- low blood pressure and temperature, with an increasingly feeble and rapid pulse rate.

### *Guidance*

- reassure and lay the casualty flat with his/her head low and feet raised
- cover and keep him/her warm but do not apply heat
- give nothing by mouth
- take and record pulse and respiration every 15 minutes
- talk to him/her and calm him/her down while waiting for medical aid to arrive.

### External bleeding

This type of bleeding is easy to see and normally requires immediate treatment:

- reassure and lay the casualty down with the affected part raised unless you think that movement would seriously disturb any fracture which may be present
- treat for shock by keeping the victim warm
- examine wound to ensure that there are no broken pieces of glass or foreign bodies that may cause further injury
- cover the area lightly with a clean cloth or first aid dressing if a foreign body is present in the wound. Apply pressure to the artery proximal to the injury, but for not longer than 15 minutes
- place a clean or sterile unmedicated or dressing pad over the wound and apply direct pressure with fingers to the bleeding part for about 5 to 13 minutes pressing hard to stop the bleeding
- bandage the pad very firmly and do not release the pressure until the bandage is complete
- keep watch on the bandage. If blood oozes through, do not remove the original dressing. Apply another pad and bandage firmly over the previous pad.

## Fracture

This is defined as a break in the bone.

### Signs and symptoms

1. **General shock**, especially at the sound of the bone snapping or sight of blood.
2. **Local** which may include:

- pain at the site of the fracture, tenderness and swelling due to rupture of blood vessels
- shortening and deformity of limb. The injured part is shorter than its opposite member
- abnormal mobility*: normally a limb moves only at a joint; but when a bone is completely broken, there may be an abnormal movement from a false joint
- crepitus*: this is a creaking vibration at the site of the fracture due to sharp ends of fragments of the bone rubbing together.

*no attempt should be made to test for these signs.

## Types of fractures

1. Simple (closed) — a clean break with the skin remaining intact.
2. Compound (open) — there is a wound from the broken bone to the skin through which infection may enter.
3. Complicated — the fracture is complicated by injury to blood vessels, nerves and vital organs.
4. Comminuted — the bone is broken in several places and there is splintering of the bone.

Other types include greenstick fractures in children, depressed fractures eg. in the bones of the skull.

## Management of fractures

### *Guidance*

The main aim is to immobilise the part as follows:
- reassure the casualty and ask him/her not to move
- treat for shock
- stop any severe bleeding at once and dress open wounds
- treat the fracture where the casualty lies and do not attempt to move him/her if there is a suspected fracture of the spine
- immobilise the fracture by using:
  - padded splint and bandage
  - soft thick padding between the two parts of the body involved, eg. legs
  - walking sticks, umbrella, broom handles, ties, stockings
- arrange for transportation of the casualty to a hospital.

## Strains and sprains

These are soft tissue injuries which may occur as clients are encouraged to take more exercise. Strains and sprains cause swelling, bruising and pain to the affected tissues. Sometimes a fracture may be suspected and must be treated accordingly.

### *Guidance*

If swelling occurs immediately after the accident:
- rest the part to avoid further damage
- apply cold compress, eg. ice to constrict blood vessels and reduce bruising and swelling. Sometimes a small pack of frozen peas is applied for 10–15 minutes, 3–4 times a day
- raise the affected part to drain tissue fluids by gravity and relieve pain
- if the swelling and pain continue, the casualty should be referred to hospital for X-ray and further treatment.

## Abrasions

A client may fall and scrape his/her arm or leg against a rough surface. This causes friction with a loss of superficial skin. The nerve endings are exposed and the area can be very painful.

### Management
- clean the wound with water or saline to remove any grit on the skin
- dry the wound and apply a suitable non-adherent dressing as a protection

## References

Bird H (1991) Sports injuries and their management. *Pract Nurse* **4**: 355–388

Holmes D (1992) Injury prevention: why warm-ups are cool. Report on sports medicine. *Pract Nurse* **5**: 233–234

Skeet M (1981) *Emergency Procedures and First Aid for Nurses*. Blackwell Scientific Publications, Oxford

Gulliver G (1991) Sticking together. *Nurs Times* June 5 **87**:74–78

Walsh M (1990) *Accident and Emergency Nursing — A New Approach*, 2nd edn. Butterworth Heinemann Press, Oxford

## Audio visual aids

### Format: VHS video

*Resuscitation*, Concord Films Council

Ref: NT 24: *Emergency Resuscitation*

Ref: 214/1-6: *CT Fractures*

Ref: Part 1: *Introduction to Fractures*

Ref: Part 3: *Fracture of the Spine*

Ref: Part 4: *Fracture of Clavicle and Upper Arm*

Ref: Part 5: *Fracture of Forearm and Hand*

Ref: Part 6: *Fracture of Pelvis and Lower Limb*

Ref: CNE4398: *Emergency Burn Treatment*

Ref: Ref: UGH4: *Burns*

Ref: 141/4CT Part 4: *First Aid Treatment for Burnt Patients*

Ref: 141/3CT Part 3: *The Lifting and Handling of Patients (advanced first aid)*

Ref: CME5720: *Airway Management: Shock in Trauma Patients*

Ref: CEAUA795: *Treatment of Shock*

Ref: CEAUA804: *EMs Vitals: Bleeding and Control of Bleeding*

Oxford Educational Resources Ltd

## Assignment

The purpose of this homework is to assist you in preparing for your Workbased Assessment of Competence. As there is no pressure on you, feel free to work at your own pace, but avoid the temptation to procrastinate. After you have read your notes and suggested references, submit your work for correction. The completed work becomes part of your Personal Portfolio.

# Health emergencies — first aid (CU1.2)

1. Define the term 'first aid' and list its aims.
2. Discuss the principles of first aid.
3. Describe what you would do if any of the following health emergencies happen when you are on duty
   a) A piece of sausage is lodged in an elderly resident's throat during breakfast.
   b) A client accidentally spills a hot cup of tea on his right thigh.
   c) A trusted resident was carving a piece of wood and accidentally cut his left thumb which started to bleed profusely.
4. A client fell out of bed, tried to get up but could not. He complains of a severe pain on his left hip. Discuss how you would manage the situation.
5. Discuss how you would care for a client who has been stung by a bee in the garden.

# Falls and accidents (CU1.3)

Accidents are chance events that occur unintentionally and without apparent cause, and may happen to any one from any age group. Care of the elderly is based on the premise that they are encouraged to control their lifestyles, take reasonable risks, dress themselves, walk or do as much as possible in order to maintain their independence. Consequently, they are also exposed to the risk of accident. Because the elderly are less steady on their feet, unexpected accidents such as falls may happen. The most common reasons given for a fall are, a 'trip', a 'turn', or 'goes off his legs'. These apparently minor incidents may lead to major injuries and even death in some cases. The number of deaths due to accidents has increased considerably, so much so that the white paper, *The Health of the Nation* (1990) aims to reduce death from accident in people aged 65 years and over by at least 33% by the year 2000.

Research has shown that most people in perfect health tend to sway and fall even when standing still. The problem is even more common in the elderly due to changes caused by the ageing process. Some residents become physically and or mentally frail and develop mobility problems. These problems may be accompanied by muscular weakness, decreased physical strength and enlarged joints. Movement is affected and, without exercise, the body becomes stiffer. It is claimed that 'trips' usually occur in the younger elderly who have been used to moving around on their own. Those over 75 years of age run the risk of 'turns' and suffer more accidental falls than other elderly people. Women particularly are at risk, because they tend to sway more than men.

### Individuals at risk of accidents

- those with a history of previous falls, bowel, bladder and feet problems
- those who are confused, disorientated, or restless; wanderers, overactive people
- people with sensory deprivation, eg. impaired hearing, vision or loss of sense of smell
- frail, very sick and helpless people with difficulty in walking or standing
- clients with dementia or other mental impairment
- passive and withdrawn people who show no interest in themselves
- overactive elderly who tend to take risks exercising their rights for independent living, ie. by walking up and down the stairs.

## Common period of occurrence

- when activity is greatest and there is less supervision and a lack of individual attention
- at night due to confusion caused by the effects of illness or use of hypnotic drugs
- getting in and out of bed and bath, when using the toilet, or undertaking exercise programmes.

## Factors which cause accidents

### 1. Physical
- muscular weakness, malnutrition, dehydration, infection and febrile conditions, stroke
- diseases, eg. hypotension, epilepsy and fainting attacks, oesteo-arthritis, stroke (CVA)
- Parkinson' disease, foot disorders, eg. bunions, corns, hammer toes, in-growing toe nails.

### 2. Psychological
- depression: this may cause a lack of awareness of hazards in the environment
- refusal to accept limitations imposed by the ageing process
- confusion and disorientation due to changes in environment, eg. admission or transfer from or to care establishments
- anxiety and hysteria: these may be in response to aggression or abuse.

### 3. Environmental
- admission to a care establishment may increase the risk of accidents in the confused elderly
- poor design in the care environment, especially if toilets are a long way from the sitting areas
- inadequate or poor lighting, awkward stairs, noise, fire
- inconveniently placed furniture, eg. chairs, small coffee and occasional tables
- lack of handrails along the corridors, in baths and toilets
- lack of mobility equipment such as lifting aids, eg. hoists
- restraint of independent movement using various methods, eg. cot-side
- poor surveillance resulting from inadequate staff level
- poor alarm system for summoning help and assistance
- unhygienic state of care environment, poor ventilation
- poor safety procedure, eg. leaving a secured door open and unattended
- doors not properly shut, especially those fitted with self-closing mechanism
- windows on floors above the ground floor left open, without any restrictive measures.

## Environmental hazards

Potential hazards in the care setting which can contribute to accidents include:
- unattended gardening equipment, such as shears, lawnmowers
- poor control or disposal of body waste, sharp objects, empty aerosol cans, broken glass
- spillage on the floor, eg. water, blood, urine
- a highly polished or wet floor, slippery rugs, frayed carpets and lino
- poor and improper use of mobility aids, eg. uncapped or worn walking sticks, frames
- ill-fitting shoes and slippers which do not grip the floor.

### 4. Medication
- incorrect administration of medication and alcohol
- accidental poisoning as a result of carelessness, poor eyesight, inability to read labels
- leaving medicine trolley unattended during routine administration of medicines.

### 5. Other causes
- open and unguarded fires and radiators may cause burns

- burns and scalds from hot drinks, eg. coffee, tea
- smoking, especially in bed with or without supervision
- below-standard performance of caring procedures, eg. bathing, lifting
- inadequate assessment and allocation of different heights of beds to clients. This may be the cause of falls and accidents when clients attempt to get in and out of these beds.

## Management of accidents

From time to time accidents may give rise to complaints, followed by claims for compensation or legal proceedings, which may call for an immediate enquiry. Such situations must be meticulously reported and investigated, not only to decide who is responsible, but also to prevent recurrence. These complaints may be on behalf of a client who has been given the wrong treatment, the result of an accident to visitors or staff such as a fall on the premises, or because of physical injury to staff during their normal course of duty. If fractures or other major injuries occur, followed by death within a few months of the accident, certain well established legal procedures will be carried out.

The starting point of management of accidents should be risk assessment of those who are prone to accidents and assessment of their functional capabilities. This should provide information to enable a care plan to be formulated. The care plan should enable a balance to be struck between safety and giving clients freedom to exercise their choice and right to live independently as far as possible. In this way, training could be given to prevent avoidable accidents, eg. smoking without supervision. Furthermore, it is important to be aware of the basic principles for managing the prevention of accidents. It involves knowledge of specific legislation, organisational policies and procedures such as:

- Health and Safety at Work Act 1974
- Fire Precautions Act 1971, Food Hygiene Act 1990
- Environmental Health Department procedures with regards to disposal of waste, spillage and hazardous items, eg. sharp objects, aerosols, bottles, chemical, dressings
- action to be taken in case of emergencies, eg. gas escapes, floods, water leakage, electrical faults, specific health emergencies, eg. epileptic fits
- staff training, eg. lifting, moving and handling people, infection control.

## Action in case of accident

### *Guidance*

If you are there when a resident has an accident which results in physical injury, take the following action:

- follow local policy on 'action to be taken in case of accidents'
- make a note of the time and events
- summon help immediately by activating the emergency alarm system
- carry out first aid, the aim of which is to make the person comfortable and contain the effects of the injury. Do not treat the injury until the person-in-charge or doctor prescribes treatment
- obtain relevant information, such as the names of any witnesses. You may be asked to make a report on any incident in accordance with local policy, eg. written statements, completion of Accident Report Book or in relation to Health and Safety at Work Act 1974. This may apply whether or not there is an injury
- retain articles or equipment involved for inspection.

## Prevention of accidents

Accidents are less likely to occur if the care setting is properly equipped and individuals or groups of clients are kept under constant observation. Many falls occur when residents are getting up or going to bed. However, restraining the person in order to prevent an accident, is seldom justified.

### *Guidance*

- develop and maintain good interpersonal relationship with all residents and demonstrate in-depth knowledge of those at risk. Be aware of their whereabouts at a given time
- observe and report regularly and legibly on any likely risk of accidents in the care environment
- ensure that heights of chairs, beds and toilets are easily adjustable to suit heights and disabilities of individual residents
- allow adequate space in the bed area so that clients can be helped without moving the furniture
- ensure that there are suitable floor surfaces to reduce damage, eg. a non-slip rug by each bed unless the floor is carpeted
- observe and report on security risks, eg. unidentified visitors, intruders or prowlers, and or defects to the security system, loss of equipment or materials
- encourage clients to participate in their favourite exercises according to their individual ability and capability
- ensure that clients maintain their individual lifestyle, but supervise those who smoke and are at risk of setting themselves alight
- encourage clients to discuss their worries, fears and concerns with the person-in-charge
- remove sharp instruments, broken glass immediately, and account for all the broken pieces of glass, razor blades, sharp tools, broken furniture, damaged lino as they may constitute a risk to the safety of anyone in the environment
- substances such as disinfectants should only be issued at the time of use, and care should be taken to ensure that bottles are not left within easy access of residents
- wipe up any spillage immediately
- ensure that residents are observed as unobtrusively as possible and be present where the majority of them congregate, especially in the lounge or sitting room
- observe and report regularly on individual clients' conditions in accordance with the care plan
- ensure good lighting to stairs and corridors, and remove obstructing furniture from the passage ways
- ensure that clients with devices, such as those that are worn like a wrist watch or round the neck as a pendant, use them as prescribed
- answer calls from clients who have difficulty in moving promptly so that he or she does not try to get up
- keep items that are used frequently close at hand, so that the person will not fall trying to reach for them
- look for obvious hazards, eg. lack of fire guards, hot radiators, loose tiles, fires
- all accidents in which residents, visitors and staff are concerned should be reported to the person-in-charge at the time, and an accident form or record completed without delay in accordance with the policy of the organisation.

## Safety of the care environment

Every member of the care team has an obligation to protect all clients in their care, by creating and maintaining a safe and secure environment, constantly looking for hazards, and reporting and taking appropriate steps to minimise or avoid them. It is, therefore, the responsibility of everyone to ensure that their particular areas of work, equipment, methods and the procedures used are safe for themselves and others, conforming with the Health and Safety at Work Act 1974, and local policies and statutory regulations relating to:

**First aid**: Ensure that boxes are stocked and fixed in appropriate sites.

**Laundry room**: Mop and keep clean. Be familiar with the operation of the washing machine and the procedure for handling soiled and dirty linen.

**Medicines**: Be aware of 'Safety of Administration of Medicines for Elderly'. Use and store cleaning materials, disinfectants in the appropriate section of the medicine cupboard.

**Floors**: Be aware of spillage and worn carpets, and take appropriate action.

**Kitchen**: Take care in the use of sharp objects, knives, fat, hot oil, ovens, storage of food.

**Glass**: Remove and account for all pieces of broken or chipped glass immediately. Wrap and put them in a plastic bag, and put in the rubbish bin. Protect, wash and dry your hands thoroughly after the procedure.

**Electricity and gas**: Ensure that you know where switches and valves are located in case an emergency situation arises.

In all cases, regular surveillance and reassurance of clients and others are of paramount importance. Low staff morale can be caused if frequent falls are recorded in the elderly; counselling sessions may be necessary to resolve the situation.

## Falling out of bed

People have many reasons for getting out of bed in the night. They may want to use the toilet, relieve pain, get some fresh air or something to drink. They may feel tired of lying in bed because they cannot sleep or feel frustrated, and want to move about. Residents who want to get out of bed should not be prevented from doing so or restrained in any way.

It is wrong to assume that making it difficult for residents to get out of bed may prevent accidents, for example by the use of cot sides. On the contrary, this action may contribute to the accidents as the person will try to climb over it. It may also cause poor personal hygiene, incontinence, anxiety and panic feelings. Tucking clients tightly in bed with bedding could have the same effect. The problem of falling out of bed should be discussed, and ways of handling it agreed by all concerned. The solution should be recorded in the person's care plan and the approach adopted should be reviewed frequently .

### *Guidance*
- Discuss the reasons for their getting up with the resident, the risks they face and how the situations should be managed. Some residents may prefer the risk of falling to restraint on their movements or a loss of privacy.
- Show clients who want to get out of bed how to proceed slowly and carefully to minimise the risk of falling. Advise them to call staff if they feel they need help or may be at risk. Respect their wishes if they prefer to get up without assistance, but be at hand should they change their mind.
- Make the environment safe for residents at risk by ensuring that hard or sharp edges and objects are kept away from their beds. Orientate them with the route to the lavatory, and place an alarm call bell within easy reach of the person so that in the event of a fall clients may call for help from the staff.
- Some elderly people require very little sleep at night. They may want to wander aimlessly from their rooms at night. In this case, night staff should be able to talk to and chaperon the client if this is acceptable to the person. A warm drink may be offered or the person may be occupied with a simple diversional activity.
- A few elderly may express fear of falling out of bed and seek protection. Cot sides should not be used, unless the person specifically asks for them. If this is the case, a single cot side may be used. But a lower

- divan bed or a mattress placed on the floor is a better option, although the person may need help in rising from the bed.
- The BT Telecare is a new monitoring system designed to provide information on the person's behaviour pattern. A sensor which detects movement is placed in the client's room. It monitors all the activities of daily living, including the temperature of the room. It is linked to the telephone and calls for help if the client cannot do so him/herself. It is useful in any situation and setting, including care in the community.

# References

Department of Health (1990) *The Health of the Nation: A Strategy for Health in England*. HMSO, London

Ironbar NO (1983) *Self-instruction in Psychiatric Nursing. Unit 5.2 Hazards of Old Age*. Bailliere Tindall, London

Mitchell RG (1984) Falls in the elderly. *Nurs Times*, January 11, 1984

## Audio visual aids

*Format: VHS video*
Ref: CNEUA834: *Treating the Elderly: Falling in the Elderly*
Oxford Educational Resources Ltd

# Assignment

The purpose of this homework is to assist you in preparing for your Workbased Assessment of Competence. As there is no pressure on you, feel free to work at your own pace, but avoid the temptation to procrastinate. After you have read your notes and suggested references, submit your work for correction. The completed work becomes part of your Personal Portfolio.

## Falls and accidents (CU1.3)

1. Discuss what you understand by the word 'accident' and how it could happen in your area of work?
2. List the categories of residents who may be prone to falls and accidents.
3. What precautions would you take to ensure that the environment is reasonably safe for the residents, your colleagues, visitors and yourself?
4. Describe what action you would take in the event of, and after a client has fallen:
   a) in the lounge
   b) in the bath room
   c) out of bed at night.
5. Discuss ways in which accidents could be prevented in your place of work.
6. An elderly client wanders aimlessly around the home night and day. How would you protect her from the risk of injury and harm?

# Care during epileptic seizures (CU1.3)

Epilepsy is a term used to describe sudden attacks, caused by abnormal electrical activity of the brain cells, which brings about physical movements of the body called seizures, fits or convulsions. Seizures may occur spontaneously at any time throughout the life of the person. It is estimated that there are about 300,000 people in Britain suffering from this condition, which affects men and women equally. It is not genetically linked. During an attack, there may be erratic disturbance of consciousness, behaviour and perception, and the person may not recall having had a seizure. Many people believe that epilepsy is a mental illness, and rarely, if ever causes learning or behavioural problems.

It is important to know if any residents in your place of work suffer from this condition. Their care plans will contain information on the frequency of attacks, and ways in which they are cared for during these attacks.

## Causes

Although the causes of epilepsy are unknown, organic brain disease, such as stroke or tumour, or injury resulting in cerebral damage, may be followed by epileptic-type seizures.

It is believed that exposure to flashing and bright lights and excessive use of television and computer games, especially by children, may lead to reflex epilepsy.

## Management of seizures

This is a medical emergency in which treatment must be rapid. Most cases are controlled satisfactorily by drugs.

## Immediate care during seizure

This requires first aid treatment which aims to prevent the person from injuring him or herself. It is important that you should have in-depth knowledge of clients with this condition as maintenance of a clear airway is crucial.

### *Guidance*
- assist the person to lie down and summon help immediately
- allow client to lie where he or she has fallen, provided he/she is not in danger
- turn the head to one side and carefully place a pillow under it
- loosen tight clothing around the neck and chest, ensure that breathing is not obstructed
- remove any nearby furniture or objects to prevent injury
- prevent the person from biting his/her tongue during fits if possible, and do not try to restrain the person, open or insert anything into his or her mouth
- protect the bed with blankets or a foam pad, and put up a cot side if the person is in bed to prevent him or her from falling out of bed
- observe what happens during the fits, eg. whether the movements begin on the right or left side, with a scream, colour of the person, passing of urine or faeces and duration of attack. Maintain an accurate record of your observations
- ensure client's dignity and self-respect at all times, especially during seizures
- provide support to other people within the vicinity and reassure them.

## Care after the seizure

When the person comes round and is conscious, he/she may be hallucinating, confused, irritable and/or restless. During this period he/she may become dangerous and carers should be able to:
- remain with the person until he/she is fully conscious. He or she may develop automatism, ie. perform various acts which the client cannot remember, ie. once the seizure is over
- help the person into bed if the seizure occurred on the floor and let him or her rest to compose him or herself
- offer a cup of tea or refreshments of choice when fully conscious
- show empathy with reassuring words of comfort and encourage the person to express him or herself
- observe and report any further seizure to the person-in-charge
- record the incident accurately in the person's care notes in accordance with local policy
- observe closely in case the person is confused or has another seizure.

## Protective measures

People who suffer from epilepsy should be encouraged to follow and maintain normal lifestyles as far as possible. However, there are certain risks where extra care is needed and clients should, if possible, refrain from undertaking these, for example operating machinery or swimming. They should be encouraged to take their medications as prescribed.

## Epilepsy clinics

Some primary health care practice teams run clinics for people with epilepsy as they do for other clinics such as asthma and diabetes. Practice nurses run the clinics supported by Epilepsy Liaison Nurses. Their aim is to identify and meet the needs of those with this condition.

# References

*Management of Protocol for Epilepsy in General Practice* (1994) Shire Hall Communications, London

Laidlaw J *et al* (1993) *A Textbook of Epilepsy*, 4th edn. Churchill Livingstone, Edinburgh

Robertson B (1992) *Study Guide for Health and Social Care Support Workers*. First Class Books Inc, USA

Taylor M (1990) Epilepsy and its diagnosis. *Pract Nurse* **3**: 29–31

## Audio visual aids

### Format: VHS video
Ref: *Label for Life*, Concord Films Council Ltd
Ref: NT 130: *Epilepsy*
Oxford Educational Resources Ltd

# Unit 3(b)
# Assist in the control of infection
# (CU1, CU2, OD1, X1, X13, Y4)

## Sources and mode of spread of infection (CU1.1, OD1)

Infection is an attack on the body by micro organisms that cause disease. When they enter the body they grow and multiply, making the person feel ill. Although medical science is advancing, infection is still a threat. There are many types of infection but the most common is cross infection. This is the spread of infection from one person to another in hospitals, nursing or residential care homes. All carers have an important role in the prevention of the spread of infection to people under our care.

### Causes of infection

Infection is caused by various types of micro-organisms, with varying modes of action. These include:

#### 1. Bacteria
These are found in air, water, soil, and food, in the cavities and bodies of men and animals, or are cultured in the laboratory. They are classified according to their shape, ie. *cocci* (round), *bacilli* (rod-shaped) or spiral and are major disease-causing organisms, through their toxins. Bacteria are parasites; some depend on oxygen (aerobic) to survive, and others can live without oxygen (anaerobic). However, some do not cause disease and are known as *non-pathogenic*. They can cause disease if they gain access to parts of the body where they do not normally live, and are then known as *pathogens*. Otherwise, they help to form part of the body's natural defence mechanism.

#### 2. Virus
Viruses are the smallest of all the disease-causing organisms (pathogenic) which can only be seen with the aid of electronic microscope. They cause diseases by reproducing inside a living cell and are responsible for diseases, such as influenza, chicken pox, mumps, measles and AIDS. They can be destroyed by the body's normal defence mechanisms although in some cases they may remain dormant inside the body cell, and may be reactivated later.

#### 3. Fungi
These are mould-like organisms – smaller than bacteria and can only be seen with the aid of an electronic microscope. They cause many local infections commonly found in the mouth and other moist surfaces of the body. Fungi cause skin conditions, such as ringworm, candida, scabies etc.

### Modes of transmission

#### 1. Direct contact
This is the spread of disease from one infected person to another. For example, sexually transmitted diseases. Others are transmitted in the air we breath. Viruses can be passed from a mother to the foetus via the placenta, eg. AIDS.

*Sexual contact*
This transmits diseases via sexual contact from one person to another.

*Inoculation*
Infection enters the body through a scratch in the skin. This may be transmitted by an instrument such as a needle or scalpel blade, which had become contaminated with blood or body fluid, as in the case of hepatitis B.

## 2. Indirect contact

This mode of transmission is by touching articles (formites) that have been near enough to an infectious person to be contaminated with bacteria, eg. carer's uniform, bedpans, bedclothes, pillows, books, eating utensils.

*Droplet*
This infection enters the body through inhaling airborne droplets via the nose and mouth. Diseases passed in this way include: the common cold, measles and tuberculosis. When breathing, coughing, sneezing, shouting, laughing or even talking, the infected person sprays germs into the air and some may fall to the floor and mix with dust.

*Contaminated Food and Drink*
Infections are transmitted by an infected food handler (carrier). A person who eats and digests such infected food or drink may have (*Salmonella*) bacterial food poisoning, eg. dysentery, typhoid.

*People*
A carrier is a person who is not affected but is harbouring disease-causing organisms, eg. typhoid.

*Animals and insects*
Animals, such as cows, monkeys, dogs and cats carry disease-causing organisms and infection can also be spread by blood sucking insects, such as ticks. On this account pets are not allowed on clients' beds in hospitals and some nursing and residential care homes.

## Body defence system (natural)

This is the mechanism by which the body resists infection. It is a group of specialised cells known as T-Cells, mainly the white blood cells which protect the body from infection. The skin is an effective barrier against disease and the acid content of skin secretions may kill or prevent the growth of certain disease organisms. The linings of the mouth and nose trap and carry away bacteria, but in ill-health the body defence mechanism breaks down and infection sets in.

## Acquired defence system (acquired)

Immunity to an infection may occur as a result of coming in contact with the disease-causing organism or a person suffering from the disease. This can take place naturally, eg. when a mother passes anti-bodies through the placenta to her unborn foetus. Another way is by immunisation or vaccination. This form of immunity lasts for specific periods and will need to be repeated. Tetanus injection is an example of this form of immunity. If a person's immune system breaks down, then infection will occur as in the case of AIDS (Acquired Immune Deficiency Syndrome). This is caused by human immunodeficiency virus (HIV).

## Factors predisposing individuals to infection

Many factors may predispose individuals to infection, for example:
- age: infants, children and the elderly are less able to resist infection because their immune systems are less effective
- nutrition: malnutrition predisposes to infection
- low temperature: this reduces the blood supply to the tissues and suppresses production of anti-bodies
- ill-health and disease: reduces immune systems of the body, increasing the risk of infection
- drugs: some drugs depress antibody production, eg. Prednisolone
- radiation: this reduces the body's ability to produce antibodies and white blood cells.

## Signs and symptoms of infection

A severe infection is the result of a battle between the defences of the body and the attacking micro-organisms. The onset is usually sudden and the person may complain of the following:
- headache and general aches and pains; a rise in temperature, pulse and respiration
- swelling and redness and discharge from the affected part, loss of function
- changes in behaviour, irritability and, in some cases, restlessness and lack of appetite.

## Care of a client with infection

This is the responsibility of the team and involves attention to the client's general health and restoring his or her strength. This may be done through ensuring cleanliness of the care environment and practising the aseptic techniques necessary to prevent cross-infection. The areas that need particular attention are the sluice, handwashing facilities, containers for removing infected matter, supplying sterile equipment and arrangements for isolation nursing.

### *Guidance*
- develop and maintain good interpersonal relationships with clients and colleagues
- encourage the client to stay in bed in a warm well-ventilated room in an upright position, supported with pillows and ensure general rest
- ensure rest of the infected area supported on a pillow or a sling together with mouth care preferably four-hourly, as directed in the care plan
- maintain individual self-respect, dignity and privacy
- offer a choice of a light, high protein diet and plenty of fluid intake
- take temperature, pulse and respiration four-hourly as directed and carry out routine care of pressure areas
- be aware of constipation and encourage the client to express his/her wishes and preferences with respect to treatment
- allow client to sit out of bed in an armchair and take gentle exercise as his/her condition improves to prevent muscle wasting and stiffness of the part/joint
- provide disposable tissues and sputum mug should a cough be present
- maintain individual's self-respect, dignity and privacy when assisting in personal cleansing and hygiene
- maintain accurate records of care, legibly written
- encourage the client to participate in diversional therapy as his/her condition improves
- assist in carrying out any routine care and treatment, eg. aseptic dressing technique.

## Precautions

### 1. Care environment
- help control infection by keeping the surroundings clean and tidy
- ensure that the environment is well-ventilated and free from unpleasant odour. If necessary, use an aerosol air freshener.

### 2. Handling linen
- hold linen away from you to prevent transferring micro-organisms
- avoid shaking or fluffing linens and keep them off the floor
- wear disposable plastic apron and gloves to handle linens soiled with blood or body fluids
- place soiled linens in proper linen bags to prevent the spread of infection
- always wash your hands thoroughly after handling soiled linens.

## References

Ayliffe GAJ et al (1981) *Control of Hospital Infection,* 2nd edn. Chapman and Hall, London

Ben RAV (1986) *Aids to Microbiology and Infectious Diseases.* Churchill Livingstone, Edinburgh

Bowell B (1992) Protecting the patient at risk. *Nurs Times* **88**(3): 32–35

Parker J, Stuckle U (1982) *Microbiology for Nurses,* 6th edn. Bailliere Tindall, London

Ward K (1992) Why not wash? *Nurs Times* **88**(24): 68–69

### Audio visual aids

*Format: VHF video*

Ref: CEAUA 132: *Bacteria and Health*
Ref: CNE4397 *Infection Control in Home Care*
Ref: 310CT: *Virus Infection of the Human Skin*
Oxford Educational Resources Ltd

## Assignment

The purpose of this homework is to assist you in preparing for your Workbased Assessment of Competence. As there is no pressure on you, feel free to work at your own pace, but avoid the temptation to procrastinate. After you have read your notes and suggested references, submit your work for correction. The completed work becomes part of your Personal Portfolio.

## Sources and mode of spread of infection (CU1.1, OD1)

1. State what you understand by the terms 'infection and body immunity'?
2. Explain six ways in which micro-organisms can enter the body.
3. Discuss factors which could predispose elderly people to infection.
4. State briefly, the signs and symptoms of infection.
5. How would you care for an elderly person suffering from infection?
6. What precautions would you take to prevent the spread of infection in your care environment?

# Management and control of infection (CU2: 1-2, OD1)

Infection is the outcome of a successful invasion of the body by micro-organisms which are present in the environment, and its control is a major concern for every member of the health care team. The basic principle of control is an awareness of the sources of infection, a local policy designed to minimise the risk factors inherent in sharing facilities, ill health and accidents, and allowing clients to recover by strengthening their body defence mechanism.

## Control of infection

Local policies should clearly state methods to be adopted for prevention of cross-infection. Successful models which have been developed can arrest the growth and spread of infection. These usually imply the strict observance by the care team of basic personal and domestic hygiene activities relating to:

### 1. Handwashing

The hands of carers, if they do not take appropriate precautions, are a major source of disease transmission from one client to another. Prevention of contamination by hands is one of the most important factors in controlling the incidence of cross-infection, since it is difficult to disinfect the hands or remove all the traces of infection from the surface of the hands. The spread of infection is greatly reduced by procedures which reduces pathogens. Hands should be washed:
- before and after client contact
- after coughing or sneezing or blowing the nose
- after handling bedpans, urinals, specimens
- after bed-making, handling soiled linens or using the toilet.

*Principles of handwashing*
- remove wristwatch and rings, use hot running water
- use correct amount of soap solution individually dispensed
- wash all areas of your hands and fingers thoroughly, and rinse off soap
- use disposable paper towels to dry hands or hand dryers.

### 2. Disinfectants

These are chemical agents capable of destroying or reducing the level of micro-organisms which are harmful to health, eg. gases, liquids, antibiotics. Look up your local policy for use of disinfectants.

### 3. Maintaining the safety and security of the care environment

This involves:
- prevention of accidents, falls and damage to the skin
- observation of basic personal and domestic hygiene requirements
- awareness of people who are susceptible or prone to infection, eg. the elderly and infants, those who are malnourished, severely ill, lack sufficient exercise and rest
- those who are persistently tired and complain of weakness
- continuing education of staff, including laundry staff.

### 4. Sterilisation

This is a method of rendering objects free from all organisms. There are various ways of sterilisation, eg. ultra-violet rays have the power to destroy most bacteria, extremes of temperature such as cryogenesis, ie. freezing and refrigeration for preserving food and heat, eg. boiling and steaming under pressure are very effective. These are alternatives to disinfectants or radiation treatment.

## 5. Legislation

Carers should show a knowledge of the legislation and local policies which relate to care of clients and safety of the environment, eg. policies of the Environmental Health Department which is responsible under Public Health (Control of Diseases) Act 1984 for:
- immunisation, notifiable diseases, hazards, eg. body waste, bottles, sharp objects
- contacting and tracing people who have been in contact with a sufferer of a notifiable disease, control of substances under Health and Safety at Work Act 1974 and Food and Safety Act 1990.

## 6. Spillage

Spillages are hazards which may result in injuries to people and must be dealt with immediately. Small spillages can be wiped up using disposable towels. Larger ones will require the use of appropriate detergent to clean the area. Consult local policy about the spillage of faeces or/and blood.

## 7. Isolation nursing

Isolation nursing is the care of a client in a separate room, and physical barriers must be placed between him or her and the rest of the care environment. Special precautions should be taken in the disposal of waste materials and movement of personnel and equipment in and out of the area. There should be local policy guidelines on the following:

**Preparation of the room:** Decisions should be made about what equipment will be necessary. These decisions should be made bearing in mind the reason for the isolation.

**Protective clothing:** Personal clothing of carers and visitors may be a source of infection. Staff uniform should be covered or changed to avoid cross-contamination. The client needs to be protected from diseases which might be carried on the clothing of other people.

**Gowns:** These are made of woven fabric and together with plastic disposable aprons which cover arms and shoulders, should be worn when in direct contact with an infected person.

**Masks:** Used to protect clients from inhaling micro-organisms released into the air by the wearer.

**Hands:** Effective hand hygiene is one way of reducing the spread of infection. Alcohol is a good skin disinfectant and effective as a hand rub after handwashing. Elbows instead of hands may be used to push open the door on leaving the isolated room.

**Gloves:** These should be used if hands are likely to become contaminated, and changed often enough to prevent the transfer of germs. As a rule, they should be changed as frequently as staff normally wash their hands.

**Supplies and waste:** Anything entering the room should be free of harmful organisms. There should be special procedures and methods for handling waste and other materials leaving the room, eg. soiled dressings, refuse, urine, faeces, laundry, used crockery and cutlery.

**Terminal disinfection:** This is disinfection following the discharge or death of the person in isolation. It is a thorough cleaning of the room under the guidance of the infection control team.

| | |
|---|---|
| **Visitors:** | The policy should say whether or not visitors are allowed inside the room. If they are, what instructions should be followed. |
| **Laboratory specimens:** | At times specimens are required for laboratory investigations, and the guidelines should be clear on procedures for collecting and sending such specimens. |
| **Transporting residents:** | The policy should state clearly what should be done if people need to attend for treatment or investigations outside the current care environment. |

## 8. Aseptic technique
This is a method of carrying out sterile procedures so that there is a minimal risk of introducing infection. The technique is achieved by using sterile instruments to avoid touching the wound or objects with bare hands. An important rule is that 'clean' procedures should be carried out before 'dirty' procedures.

## 9. Food handling
Clients may run the risk of contracting food poisoning if the process is not handled safely and in accordance with the Food and Safety Act 1990.

## 10. Storage of food
Food may become infected, contaminated or decomposed if is not stored under the following conditions:

| | |
|---|---|
| **Clean:** | The kitchen should be kept clean including storage spaces, especially the refrigerator. |
| **Cool:** | It is essential for food to be stored below 5°C in the refrigerator. Food should be dated and stored for no more than 24 hours from the time it was purchased. If still in its original wrapper, store only until the sell by or use by date. Raw meat, fish, poultry or eggs should not be stored with cooked food. |
| **Covered:** | All food must be covered and sealed, eg. in a resealable plastic box. Label the box with the client's name and date. Once food has been served, it must be disposed of if not consumed. Waste bins must be covered at all times with a well-fitting lid. |

## 11. Sharp objects
Accidental inoculation, especially with needles, is a minor risk leading to infection. Check local policies regarding handling and disposal of sharp objects as, if this is ignored, it may become a major risk. Dispose of needles and other sharp objects in the proper containers.

## 12. Special precautions
The following actions may help to prevent the spread of infection.

### Guidance
- be aware of local policy on waste disposal as a matter of good practice
- take care in handling soiled linen contaminated by secretions, discharges and excretions
- maintain good personal hygiene at all times. Hands should be washed regularly with soap or detergent and water, and followed by rinsing between routine contact with clients
- keep nails short and hair pinned up under a cap
- handle bedclothes and pillows carefully so that dust is kept to a minimum
- take care after contamination of client's personal clothing and that of your own. Follow local policy on routine precautions for handling soiled linen and clothing
- take all necessary steps to minimise the risk of accidents to patients and staff

- be aware of potential hazards in the working environment
- show knowledge of the patients/residents especially those who are vulnerable to falls
- take care not to wear the same uniform for clean and dirty duties. Use protective and disposable aprons at appropriate times and discard after use
- be aware of the requirements of the Health and Safety at Work Act 1974 and the Food and Safety Act 1990
- wear protective equipment, such as a mask, apron or gown or the potential for exposure to blood, body fluids, skin rashes, bleeding or open wounds, broken skin is possible
- remember that infection applies both ways. Carers are equally at risk of contracting an infection from the work environment, or if they skimp on cleanliness routines. Take regular outdoor exercise to maintain maximum fitness
- eat a nutritious diet and ensure that your rest and sleep are adequate.

## References

Ayliffe GAJ et al (1982) *Control of Hospital Infection,* 2nd edn. Chapman and Hall, London
HMSO (1990) *Food and Safety Act 1990*. HMSO, London
Gidley C (1987) Now wash your hands. *Nurs Times* **82**(29): 41–42
McCulloch M (1992) Control of infection: points to remember. *Nurs Times* **6**(27): 28–30
Palmer MB (1984) *Infection Control*. Saunders Blue Book Series. WB Saunders, London

**Audio visual aids**

*Format: VHS video*
Ref: LPLM 338: *Clean Hands Save Lives*
CNE4397: *Infection Control in Home Care*
Ref: 301CT: *Clean Food*
Ref: 313 CT: *Hazards of Disposal*
Ref: PYR89: *Infection Control for Health Care Workers*
Ref: PYRR64: *On Guard: Infection Control for Safety and Health Care Workers*
Oxford Educational Resources Ltd

## Assignment

The purpose of this homework is to assist you in preparing for your Workbased Assessment of Competence. As there is no pressure on you, feel free to work at your own pace, but avoid the temptation to procrastinate. After you have read your notes and suggested references, submit your work for correction. The completed work becomes part of your Personal Portfolio.

## Management and control of infection (CU2: 1–2, OD1)

1. State your understanding of the term 'infection control'?
2. List 12 methods in which infection can be controlled.
3. Discuss factors that could predispose elderly people to infection.
4. State your understanding of isolation nursing as a means of infection control.
5. Discuss the principles of handwashing.

6. Explain the principles of storage of food in relation to the Food Hygiene Act 1990.
7. Discuss what special precautions you would take in the control of infection.
5. How would you care for an elderly person suffering from infection?
6. What precautions would you take to prevent the spread of infection in your care environment?

# Infestations

About 20 years ago, infestation, especially with head lice, was regarded as a feature of poverty and unhygienic living conditions. Of late, however, the phenomenon has reappeared even among more affluent populations. Current observations note that such infestation can spread through contact with a source or by wearing clothes containing unhatched eggs. This should not be regarded as shameful or embarassing, but appropriate remedial action should be instigated.

## Scabies

This is a contagious skin disease caused by itch mite. It is believed that scabies has been a common condition for at least 3,000 years. In the past scabies was prevalent in homes and institutions where overcrowding was a problem, and for this reason is associated with cramped, dirty conditions and is viewed as a disease of dirty homes. It is important to treat and cure scabies as quickly and effectively as possible.

### *Mode of transmission*
Scabies is transmitted by close skin to skin contact when the female mite burrows beneath the skin and deposits eggs. The sites affected are chiefly between the fingers and toes, the axillae, the buttocks and groin. However, should an outbreak occur within a nursing home for elderly people, the stigma associated with scabies may be such that clients will refuse to stay or visit such establishments. It is important when dealing with a single case or an outbreak, to ensure that both the psychological and sociological factors are considered, steps are taken to overcome associated problems that may arise and treatment of the disease is carried out as soon as possible.

### *Signs and symptoms*
After invading the body, the itch mite lives and sucks the host's blood after biting the skin. The itching is at its worst in a warm bed, or when the body is warm, eg. at night, after exercise or in a warm bath. The most common signs and symptoms include:
- a general feeling of tiredness
- constant disturbance due to intense itching and scratching which may damage, cause inflammation to the skin, and swelling which may result in impetigo
- burrows and rashes causing red papules (small pimples on the skin), vesicles, pustules, crusted lesions and eczematous patches
- bleeding as a result of scratching, which may lead to anaemia.

### *Burrowing*
The earliest lesions are burrows about half an inch long, and the margins are rough and may collect dirt so that they often appear as dark streaks. Burrows can be seen on the hands and wrists, at the sides and between the web of the fingers, elbows, back of the knees, buttocks, under the breasts, arm pits, groin, on the penis and around the umbilical region. Scabies can affect most parts of the body. In adults, the head is usually spared, whereas in infants the rash may be generalised.

### Principles of care

The aim is to break up the roof of the burrows to expose the itch mites' eggs by washing and applying scabicide as prescribed. All residents and known contacts will be examined and assessed for the presence of burrows, excoriated, crusted or vesicular lesions on the skin.

### Care plan

An action plan should be agreed and should cover the following points:
- treatment methods
- plans for briefing all staff on the treatment of scabies
- a day should be set aside for start of the treatment and a sufficient workforce should be available
- ensure that there is a correct and sufficient quantity of scabicide for the care
- time of treatment, eg. when there is least disruption ie. if applied before bedtime.

### General preparation

#### Guidance

- maintain good relationship with clients, encourage independence, self-respect, privacy and dignity
- be aware of how the infection is transmitted and the actions which should be taken to limit the risk of infection, eg. effective handwashing
- demonstrate a knowledge of statutory requirements for reporting and tracing contacts, eg. the Public Health Act 1984
- explain to clients precautions or special measures which need to be taken to prevent cross infection, eg. wearing of special clothing, aprons
- demonstrate a knowledge of the methods used to control the risk of personal infection without restricting clients' movements or freedom too much
- display a knowledge of local policy for protecting clothing, disposing of soiled linen, and preventing cross-infection and re-infection.

### Implementation of care

- check the list for items which may be required, eg. gloves, apron, cottonwool, bowls, socks for frail, elderly clients
- apply the prescribed lotion, eg. scabicide, from the neck downwards to all areas, paying special attention to the hands, feet, under the nails, breasts, armpits and genitalia
- apply scabicide to cool, dry skin. A hot bath and skin scrubbing is not recommended
- use cotton wool soaked with lotions and creams using the bare hands
- offer an explanation and constantly reassure clients because of the associated guilt
- watch for and report any signs of hypersensitivity to treatment
- apply and reapply scabicide to hands every time they are washed during treatment
- encourage clients to maintain good personal hygiene.

One of the principles of managing scabies is tactfulness and a realistic approach, especially if a client has a mental health problem. Remember, **everybody should be treated equally**.

### Lice

There are different types of lice which live in different parts of the human body. They range from 2–4mm in length and their bites cause intense itching. There is an increasing problem because some lice are resistant to treatment and can cause considerable embarrassment.

## Types and management of lice

### 1. Head lice (pediculosis capitis)

Minute white eggs from the lice attach themselves to the hair, usually on the scalp at the back of the head and behind the ears. Close contact between children at play increases the opportunity for the lice to spread from child to child. The eggs are usually stuck firmly together and to the hair and cannot be removed by washing with an ordinary shampoo.

*Guidance*
- part the hair and comb outwards with a fine tooth comb
- wash with special shampoo or apply a lotion or oil to detach the eggs and kill the live lice
- disinfect hair brushes and combs.

### 2. Body lice

These do not live on the body but in the fibres and seams of clothing and only move to the skin for sustenance. They live on people who wear the same clothes continuously and who do not take them off to wash.

*Guidance*
- bathe the client
- apply insecticide powder or spray
- remove and incinerate affected clothes
- wear protective clothing, plastic disposable apron and gloves while carrying out the treatment
- maintain good standards of personal hygiene
- change and launder your uniform.

### 3. Fleas

In the past human fleas were very common and men used to shave their heads and wear wigs to reduce infestation. Fleas used for entertainment in flea circuses were once commonplace, but nowadays people are more likely to be bitten by fleas from animals, eg. dogs and cats. If this happens, the animal and soft furnishings it has been in contact with will have to be treated.

## References

McMahon CA, Harding J (1993) *Knowledge to Care: A Handbook for Care Assistants*. Blackwell Scientific Publications, London

Flack M, Johnson M (1986): *Handbook for Care*. Beaconsfield Publishers Ltd, Bucks

Hinchliffe SM *et al* (1993) *Nursing Practice and Health Care*. Edward Arnold, London

Pankhania B (1993) *Scabies Management*. North West Surrey Public Health Department, Frimley, Surrey

### Audio visual aids

*Format: VHS video*
Ref: UP293: *Scabies*
Oxford Educational Resources Ltd

# HIV/AIDS and hepatitis B

AIDS is defined as an unusual infectious illness in which the AIDS virus attacks the immune system of people who previously enjoyed good health. The virus also attacks the brain cells, leading in many cases to dementia. AIDS cripples the body's natural defence against disease and the person eventually dies from infections. It is, therefore, reasonable to assume that everyone infected with this virus would eventually suffer some form of ill health as a consequence.

## Normal immune system

Immunity is the power of the body to resist the toxins of invading micro-organisms shown in the blood by the presence of neutralising antitoxins. Its purpose is to prevent pathogenic infection.

## Types of immunity

These are:

**Natural:** that which is inherited (innate) and it can be racial or familial.

**Acquired:** that which is produced naturally through an attack of the disease or by repeated small infections by organisms.

**Artificially acquired:** that which is produced by an injection of toxins or vaccines.

**Active:** by the introduction of sera (passive).

## Human immunodeficiency virus (HIV)

This virus belongs to a sub-group known as lentiviruses, 'slow virus' with a long incubation period, ie. the time the individual is exposed to infection to the day he/she becomes clinically unwell may be in excess of eleven years. Although it is now known that most people with HIV infection will become ill, there will be some who will never show any clinical symptoms of the disease.

### *Modes of transmission of HIV*

HIV is a blood-borne virus and has been isolated from blood, semen, saliva, tears, breast milk and cerebrospinal fluid. It is principally transmitted sexually, but can occur through contact with blood, blood products and other body fluids.

#### *Sexual*

The chief route is via sexual intercourse when infected semen and small amounts of blood are present (common in penetrative rectal intercourse). It is more common in homosexual or bisexual men, due to the practice of anal sex and taking multiple sexual partners. Female to female transmission is extremely rare.

#### *Blood and blood products*

HIV has been transmitted following transfusion of whole blood, blood components and the administration of concentrated Factor VIII manufactured from pooled plasma and used in the treatment of haemophilia.

#### *Injecting substance misuse*

Individuals who misuse injectable drugs. HIV is transmitted by sharing blood contaminated needles and syringes.

#### *Organ transplant*

Donors of organs (kidneys, corneas, hearts) are at potential risk.

## Transplacentral and perinatal

Children have contracted HIV infection as a result of receiving a blood transfusion or concentrated Factor VIII for haemophilia, or more commonly as a result of having a parent infected with HIV. Infection may be contracted in the uterus of infected mothers, at birth or in the neonatal period.

## Other modes of entry

HIV can enter the body through:
- puncture wounds from infected needles or broken glass
- cuts or open sores
- mucous membranes (nose, mouth, eyes).

## Symptoms

When people are infected with HIV they are carriers for life. Some carriers never show symptoms, but can transmit (pass on) HIV to others. In the early period of the disease, some individuals may develop mild symptoms within a few days of infection, often giving a history of 'flu-like' symptoms such as:
- dry unproductive cough, chest pain
- fever and chill, dyspnoea (difficulty in breathing) and extreme distress
- swollen glands, night sweats, rash, fever.

These symptoms may go away, but the HIV remains in the body. There is no cure although a number of preventive measures may reduce the likelihood of full blown AIDS developing. A vaccine for HIV/AIDS is now undergoing clinical trials, but its success rate is unknown. In advanced cases, when the disease becomes known as Auto Immune Deficiency Syndrome (AIDS), between 5 to 15 years, individuals may develop and show the following symptoms:

## Physical
- deterioration in self-care and attention to personal cleanliness
- seizure disorders
- weight loss
- diarrhoea
- diseases, such as Karposi's sarcoma, pneumonia etc.

## Social
- social withdrawal, embarrassment and anti-social behaviour.

## Psychological
- loss of memory with an inability to concentrate and to learn
- slowness and difficulty in thinking and making rational judgement
- anxiety, depression, frustration, irritability, mood changes
- demanding behaviour and altered interpersonal relationships.

## Hepatitis B virus

Hepatitis is the term used to describe inflammation of the liver by the B virus. Transmission is through irregular contact with infected blood or blood products and certain body fluids occurring one to six months after the initial infection by the hepatitis B virus. This is often seen in drug addicts and can be fatal.

## Modes of transmission

The virus is transmitted primarily through:
- fluid and breast milk

- semen and amniotic fluid
- unprotected sexual intercourse
- vaginal secretions
- administration of unscreened blood/blood products
- sharing of contaminated syringes and needles
- mucous membrane (eyes, nose, mouth)
- damage to the skin by cuts, rashes, dry skin
- contact with infected blood or blood products
- body fluids, urine, faeces, semen, tears, saliva.

## Signs and symptoms
- fatigue, mild fever, muscle and joint pain
- nausea, vomiting and loss of appetite.

## Care of clients with HIV/AIDS and hepatitis B virus
There is no known cure. A blood test is the only way to find out if a client is infected. The aim of carers should be to:
- maintain a safe environment in which the client can recover
- prevent complications from infection
- maintain vital functions, eg. airways
- provide support to the client, his or her family and friends
- assist the client to regain maximum independence
- assist the client to meet self-care requisites.

## Prevention of HIV/AIDS and hepatitis B
Prevention should aim to:

### Promote health education
- encourage exercise, mobility, healthier diet, sleep/rest, recreation
- assist client to participate in leisure and educational activities.

### Reduce harmful situations
- reduce drug intake, both legal and illegal, eg. nicotine, caffeine, heroin, cocaine
- reduce alcohol, stress, risk of contamination by body fluids, encourage safer sex
- do not re-use needles
- maintain healthy skin and cover all cuts with waterproof dressing
- counsel and advise on reducing the number of sexual partners.

### Limit the spread of infection
- educate and counsel all infected people, families and sexual partners
- promote social cleanliness, eg. handwashing, safe handling and storage of food. Be aware of approaches to the management of infection.

# References

Department of Health (1988) *AIDS: HIV Infected Health Care Workers: Protection Against Infection with HIV and Hepatitis B Viruses*. Expert advisory group on AIDS. HMSO, London

Department of Health (1990) *Guidance for Clinical Health Care Workers: Protection against Infection with HIV and Hepatitis Viruses*. Recommendations of the Expert advisory group on AIDS. HMSO, London

Health Education Council (1986) *AIDS: What Everybody Needs to Know*. AIDS Unit, Department of Health

Pratt R (1991) *AIDS: A Strategy for Nursing Care*. Edward Arnold, London

**Audio visual aids**

*Format: VHS video*

Ref: 8192: *Facts about AIDS*
Ref: 5530: *Management of AIDS*
Ref: CME: 5507: *Management of Hepatitis*
Ref: CNE 4334: *Universal Precautions: AIDS and Hepatitis B Prevention for Health Care Workers*
Oxford Educational Resources Ltd

# Assignment

The purpose of this homework is to assist you in preparing for your Workbased Assessment of Competence. As there is no pressure on you, feel free to work at your own pace, but avoid the temptation to procrastinate. After you have read your notes and suggested references, submit your work for correction. The completed work becomes part of your Personal Portfolio.

## HIV/AIDS and hepatitis B

1. Discuss what you understand by the terms 'HIV/AIDS and hepatitis B'.
2. What do you understand by normal immune system and list types of immunity?
3. State six ways in which HIV/AIDS and hepatitis B infection can be transmitted to other people.
4. List symptoms of these infections.
5. One of the residents in your place of work is diagnosed as suffering from hepatitis B. Explain the care of this person.
6. Discuss ways in which both the AIDS/HIV and hepatitis B could be prevented.

## Wound care — aseptic technique (CU1.3, X13.1, Y4.1)

A wound can be described as a break in continuity of the tissue which may occur suddenly as a result of injury, harmful agents, or a surgeon's knife. It should heal within a relatively short period of time when the edges of the skin are brought together in close proximity, and made to function in unison. This healing process may be delayed in the presence of harmful agents, such as bacteria or viruses. Other factors may affect the wound's healing, such as drugs, radiation, stress, nutritional state and the lifestyle of the individual.

### Types of wounds

People in nursing and residential care homes may have any of the following wounds: surgical, pressure sores, burns, leg ulcers — arterial and venous, lacerations, superficial wounds, granulating wounds, fungating wounds, infected wounds, sinus and fistula (cavity wounds). All wounds can be divided into two of the following basic categories:

### 1. Primary intention
Wounds where the edges are brought together for repair are known as primary intention. They are usually acute surgical wounds which are closed at the time of operation with clips, sutures, glue or dressings, in an attempt to minimise the chance of infection. Other types include simple cuts, grazes, and abrasions. They are all expected to heal rapidly because new cells do not need to migrate and there is less risk of the wound becoming infected as closure provides an immediate barrier against invading bacteria.

### 2. Second intention
These are open wounds that are closed by granulation. Wounds which heal by this process are infected ones which are left open, to allow gradual filling with granulation tissue. They are chronic wounds such as leg ulcers, pressure sores.

## Factors that may influence healing

Many situations may influence the healing of wounds:
- ageing due to changes in the cell activity
- malnutrition, including a reduction in vitamin C
- psychological factors, such as anxiety and depression
- infection due to the presence of bacteria, slough and dead tissue
- recurrent trauma which may cause persistent disturbance of the wound
- drugs which may reduce the efficiency of the immune system
- smoking: it is believed that nicotine inhibits the formulation of epithelial cells over the wound surface.

## Infection of wounds

The sources of infection may be regarded as:
- endogenous: which can be from the person's own nasal passage or mouth, skin or bowel and poor personal hygiene
- exogenous: as a result of cross-infection from the environment or equipment.

## Management of wound infection

### Guidance
The aim of wound cleansing is to remove foreign bodies, debris, necrotic tissue and excessive slough. The mechanics of cleansing will reduce the microbial load and in nursing and residential care homes, management of wounds is based on:

### 1. Assessment of wounds
Each wound is as individual as the patient and must be treated as such. This assessment is repeated and recorded at each dressing change so that progress may be monitored. The aim is to enable suitable dressing material to be applied. Considerations for assessment are:
- the stage of healing
- the depth of the wound
- the presence and amount of exudate. An open wound should have the surface area accurately measured and monitored weekly.

### 2. Role and responsibility for wound care
The person-in-charge is responsible for the total care of clients and their needs. This involves:
- assessing the wound and selecting cleansing agents, dressing and bandages that will cause no damage to newly formed tissue

- managing the wound within the framework of total patient care
- understanding and applying the principles of asepsis together with knowledge of the wound healing processes
- assisting healing by using appropriate wound care products, and monitoring wound healing by documented evaluation.

## The role of care assistants

With the advent of the NHS and the Community Care Act 1993, care assistants are being trained to assist in caring for elderly people living alone in their own homes. In nursing homes and residential care settings, and in accordance with local policy, care assistants may be asked to assist by the person-in-charge who should have an updated knowledge of wound care. If this is the case, it is important to be aware of the suggested guidance in conjunction with agreed practices.

## Guidance for implementation of wound care

- clean wounds should be redressed before infected ones and changed as infrequently as possible
- dressing material and procedures should be based on research findings
- observe and report on any sign of infection, eg. pain, swelling, redness and pyrexia as swabs may be taken for laboratory examination.

### 1. The client
- maintain a good interpersonal relationship by explaining the procedures and seeking his or her consent or co-operation
- make the person comfortable in bed or sitting on a chair with the limb raised
- ensure that he or she is adequately protected and that his or her self-respect and dignity are maintained
- reassure him or her at all times during the procedure.

### 2. Environment
- all domestic dust-producing activities should cease at least an hour before dressing commences to allow dust to settle out of the atmosphere, eg. bedmaking or dusting
- the room environment should be well-ventilated, clean and dry. The bed may be screened if necessary.

### 3. The dresser
- the staff undertaking the procedure should not have any form of infection or sore throat
- cuts and abrasions must be covered with a waterproof dressing
- nails should be kept short
- wash and dry hands thoroughly before and after the procedure
- wear a clean uniform and change when it is soiled; wear protective clothing if necessary, eg. plastic disposable apron, gloves.

### 4. Equipment
- clean the dressing trolley with hot water and detergent and dry thoroughly. Wipe with 70% alcohol or a clear soluble phenol disinfectant
- examine the cleansing packs to ascertain that there is no damage to the outer layer and that the sterile indicator tape is dark brown
- discard all damaged and out-of-date products
- ensure that only sterile equipment and lotions come in contact with the exposed wound and areas around the wound.

## 5. Aseptic technique

This is a technique for carrying out sterile procedures so that there is minimal risk of introducing infection. Dressings are changed by using sterile equipment and non-touch techniques. The current approach is hand or glove technique. Once the wound has been assessed, the most suitable dressing is chosen and cleansing is carried out in accordance with locally agreed policy.

## Procedure

The procedure may be carried out either in clients' rooms or in a designated room in the home. A care plan should be consulted for individual clients. The carer should:
- maintain a good interpersonal relationship with clients and colleagues
- prepare clients
- prepare a dressing trolley or tray in accordance with agreed practice
- wash and dry hands thoroughly before and after the procedure
- carry out the procedure
- dispose of clinical waste immediately after use in accordance with locally agreed policy
- report the condition of the wound to the person in charge.

## Surgical wounds

After an operation, surgical wounds are usually sutured and covered with a non-adherent island dressing or film dressing in spray or sheet form to prevent infection. As a rule, these wounds are not disturbed, except if a client complains of pain and there is a rise in temperature and pulse. Change of dressing increases the risk of infection. But, checking the dressing and area around the wound forms part of post operative observations. Depending on the extent of surgery, a wound drain may be inserted to drain the blood or serum. It should be observed together with the dressing and any unusual drainage should be reported. Sometimes surgical wounds may be left open to heal from the base upwards, eg. pressure sores.

## General after care of wounds

The successful healing of wounds depends upon a variety of factors, including the nutritional status of the client. A conducive environment will also influence this healing process and prevent the onset of infection. The following factors should be considered when formulating clients' care plans.

### Diet
A diet should include a wide variety of foods which are acceptable to the client to meet his nutritional needs. A well balanced diet containing adequate amounts of fluids, protein, carbohydrates, fats and vitamins plays a vital role in the repair process and promotes rapid healing with the formation of white blood cells and fibroblast. Vitamins are also essential, especially vitamin C, as deficiency may impair the fight against infection and the production of fibroblast.

### Rest
Large wounds require rest and heal best if left relatively undisturbed for several days. Wounds should never be tightly packed and bandaged except to arrest haemorrhage, and changed when necessary.

### Exercise
Gentle exercise should be encouraged according to individual ability in order to improve blood supply to the injured area. Exercise could also prevent muscle wasting and stiffness which may be due to top scar formation. This will depend upon the site.

## Education

Explanation and advice should be given to clients on simple care of the wound. He/she should also be encouraged to observe and report on exudate, pain and application of bandages.

## References

Cutting K (1994) Factors influencing wound healing. *Nurs Stand* **8**(50): 33–36

Draper J (1985) Making the dressing fit the wound. *Nurs Times* **81**(4): 32–35

Hateley P (1993) Cleansing agents. *Nurs Times* **89**(45)

Johnson A (1988) Cleansing ethics. *Nurs Times* **84**(6): 9–10

Morgan D (1991) Practice in nursing homes. *Nurs Times* **87**(49)

Roberts G (1988) Nutrition and wound healing. *Nurs Stand Special Edition* **14**: 8–12

Thomas ST (1989) Pain and wound management. *Nurs Times* (Community Outlook Supplement) **85**(28): 11–15

Turner TD (1985) *Which Dressing and Why? Wound Care.* Heinemann, London

Bree-Williams F (1996) Use of gloves in aseptic technique for wound care. *Nurs Times* **92**(5): 24

### Audio visual aids

*Format: VHS video*

Ref: 125/CT 3: *Cross-infection — Sources of Wound Infection*

Ref: 125/CT 4: *Cross-infection — Prevention of Wound Infection*

Ref: LPLM338: *Clean Hands Save Lives*

Ref: 296/1-3 CT: *Surgical Dressing in the Home*

Ref: CNE4266: *Scrubbing, Gowning and Gloving*

Oxford Educational Resources Ltd

## Isolation nursing (CUI: 2–3, XI: 1–3)

Infection is one of the common causes of death, and its control is the carers' major concern. Some people who develop an infection are at risk of infecting others, and so isolation or barrier nursing may be required. People suffering from smallpox, tuberculosis and other infectious diseases may be isolated to prevent the spread of infection to other people. If a client or a number of people have already been affected, it is necessary to take immediate action to investigate and control the outbreak.

The starting point is to identify the source and isolate either the client or the site of infection, for example, the wound. Clients with tuberculosis may be isolated in an attempt to prevent the spread of infection to others. It is also important that the infected client is not exposed to another infection acquired through the home or hospital conditions — termed cross-infection. Crow (1989) states that the aim of isolation is to restrict the growth and obstruct the movement of disease-causing organisms. The outcome is an environment free of these organisms, preventing the spread of infection to others, including carers.

### Methods of control

In order to control the infection, it will be necessary to take precautions such as isolation of infected patients or clients, closure of ward or nursing homes, restriction of staff movements, surveillance of contacts, examination of all staff and clients/patients for carriers, survey of procedures and practice, bacteriological examination of specimens, equipment and buildings.

## Isolation techniques

The method used for each communicable disease may include barrier nursing in the open ward, barrier nursing in a cubicle and isolation in an infectious disease hospital or unit. But the appropriate methods of isolation necessary to prevent the spread of infection from one person to others will depend on the nature and severity of the infection, the mode of transmission, and the ability of other patients and carers to withstand the infection.

Whatever method is used, the aim is to confine the organisms and stop their spread. This is achieved by assessing each individual client with a communicable disease, and planning the care to meet his/her needs. The system of client allocation could be used to control the number of staff who come in contact with the person, thereby reducing the risk of individuals contacting an infection.

Apart from clients who are infected, isolation techniques can be used for those receiving special drug treatment which greatly reduces their natural ability to produce antibodies and protect immune defence mechanisms. These clients are prone to infection from any source they may come into contact with. There should be a local policy and guidelines reflecting relevant legislation on the following:

### *Accommodation*

A single room is necessary when the client has an airborne disease or when the person cannot confine and contain his body fluids. The room should contain a sink for handwashing as well as toilet and bathing facilities. Clients with airborne infections such as tuberculosis should be nursed in separate rooms with good ventilation systems — extractor fans to prevent contaminated air from entering other parts of the home. To help reduce the feeling of isolation, the room should preferably have a good outlook with glass partitions between the room and the rest of the ward.

All staff entering the room must wear appropriate protective clothing, gloves and masks. Signs should be posted on the door requiring visitors to report to the person-in-charge before entering. Depending on the type of infection, protective clothing, gloves and masks may be required.

All supplies and equipment for care should be stored in the room. Always gather any additional equipment before putting on a gown or entering the room. Provide diversional therapy, eg. puzzles or other forms of amusement to occupy the client.

### *Protective clothing*

The use of articles of protective clothing required for individual cases, is entirely dependent on the way the particular infection spreads, the type of care being given and the client. For example, when entering a room to talk to a patient with salmonella there is no need to put on gloves and apron, but if the same patient requires help with using the toilet, then such items should be worn to prevent risk of cross-contamination.

### *Gowns and plastic aprons*

Transfer of organisms from staff clothing is possible but not a major problem. The wearing of gowns or disposable plastic aprons is accepted as part of isolation nursing technique, particularly when handling infectious material. A plastic apron offers better protection than a cotton gown because it is cheap, cannot be penetrated by organisms and water and is easy to put on. Bab *et al* (1989) state that the apron can be reused without a significant rise in the load of bacteria, provided that it is allocated for use with one particular client and it is dry and the ties are intact.

## Masks

It is generally considered that masks contribute very little to the safety of patient or staff. Carers with colds do not need to wear masks to protect patients — they should not be on duty. Clients with measles or chicken pox should be cared for by staff who are immune to these diseases and do not need to wear a mask. If a mask is necessary, it should be the same type as that used in theatre, ie. an efficient filter type.

## Gloves

Wearing gloves plays an important role in the prevention of spreading infection. It is believed that gloves prolong the effect of hand disinfection as well as reducing cross-contamination of the hands from the infected site and equipment. A pair of well-fitting latex gloves should be used. They should be comfortable and not split or slip off during procedures such as bedmaking. Unless, the procedures are aseptic, there is no need to wear sterile gloves. They are no substitute for handwashing, and should be disposed of after use.

Always wear gloves when in contact with:
- people with open wounds, pressure sores, skin rashes or broken skin
- blood or other bodily fluids
- soiled and contaminated linen

*Putting on gloves*
- check for cracks, punctures, tears or discoloration and dispose of if damaged
- check for proper size and fit
- pull the gloves over gown cuffs if a gown is worn.

*Removing gloves*
- hold at the cuff and pull inside out
- fold the second glove off the hand over the first glove, and enclose the first glove within the second
- dispose of gloves using the designated bin for infected waste
- wash and dry your hands thoroughly.

## Uniform

It is uncommon for the shoulder of the uniform to become contaminated, but the area of maximum contamination is the front of the uniform at bed height. Use disposable plastic aprons and change uniform whenever necessary.

## Handwashing

Hands play an important part in the spread of infection by contact, and disinfection is the most effective method of preventing the spread of infection. Research shows that there is a great variation in both quality and frequency of handwashing practices. Despite understanding the importance of handwashing, the number of times that staff report that they have washed their hands is often well above the frequency actually observed.

Phillips (1989) believes that there are three types of handwashing: social, using soap and water; antiseptic, using an antiseptic detergent solution or an alcohol hand rub; and surgical, requiring washing for a total time of three minutes using an antiseptic detergent. Following contact with known or suspected contaminated surfaces and materials, staff should use an antiseptic detergent solution or alcohol hand rub. Research has shown that infrequent handwashing and poor techniques continue to cause infection to spread via hands.

## General principles

There are many views on the act of handwashing, but many people follow Ayliffe *et al* (1982). Their technique is:
- remove wristwatch and jewellery
- use hot running water to dampen your hands
- use the correct amount of individually dispensed soap solution
- wash all areas of your hands and rinse off soap
- dry your hands thoroughly with disposable towels.

Gibley (1987) agrees with Feldman's criteria for handwashing in that:
- lather of soap should be visible and there should be continuous running water
- hands should be held down so that water drains from fingertips into the sink
- splashing clothing or floor should be avoided
- friction should be used on all surfaces — back of hands, the thumb and between the fingers
- hands should be held down to rinse and all surfaces of the hands should be dried thoroughly
- taps should be turned off with paper towel.

As a rule, treat everyone with caution because you do not know who is infected or not. Hands should be washed and dried before and after contact with clients and carrying out any caring procedures.

### Equipment

Over the years there has been increasing awareness of the need to dispose of equipment which has been in contact with blood or other body fluids or used on or by patients in isolation. The Health and Safety Act 1974 (DHSS, 1987a) states that 'manufacturers are required to ensure that their employees are not put at risk, for example, by handling items that may be contaminated as a result of their use in health care or in a laboratory'. Managers have a similar duty of care towards their employees and have a responsibility to ensure that neither clients nor staff are put at risk from inadequately cleaned and contaminated equipment.

Disposable or autoclavable equipment should be used whenever possible and the amount of equipment taken into the room kept to a minimum. Certain pieces of equipment, eg. stethoscopes should be used exclusively for the patient and kept in the room until discontinuation of isolation precautions. Locally agreed policy should provide guidance on methods of disinfection as recommended by the control of infection team. Advice should include the method of decontamination to be used, eg. chemical, low temperature steam, autoclaving.

### Waste disposal

HIV infection has raised public concern with regard to the disposal of clinical waste, in particular the disposal of contaminated sharp objects. Although clinical waste, excluding contaminated sharp objects, does not necessarily present a greater infection risk, it is recommended that waste from clients with some types of infection should be double-bagged. This technique involves placing waste in yellow coloured plastic bags which are of a minimum gauge of either 800 if low density or 400 if high density. These bags of waste must be disposed of in approved boxes for sharp objects for final disposal by incineration.

Infected linen should be enclosed in totally water-soluble bags, or bags with a soluble strip, at the bedside to prevent the dispersal or transference of organisms. The bag is designed so that it remains intact until placed unopened in a washing machine, where part or all of the bag will be dissolved to release the contents.

## Care of residents in isolation

The needs of clients depend on the reasons for their isolation. It should be remembered that it is the micro-organism that is being isolated and not the person. So, there is a need to assess not only the physical but psychological and social needs as well. Clients will feel depressed, anxious and frightened about the outcome of the disease.

## Management of the problems

### Guidance

- develop and maintain a good interpersonal relationship with the individual
- sit down and spend time with the person and share your thoughts with him or her
- listen to what he or she says and encourage the person to express his or her views, wishes and ideas and offer reassurance by touching and holding hands with the individual
- encourage simple diversional therapy, eg. sketching, in the understanding that the finished product may be destroyed as part of the procedure of terminal care
- offer relatives similar care should they seek your help or refer them to the person-in-charge.

### Information

Leaflets should be available explaining why isolation is required and what precautions are needed with particular emphasis on handwashing.

## References

Ayliffre GAI *et al* (1982) *Hospital-acquired Infections. Principles and Prevention*, 1st edn. John Wright, Bristol

Babb JR *et al* (1983) Contamination of protective clothing and nurses' uniforms in an isolated ward. *J Hosp Infect* **4**: 149–157

Bagshave KD *et al* (1978) Isolating patients in hospital to control infection. Part 1: sources and routes: Part 4: nursing procedures. *Br Med J* **2**: 609–612, 808–811

Crow RA (1989) *Asepsis, The Right Touch*. Everett Companies, Louisiana, USA

Department of Health and Social Security (1988a) *Public Health in England. Report of the Committee of Inquiry into the Future. Development of the Public Health Function*. HMSO, London

Gibley C (1987) Now wash your hands. *Nurs Times* **83**(29): 41–42

Phillips C (1989) Hand hygiene. *Nurs Times* **85**(37): 76–79

## Audio visual aid

### Format: VHS video

Ref: CNE4266: *Scrubbing, Gowning, and Gloving*
Oxford Educational Resources Ltd

# Unit 4
# Contribute to the protection of individuals from abuse (Z1, Z18)

## Protect individuals from risk of abuse (Z1: 1–3, Z18: 1–2)

Abuse can be defined as the use of power over someone in such a way that it causes that person undue stress and discomfort. This abuse is varied and can be inflicted repeatedly by those in close, caring relationships or by a stranger. It can be premeditated or spontaneous, aggressive or passive. The incidence of abuse has been more commonly associated with children because of the longstanding and close relationships between the abuser (often a parent or guardian) and the child. This abuse is more easily recognised and detected because children are periodically examined and checked, either in the clinic or at school.

However, society has difficulty in accepting the incidence of the abuse of older people owing to the lack of a common framework or understanding of the subject; the main cause for this lack being that, unlike children, elderly people were not subject to regular health checks. Even if evidence of such practice existed, it would be denied for fear of social and family stigma. In essence, the abuse and neglect of older people is a reality and common practice. It was not until the mid 1970s that recognition of the incidence became widespread. As it primarily involved elderly women, it became known as 'granny-bashing'. In 1992, a social services report showed that abuse of elderly people was most likely to be carried out by an adult child who was the principal carer, and who shared a residence with the older person.

### Reasons for abuse

Abuse and neglect of the elderly may be carried out by members of their families who are informal carers, and professional carers in clinical settings. It is claimed that the problem for family carers may be due to deteriorating family relationships, especially if there is little respite care. In the health care setting, it is believed that caring for a high level of physically- and mentally-dependent residents increases the level of stress in staff, and is related to the way in which carers respond to aggression and violent behaviour. In retrospect, the subject of abuse is one of the most difficult to detect and control, because few people are willing to admit to their actions as the consequences may lead to social isolation, criminal proceedings or disciplinary action. The reasons for abuse by carers are many and varied, and include the following:

- feelings of hopelessness or helplessness
- poor relationships, especially if there are no friends or relatives to act as advocates for the person
- isolation
- overcrowding
- stress of caring or doing the job and a lack of adequate supervision
- poor staffing levels with no back up or supporting system
- lack of in-service training, induction or orientation programmes
- prejudice and discrimination combined with a lack of moral sensibility

- anxiety due to a previous history of abuse
- deterioration in the physical and mental health of the carer
- tiredness due to lack of adequate rest and sleep.

## People at risk of abuse

Every client in care is unwittingly exposed to abuse during the process of carrying out the caring procedures which are related to activities of daily living. The majority of clients at risk of neglect and abuse are those who are seriously ill and the frail dependent elderly who are vulnerable. These are usually people with:
- communication difficulties, such as those who are hard of hearing or have poor eyesight
- mental health problems and learning difficulties who may have difficulty in living independently and communicating.

## Forms of abuse

Clients may be abused in a number of ways. These include: sexual and environmental abuse; physical assault; administration of inappropriate drugs; deprivation of prescribed drugs or nourishment; emotional and verbal abuse; deprivation of help in performing activities of daily living.

### 1. Physical abuse
- rough handling, punching, slapping, kicking
- use of violent and aggressive behaviour.

The abused individual may display signs of malnutrition, poor personal hygiene, including unexplained bruises and cuts on the face, lips, mouth, back, buttocks and thighs at various stages of healing.

### 2. Psychological abuse
- verbal abuse, shouting, causing emotional distress by insulting, demeaning or coercive behaviour
- bullying, intimidating, making someone perform acts which are personally distasteful.

The abused individual may display a pattern of passive behaviour, such as withdrawal from contact, with little or no interest in care. He or she may seem anxious, depressed, tense and fearful, avoiding contact with carer. He or she may be submissive with low self-esteem and have poor communication skills. At visiting time, if the abuser is a relative or an unwanted visitor, the client may seem distressed.

### 3. Deprivation *(deliberately withholding basic rights and comforts)*
- such as food, light, heat, personal hygiene
- denying the person contact with others and opportunities to express his or her feelings
- such as beliefs, lifestyle, choice, ability to take risks or manage their own affairs as far as possible.

The abused individual may display signs of malnutrition, loss of weight, dehydration and low self-esteem.

### 4. Sexual abuse
This involves forcing or promoting unwelcome sexual attention on the individual, eg. rape. Signs of abuse may include:
- difficulty in walking or standing, torn, stained or bloody underclothing, pain, itching
- bruises or bleeding in external genitalia or anal areas.

***Misappropriation of personal effects*** *(stealing)*
- money, valuables, articles with sentimental attachments
- any other items of clients' personal belongings, eg. stamp collections, clothes, shoes.

It is important to keep a regular check on clients' personal belongings in accordance with organisational policy and report any discrepancies.

### 6. Institutional abuse
This may be in consequence of:
- inadequate staffing level, low standards of staff training, few qualified staff
- lack of supervision resulting in a substandard quality of care
- a large number of part-time and temporary staff who may fail to comply with safety standards or offer adequate mental stimulation and personal hygiene to residents
- failure to comply with safety standards which could result in an unhygienic care environment
- inadequate attention to incontinence which could result in a dirty home environment
- out-dated regime and practices and accommodation without basic facilities.

## Management of problems

It is reported that the detection rates of abuse and neglect are low because little attention is being paid to developing policy. Hence, care assistants lack confidence in their approach and should be made aware of approaches available for tackling the detection of abuse.

### 1. Organisational policy
Managers should be able to formulate local policy and guidelines on how to deal with the problem. This policy should aim to:
- assess or screen all residents at risk of abuse and place their names on the 'at risk' records maintained by the health care staff. These should be reviewed at predetermined intervals.
- provide support systems for the residents and their families which, if necessary, include legal intervention.

### 2. Staff support system
There is a need for an occupational health system which identifies the mental health and behavioural problems of the staff, and offers a professional counselling service within the Health and Safety at Work Act 1974, as recommended in the case of the Alitt Enquiry (1994). This should include:
- internal support measures, such as counselling for the abuser
- review of conditions of service in relation to the hours of duty and review of the staff/client ratio.

### 3. Education and training
In-service education and training programmes should include:
- recognition of cultural influences in alleged abuse situations
- methods of recognising and handling the incidence of abuse
- induction and orientation of all staff
- local research on possible causes
- respite facilities in the work area
- the right to consult residents, their families and the authorities as necessary
- investigation and reporting so that the abused people can be protected.

### 4. Investigation of abuse
Local policy should provide information on procedures for investigation of alleged cases of neglect and abuse.

### Guidance
If there is suspicion of abuse, carers are ethically obliged to assist in making a thorough assessment of clients and the situation. Assessment of injuries must be made and findings accurately recorded. Where the person-in-charge feels that an abuse has occurred, appropriate authorities should be informed in accordance with local policy. The abused person should be reassured at all times and left quietly in a 'sterile' environment pending further instruction. But on no account should any item of the personal clothing worn at the time of the alleged incident be removed, or the abused person be allowed to have a bath or given a shower. It is important to maintain an accurate record of the incident as follows:
- time of the report or observation of the incident
- location of the incident
- any witness at the time of the report or observation, and the action taken
- condition of the client — anxious, frightened or weeping.

## 5. Legislation
Certain acts of parliament are designed to protect those at risk of abuse, eg. the Children's Act 1986; the Mental Health Act 1984; the Health and Safety at Work Act 1974.

## 6. Preventive measures
The following are some of the measures which may be taken to protect clients in long-term care:
- review of accommodation to prevent isolation, lack of privacy and dignity
- periodical review of clients' personal possessions, including money
- security of care environment and good support for clients, relatives and staff
- early identification of staff health problems and an induction programme for new staff
- modify routine care, eg. time of retiring to bed, activities in the absence of supervision.

### Guidelines
The ability to develop and maintain good interpersonal relationships, especially by being assertive and acting as an advocate for the rights of your clients, is very important. You should also be able to:
- show an in-depth knowledge of all clients at risk of abuse and their whereabouts at any given time
- be aware of organisational policy and guidelines for dealing with problems
- observe and report accurately signs of abuse or untoward incidents when carrying out procedures, such as bathing, dressing, feeding, helping clients in and out of bed
- encourage clients to express themselves and be alert to what they may have to say
- know all visitors to the home and individual clients' relatives
- be aware of prowlers and intruders to the home and report any suspicious circumstances
- demonstrate a knowledge of the security of the care environment and be familiar with guidelines for reporting and dealing with complaints
- be aware of the list of unwanted visitors which may be maintained in the home, and bring to the attention of the person-in-charge the presence of any stranger.

It is acknowledged that various people who have access to clients can mistreat them while in the care environment. This includes: their friends, relatives, spouses, strangers, visitors and, in certain circumstances, the clients themselves. It is important to recognise the usual locations of injuries.

These include:
- eyes and ears as a result of a slap or punch
- upper arms and under the arm where excessive force or pressure might have been applied, ie. if the client was lifted or restrained
- bruises to the shoulders usually occur when the elderly person is pushed or falls against an object.

A comprehensive knowledge of individual clients, their visitors and colleagues, together with constant observation and accurate reporting, are some of the requirements which may contribute to the prevention of neglect, mistreatment or abuse of older people.

## References

Clotheir C (Chairman) (1994) *The Alitt Enquiry.* HMSO, London

DOH/SSI (1992) *Confronting Elder Abuse: Department of Health/Social Services Inspectorate.* HMSO, London

Eastman M (1984) *Old Age Abuse.* Age Concern, London

Fagg J (1994) Detection of abuse. *Nurs Times* **90**(37): 67–68

Glen G (1994) Joint approach: Abuse of older people research. *Nurs Times* **90**(37): 69–71

Homer A, Gilleard C (1990) Abuse of elderly people by carers. *Br Med J* **301**: 1359–1362

Phillips L (1983) Elder abuse — what is it? Who says so? *Ger Nurs* **4**: 167–170

RCN (1996) *Combating Abuse and Neglect of Older People. RCN Guidelines for Nurses.* Royal College of Nursing, London

### Audio visual aids

*Format: VHS video*

Ref: CNEUA336: *Elder Abuse: A Family Secret*

Ref: PATUA 336: *Elder Abuse*

Oxford Educational Resources Ltd

## Assignment

The purpose of this homework is to assist you in preparing for your Workbased Assessment of Competence. As there is no pressure on you, feel free to work at your own pace, but avoid the temptation to procrastinate. After you have read your notes and suggested references, submit your work for correction. The completed work becomes part of your Personal Portfolio.

## Protect individuals from risk of abuse (Z1: 1–3, Z18: 1–2)

1. What do you understand by the word 'abuse'.
2. Mention six ways in which clients could be abused.
3. Discuss common reasons for clients 'at risk' to be abused by:
   a) a member of his or her family
   b) a member of the caring staff.
4. State how you would protect the right of a client who tells you in confidence that he or she has been abused by one of your colleagues.
5. List five acts of legislation designed to protect those who are at risk of abuse.
6. Discuss ways of monitoring clients at risk of abuse in your care environment.

# Section IV: The delivery of care — option group A

At the end of this section, candidates should be able to demonstrate an understanding of the basic principles of delivering care defined by the following units.

|  | Units and elements of learning |  |
|---|---|---|
| **Unit 5: Assist clients adjust to changes in care** | **W2, W3, Y5** | 145 |
| o Admission, transfer and discharge | W3: 1–2, Y5: 1–2 | 145 |
| o Clients' contact with family and significant others | W2: 2–3 | 153 |
| **Unit 6: Promote communication in care through physical contact** | **CL2, CL6, S11** | 157 |
| o Clients with sensory deprivation | CL2, CL6, S11: 1–3 | 157 |
| o Hearing loss |  | 157 |
| o Deafness |  | 158 |
| o Visually impaired people | CL2: 1–2, CL6.1, S11: 1–3 | 162 |
| o Clients with dysarthria, aphasia and mental problems | CL1.1 | 167 |
| **Unit 7: Enable clients to achieve physical comfort** | **Z19** | 170 |
| o Nature and purpose of breathing | Z19: 1–2 | 170 |
| o Help clients to rest, relax and sleep | Z19.2 | 176 |
| o Helping clients to sleep | Z19: 1–2 | 179 |
| **Unit 8: Enable clients to eat and drink** | **NC12, NC13** | 184 |
| o Eating | NC12: 1–2, NC13: 1–2 | 184 |
| o Helping clients to eat | NC12: 1–2, N13: 1 | 189 |
| o Helping clients to drink | NC12: 1–2, N13: 1–2 | 193 |
| o Therapeutic and special diets |  | 198 |
| o Food Hygiene Act 1990 |  | 202 |
| o Diabetes |  | 204 |
| **Unit 9: Assist clients to access and use toilet facilities** | **Z11** | 208 |
| o Principles of elimination | Z11: 1–2 | 208 |
| o Constipation |  | 210 |
| o Diarrhoea |  | 211 |
| o Care of the bowels | Z11: 1–2 | 213 |
| o Promotion of continence | Z12: 1–2 | 217 |
| o Care of the catheter and drainage bag | Z12.2 | 222 |
| **Unit 10: Assist clients with personal hygiene and appearance** | **Z9** | 227 |
| o Personal grooming and dressing | Z9: 1–2 | 227 |
| o Care of face, ears, eyes and prosthesis | Z9: 1–2 | 231 |
| o Care of the mouth, teeth and dentures | Z9: 1–2 | 233 |

- o  *Personal cleanliness (bathing)*      Z9: 1–2      238

**Unit 11: Assist clients to move, exercise and maintain desirable posture**      **CU6, Z6, Z7**      243

- o  *Positions used in care*      Z7: 1–2      243
- o  *Moving and handling clients*      Z7: 1–2      245
- o  *Exercise and passive movements of limbs*      Z6: 1–2      250
- o  *Prevention of pressure sores*      Z7: 2–3, Z19:1–2      252
- o  *Care of mobility aids*      CU6:1–3, Z6: 1–2      259

# Unit 5
# Assist clients adjust to changes in care (W2, W3, Y5)

## Admission, transfer and discharge (W3: 1–2, Y5: 1–2)

If an elderly person becomes ill and admission to a hospital or a nursing home is necessary, especially for the first time, this can be a very difficult and stressful time for the person and his or her family. Some live alone in their own homes and their needs are so many and varied that a single profession cannot meet them. The solution is to admit them to a care institution where special clinical and social skills, and experience are readily available. However, giving up their own homes to enter residential care is a major upheaval and must be undertaken with careful planning and sensitivity.

### Sources of referral

Clients may be referred by their own general practitioners in consultation with members of the primary care team in the community, ie. district nurses, community psychiatric nurses and social workers. A comprehensive history of the client's life prior to admission will assist in the planning and continuity of care. The matron or person-in-charge should then visit the client in his or her current accommodation and carry out a basic initial assessment to confirm that the accommodation to be provided will be suitable for the person and to establish contact with the client and his or her family.

### Pre-admission visits

Admission to nursing and residential care homes is a matter of choice. In most cases, the client and his or her relatives will visit several homes before making a final decision about the one that will best meet his or her needs and where he or she will feel most comfortable. This visit may help the person start to adjust to the new environment before admission, and reduce the level of anxiety associated with the transfer. It also means that the family can be involved in care.

The financial aspect is a sensitive area which requires tactful handling and explanation to ensure that the people involved receive the correct advice on fees and benefits. This need is usually discussed by a responsible person and agreed with clients and relatives prior to admission.

### Contract of care

The client is presented with a copy of the contract of care which sets out the agreement relating to fees, accommodation and general provision of care, after prior discussion and understanding with the client and his or her relatives. A copy of the local Patient's Charter is presented as well.

### Admission of elderly people for care

The NHS and Community Act 1993 sets out information on the rights of individuals with respect to the length of waiting time for an operation. It requires the local authority to provide a cost effective service for keeping elderly people in the community, and in their homes, to ensure that there are sufficient resources to target all those who are in greatest need. It may not always be possible for the client to remain in the community as he/she may be in need of long-term care in a hospital or nursing home. The local authority then has responsibility for purchasing nursing and residential home care from the owners of these homes.

**Factors leading to admission**

A significant number of elderly people will be frail prior to admission or suffer from disabling conditions; and those who live alone may have limited means and capability for self-care. When an elderly person becomes ill, the problems may present themselves in a number of ways, but often include deterioration in physical, psychological and social health. Any one or any combination of these conditions may lead to admission and accounts for about 80 percent of emergency admissions. Factors may include:

**1. Immobility and falls**
Falls and immobility are among the most common reasons for admission to a nursing home or hospital.

**2. Dehydration**
Elderly people often do not drink enough because of an impaired sense of thirst. They may not feel thirsty and so become weak and averse to drinking. The fear of being incontinent may cause a reluctance to drink for fear that the intake of fluid could increase their incontinence. The confused elderly may refuse nourishment yet continue to lose fluid in urine and sweat, thus becoming dehydrated.

**3. Confusion**
The function of the brain is easily upset by any form of physical disturbance, and a sudden onset of confusion is one indication of illness in old age. Confusion is also a side-effect of numerous drugs such as hypnotics, tranquillisers and antidepressants.

**4. Reaction to drugs**
The older person is very sensitive to drugs and harmful side-effects are common. Drugs are metabolised more slowly in the liver and excreted more slowly by the kidneys. Therefore, medicines should be given in smaller doses.

**5. Temperature regulation**
The rise in body temperature in response to infection is frequently less severe. Rigors (a shivering attack) may be an indication of a urinary or gall bladder infection. If the elderly person seems unwell, a normal temperature should not be taken as an indication that she/he is not ill. Pulse and respiration is often a better guide to his/her condition. Impaired temperature regulation is a reaction to cold, and body temperature may fall below normal, ie. hypothermia.

**6. Loss of pain and sensation**
Pain in the elderly person may be less severe, which makes life less uncomfortable but increases the risk of injury. For example, he or she may burn his/her skin by sitting too close to the fire, or may bruise a leg against a bed cradle. Even serious injuries like fractures which cause severe pain in younger people, may be less obvious in the elderly.

*7. Inability to cope*
Quite often the individuals are presented either by themselves, neighbours, friends, home helps or other people in terms of 'it takes him over two hours just to get dressed' or 'he does not know day from night', 'he cannot recognise me any more', 'his room smells of gas and I am afraid he cannot look after himself and may put other people at risk of explosion'. The elderly person may also suffer from incontinence and when these circumstances are combined, the need for help is urgent.

**Reasons for admission**

The person may be admitted for a variety of reasons. The onset of illness may be acute or insidious; it may be chronic or progressive causing the person to become gradually less active. Consideration should be given to the effects of ageing because of the complexity of the elderly person's need for:
- a comprehensive assessment of physical, social and psychological well-being
- assessment of functional ability in relation to activities of daily living
- use of specialist resources for analysis and protection of the individual from harm and abuse
- relief for the family caring for the elderly relative
- convalescence, rehabilitation and respite care.

On admission and away from familiar surroundings, the person may be disorientated, with an increased risk of anxiety and mental confusion. For many, this is a stressful period, and if a change of home is to become permanent, some may pass through the classical stages associated with bereavement and grieving. The elderly person must be suitably prepared for any change of home, especially a change for which he/she is an unwilling participant. This change involves the whole of the multidisciplinary team.

**Admission procedures**

One of the most important aims of care is to promote independence as soon as possible. Also, first impressions of the home are important and may affect the way in which the new resident settles. A sensitive approach is essential to ease the anxieties of the client and his or her relatives.

**Guidance**

*1. Preparation of client's room*
- check that the client's room contains the necessary facilities for his or her use, and that these are in good 'habitable' and working order, eg. the alarm call bell, television, hot and cold water taps, the wardrobe and bedside lockers are clean
- read relevant information about the client and identify how he or she would like to be addressed, eg. by christian name or a more formal title
- be aware if the person is admitted under the Mental Health Act 1983, as appropriate to the care environment.

*2. Reception of client*
The way in which the person and his or her relatives are received is very important, and may affect the way he or she settles in. It may take some people several days to feel at home. Therefore, the first impression is very important, and requires the use of social skills, ie. greetings, salutation and introduction to allay associated anxiety and stress.

> *Guidance*
> - demonstrate your social skills (interpersonal relationships) by receiving the client and his or her relatives with courtesy, dignity and friendliness. Introduce yourself and other members of staff
> - make the client and his/her family feel that they are expected, and report their arrival to the person-in-charge

- provide additional information about the new surroundings, eg. the location of the lounge, toilet and washing facilities and the daily routines of the care establishment
- escort the client and his/her relatives to his or her room and spend some time with them there
- introduce the person to other residents who may be within the immediate vicinity or next beds, if this is considered appropriate. It may help to relax the person and relieve tension
- encourage conversation and answer any questions tactfully
- show the client how to use the nurse call system to summon help if necessary
- introduce the client to other residents and staff at the appropriate time
- offer practical help and reassure the client and his or her relatives
- offer refreshments at an appropriate time if necessary
- help the client to put personal belongings away if he/she would like you to do so
- leave the room with a welcoming remark, eg. 'I hope you will be happy here', and pass on any relevant information to the person-in-charge.

## 3. Personal belongings

These are everything the person brings into the home, including what he/she is wearing. All belongings should be checked, preferably by two carers, noted in the appropriate record and duly signed. Valuables must be accurately recorded in an appropriate property book or record, and jewellery should be described, eg. rings as either a yellow or white metal, money, personal mementoes and ornaments. Medicines, sharp objects, eg. razors and knives, brought in by the client should be reported to the person-in-charge who may retain them for safekeeping. All articles retained by the client or taken away by the relatives must be recorded properly in the appropriate document and witnessed.

## 4. Assessment

### Needs or nursing problems

A client may have disorders or disabilities which have developed over a period of time. The situation may be complicated further by the effects of ageing, social and economic problems. The overall framework for assessment is for members of the health care team, relatives and the advocate to establish additional resources of support, such as paramedical services, and their input in the care, eg. dietary need. Assessment should be on an ongoing basis, to extract information that will help staff to make informed decisions about the care, and to ensure that it is delivered appropriately and promptly.

### Risk-taking

Before or after admission, information should be gathered about the resident's realistic limitations, and an individual care plan with regard to risk-taking should be agreed by those involved in the care place, ie. residents, relatives and advocate(s). This must include statements on the levels of risk and how decisions are to be taken on a day-to-day basis. The aim is to balance the client's safety requirements and need for independence.

### Observation and reporting

Collection of information for formulating an individualised care plan (nursing process) by observing and reporting is the inital requirement and involves every member of the care team. The following areas should receive attention during and after admission.

## Guidance

*Physical state*
- height and weight, conversation, memory
- condition of the skin, eg. evidence of pressure sores, bruising
- temperature, pulse, respiration and blood pressure
- routine urinalysis for sugar, albumin.

*Social state*
- information on home situation, family, next of kin, funeral arrangements.

*Psychological state*
- ability to concentrate
- the degree of alertness and insight
- memory and intellectual functioning
- personality characteristics affecting behaviour and motivation.

## 5. Care plan

The care programme should include:
- medical treatment
- individual clients' needs in relation to activities of daily living
- treatment to restore physical mobility
- diversional activities to maintain or restore interest in activities of daily living
- regular review and reassessment of functional abilities and rehabilitation
- relatives, significant others, advocates and social workers
- risk-taking assessment and the rights of individuals to take risks.

## Rehabilitation

As part of assessment, the future pattern of a client's care is provisionally determined, and a common goal set towards which the person, his or her relatives and members of the health care team can work to achieve. The aim is to determine a goal for either one of the following outcomes:
- a return home with the support of community services or acceptance by a relative
- warden-controlled or supervised settlement or local authority residential care home
- continuing care in the hospital or residential care homes.

It is important that a newly admitted client should be observed discretely and approached in a quiet, calm and confident manner, with sensitivity to his or her needs. Attention should be paid to verbal and non-verbal behaviour and any unusual observations reported to the person-in-charge. Such information will help towards a more comprehensive assessment when planning and implementing care.

## Helping a client adapt to a new environment

One of the important roles of care assistants is to help a newly admitted person to settle in as soon as possible, and assume responsibility for his or her own welfare. This requires the use of empathy (displaying insight into others' feelings). It is recognised that clients entering a home may become dependent and assume the patient or client role, with the carers assuming a dominant role. This in turn increases the person's dependency.

After admission and when relatives have left, the client should be encourged to arrange his/her personal belongings and take control of the management of his/her room and lifestyle. This provides a framework and an opportunity for the continued use of social skills to develop interpersonal relationships. Ornaments or family photographs may prompt conversation. The care environment can be a social 'centre' for people to interact with one another. The new resident could be encouraged to meet and socialise with other residents in the lounge or dining room. Introduce him or her to someone who is reasonably well and friendly so that they can sit and talk together at the dinner table. This will help the client to adjust to his/her surroundings. Afer the meal, they may spend the evening together in the lounge. Sit with the person offering information about routine programmes of social and recreational activities before he or she retires. Advise him/her what time to rise in the morning and ask whether he/she would like a night-cap.

## Effects of admission

### 1. On the client/patient

It is recognised that a change of environment can be a frightening experience for some clients and their relatives, especially if it is the person's first admission. This experience may bring about changes in the individual's personality and attitude, which may require immediate use of essential supporting skills, such as counselling and advocacy to help the person to adjust to his or her new surroundings. Also, experience of previous admission(s) may help the individual to settle in quickly. However, some people may feel anxious, distressed, depressed or even display hostility in response to:

- loss of independence and freedom due to unfamiliar surroundings and people. Occasionally there is an unconscious attempt to reject the present situation
- unfamiliar activities and routines and inadequate standards of care
- separation from family, friends, familiar faces and places
- loss of home, savings, personal belongings, pets and contact with a familiar environment
- feelings similar to those of bereavement, such as anger, grief, disorientation, depression and frustration
- fear that responsibility for managing his or her own life will be lost. This can result in uncooperative behaviour
- belief that someone may make an unwarranted attack on his or her personal liberty
- change of role, for example, no longer being the breadwinner, and loss of personal faculties.

The few weeks following admission are a crucial period for those involved. Plenty of reassurance and support should help the person to accept the situation and reconcile him/her to the prospect of permanent care in an institution. During this period, he or she may become depressed and could attempt self-harm or suicide.

### *Guidance*

- maintain continuing support and discrete observation. Be aware of the client's whereabouts and use diversional therapy to divert his/her attention
- listen attentively to what he/she may say and report any remark which suggests self-harm, such as 'this is an awful place' or 'I wish I could die', to the person-in-charge.

### 2. On relatives

The family of the client may have a mixed reaction to a previous experience of admission and the current admission may induce feelings similar to those caused by bereavement. These may be:

- feelings of guilt at not caring for the client during the illness or feelings of failure due to the admission
- indifference or secret pleasure at not having to look after him or her, or relief at no longer having to bear the responsibility of the client's care
- resentment at the loss of the additional income earned by looking after the person
- stigma that admission may reflect badly on the family.

These ambivalent feelings may lead relatives and others to:
- complain about trivial or imaginary shortcomings in an attempt to demonstrate their continuing interest and support. They may feel that this attitude will reassure their relative that he/she will be properly cared for and that everything possible will be done to ensure his/her comfort and safety
- depend upon the care establishment as a source of constant reassurance that they 'did the right thing' in having their relation admitted
- blame others, including the general practitioners and community nurses, for a lack of initial information or care which they feel may have caused the illness or situation that led to the admission.

## Transfer

This usually follows a set procedure, comparable to that of admission, and requires careful preparation involving both the client and his/her family. Clients may be transferred in response to a need for investigation and treatment for the person's physical, social or psychological well-being. In all situations the person-in-charge is responsible and delegates the tasks.

### *Guidance*
- everything should be done to ensure that the client leaves the home in a happy frame of mind
- the carer's attitude to the procedures of transfer are as important as his/her attitude to admission procedures
- check personal belongings including valuables and medicines, and ensure that nothing is forgotten
- arrange an escort and transport and prepare relevant documents to accompany the client
- inform relatives as soon as possible, preferably before the transfer takes place. Ensure that information is given on the administrative situation regarding fees.

## Discharge from the home

The event should be properly planned and coordinated as many elderly people may be returning to isolation and loneliness. The care team should liaise with social services staff to ensure that adequate resources are available in the community to support and enable the individual to live as independently as possible. Planning for discharge should include asessment of specific needs, such as heating and food. Check that help is available and that drugs, exercise and medical regimes are thoroughly understood and practised before discharge. In some cases a 'discharge package' should be prepared.

## Discharge arrangements

### *Guidance*
It is important for everyone involved in care to be familiar with the organisation's policy on discharge. The policy changes from one care establishment to another, but the most important requirement is that the resident or/and his/her relatives must agree to the discharge. The health care team should be able to:
- decide when the person should be discharged and determine the date on which he/she will be returned to his/her previous address. Information about the home is essential
- consider assessment previously carried out to see if home acommodation is adequate or whether other accommodation should be arranged, eg. a warden-controlled home or another nursing home
- educate the client and consult relatives about self-care, especially self-administered medication
- make arrangement for independent living in the community and communicate with the appropriate support agencies, such as general practitioners or community nurses on the provision of an adequate rehabilitation regime
- arrange for an escort and transport to complete the discharge arrangements.

**Procedure**

The person-in-charge should organise the discharge plan ensuring that:
- special legal documents are completed in accordance with statutory requirementrs, such as the Mental Health Act 1983
- case notes, medical notes and nursing notes are completed
- personal belongings, valuables and money are collected and handed back to the client or his/her relatives
- information is given regarding help in the community with food, drugs, finance, exercise and any other facilities that are required.

Most residents in private nursing and residential care homes may not be well enough and sufficiently rehabilitated to be discharged back into the community. This should be considered as part of the admission process and forward planning of care should be initiated if necessary.

# References

Department of Health (1984) *Nursing Homes and Mental Nursing Homes Regulations*. HMSO, London

Faulkner A (1996) *Nursing. The Reflective Approach to Adult Nursing Practice,* 2nd edn. Chapman and Hall, London

Jacques I, Monkman J (1993) The right fit. *Nurs Times* 89(4): 40–42

McMahon CA (ed) (1993) *Knowledge to Care. A Handbook for Care Assistants*. Blackwell Scientific Publications, London

Savage J (1992) *Caring for People*. Macmillan Publications, Basingstoke

## Audio visual aids

### Format: VHS video

Ref: *Welcome to our Home: Admission of Patients*. The Registered Nursing Home Association

Ref: PAT 0417: *Geriatric Discharge Planning: What to Know before Leaving*

Ref: PAT 0419: *Geriatric Planning: Long-term Home Health Care*

Ref: PAT 0420: *Geriatric Discharge Planning: Rebuilding your Health*.

Ref: NT3: *Principles of Admitting Patients*

Oxford Educational Resources Ltd

# Assignment

The purpose of this homework is to assist you in preparing for your Workbased Assessment of Competence. As there no pressure on you, feel free to work at your own pace, but avoid the temptation to procrastinate. After you have read your notes and suggested references, submit your work for correction. The completed work becomes part of your Personal Portfolio.

## Admission, transfer and discharge (W3: 1–2, Y5:1–2)

1. Discuss the sources from which clients may be admitted into your care environment.
2. A new client is expected for admission when you are on duty:
   a) discuss your role in these procedures
   b) what observations and reports would you make to the person-in-charge?

3. Describe how you would prepare a client for a smooth transfer to another care environment.
4. Discuss effects of admission, transfer and discharge on clients and their relatives.
5. Discuss how you would help a newly admitted client to settle in, and assume responsibility for his or her lifestyle.

## Clients' contact with family and significant others (W2: 2–3)

In any society, the family is the basic unit. Almost every resident in nursing or residential care homes has been or is a member of a family; any change in circumstances of one member has the potential to affect other members of the family. A family is defined, in the broadest sense, as a permanent group of people who relate to each other in a meaningful way, especially by birth, and share intimate day-to-day routine living activities. Members of the family provide a network, and support one another in order to maintain a tradition of their own making. In the care setting, they are generally known as the next-of-kin, who seek to maintain a continuous and untiring interest in their relatives' welfare.

There are also other people who may show a similar interest, but relate to clients in a different way, either professionally or socially, and to whom clients would allow access in order to maintain contact while they are in care. These people are generally known as *significant others,* and may be clients' partners, friends, religious leaders, solicitors, neighbours, pets, ex-spouses and named others in the community. So, it is essential to see the residents, not as isolated individuals, but as members of a family, and explore how the family and others in such a close relationship can help in their care.

### Role of the family in care

When a client is admitted into a hospital or a long-stay care institution for treatment, the person feels isolated from loved ones and from his or her familiar environment. An attempt should be made to help the person maintain contact with members of his or her family, significant others and to maintain a link with his or her local community. This will reassure the person that everything possible is being done to put his/her mind at rest, and hasten the healing process.

### Methods of maintaining contact

There are many ways in which clients could be encouraged to maintain contact with their families and others significant to them, especially in this advanced technological age. Letter writing and telephone calls are the most common means of contact. The use of audio visual aids such as video tapes, fax, cassette tapes, computer are fast becoming popular and are being used to maintain contact. Relatives, who have to travel some distance to visit relatives in residential homes, might require travel information or details about nearby accommodation. Information about facilities in the home or a neighbouring guest house or hotel would be appreciated. Also, sending messages by word of mouth through friends and other acquaintances provides an additional means of contact.

### Visits

Several research studies have shown that clients value and always look forward to visits from their loved ones, be it in hospitals, nursing homes or prison. Visits of this nature are important because they break the monotony of seeing the same people day in and day out. Members of families should be encouraged to visit as frequently as possible, and made to feel welcome. They should be given information on the aims and philosophy of care, with an explanation as to how they can participate in the treatment and subsequent rehabilitation of their relatives. But, the most reassuring and commonly used means is personal contact through visiting.

**Benefits of visits to clients**

Visits have a therapeutic effect by providing residents in care homes with:
- relief that their relatives care for them and have their best interests at heart
- a feeling of confidence that hospitals or nursing home personnel will provide them with the best possible standards of care, because their relatives as advocates, will be seeking information to ensure that this happens, on their behalf
- information on events which allay their anxiety, especially worries relating to their homes, local community and neighbourhood
- an opportunity to talk in confidence about their feelings on personal matters, eg. finance, birth or death of close friends, progress of business interests
- emotional support and social relationships so that elderly people feel cared about rather than just cared for.

One of the most important aspects of these visits is that some clients are frequently taken out for a drive, picnic or even visit their homes in order to sustain their morale. Clients should be prepared before the arrival of their relatives for this outing, and checked for any untoward signs of distress on their return.

**Benefits to staff**

Experience has shown that staff always look forward to visiting times, especially in long-stay care environments, as the occasion provides a change for clients and staff, and forms an integral part of the rehabilitation programme. Good interpersonal relationships are established and relatives are made to feel part of the team. The outcome is that staff are provided with:
- an opportunity to develop a greater insight into their clients' personalities and characters
- information for assessment of clients' total care needs and subsequent discharge
- support through the visitors physical presence in the care environment, giving a flow of information and advice which could be shared with other members of the health care team, especially at case conferences
- a system of additional emotional support for clients
- an additional 'pair of hands' in actual caring skills, and organising and participating in social and recreational activities such as coach outings, Christmas parties, fund raising events and other forms of entertainment on behalf of the care environment for their relatives
- an opportunity to use the family as a natural support system for clients.

**Promotion of family contact**

The contact of clients with their families and those significant to them, is a very rewarding task and requires the use of good interpersonal relationships skills. Some care establishments have policy guidelines on visiting, and it is advisable to find out what these are. It is also necessary to issue instructions regarding the people likely to visit a particular client. However, the following guidelines may be useful.

> *Guidance*
> - demonstrate a knowledge of local policy and procedures for admission, assessment of individual clients' needs and implementation of care. Also, be aware of the people who may be significant to them, and be able to identify them individually

- check and report on any changes in a client's physical, social and psychological well-being which may prevent the person from receiving visitors. It may be necessary to check with the individual concerned or with the person-in-charge
- be friendly and promote effective communication with relatives or visitors. Give them time and an opportunity to discuss their feelings with you. Observe and report any difficulties or lack of support in their relationship to the person-in-charge
- encourage families, visitors or friends to participate in an individual client's care plan
- observe and report any signs of abuse or neglect of clients at risk during and after visits
- be aware of your local policy and procedures for managing stressful situations which may be encountered in your work. Also be aware of personal relationship problems and ways of coping with stress or distress associated with caring for clients
- be aware of sources of support from outside for individuals — self-support groups and relief agencies, such as MIND, Age Concern, Help the Aged
- be aware of organisational policy and procedures for reporting complaints, and of facilities available to visitors, eg. accommodation, and be able to explain ways of obtaining help for them. It is important to inform the person-in-charge of a need for these additional facilities
- pass on any messages received on behalf of a client promptly and maintain any confidentiality of information as may be necessary
- know that some clients have personal attachment with a few selected people or toys as part of their emotional development. This is known as affectionate bonding and any attempt to interfere with this relationship may lead to problems. Always check with the person-in-charge if you have any doubts about any visitor.

# References

Irvine RE *et al* (1986) *The Older Patient. An Introduction to Geriatric Nursing, Families and Carers.* Hodder and Stoughton, London: ch 5

McMahon CA, Harding J (1994) *Knowledge to Care. A Handbook for Care Assistants.* Blackwell Scientific Publications, London

**Audio visual aid**

*Format: VHS video*
Ref: NCE 7628: *Ageing Population: Caring for the Family*
Oxford Educational Resources Ltd

# Assignment

The purpose of this homework is to assist you in preparing for your Workbased Assessment of Competence. As there is no pressure on you, feel free to work at your own pace, but avoid the temptation to procrastinate. After you have read your notes and suggested references, submit your work for correction. The completed work becomes part of your Personal Portfolio

## Clients contact with family and significant others (W2: 2–3)

1. Discuss the role of families in a client's care.
2. List individuals who may be significant to clients and their role in his or her care.

3. Discuss the advantages that the family and significant others could make to the care programme regarding:
   a) the clients
   b) staff
   c) care environment.
4. A man who claims to be a nephew of a confused elderly resident, telephoned and arranged with you to take his aunt out for the day:
   a) how would you establish his relationship with the resident?
   b) describe how you would prepare the elderly person for this outing.
   c) state briefly what observations you would make and report on the resident's return from the outing.
5. Discuss how you would help an active elderly person to maintain contact with a member of his or her family.

# Unit 6
# Promote communication in care through physical contact (CL2, CL6, S11)

## Clients with sensory deprivation (CL2: 1–2, CL6: 1–2, S11: 1–3)

As people grow older, they may experience sensory loss caused either by accident or the normal ageing process. This may affect their ability to live independently and cause some of them to depend on other people for help. Some elderly people live alone in their own homes, some with relatives, and others are in nursing or residential care homes. Because of their sensory deprivation, they may become dependent on others and could be isolated through a lack of ability to communicate their needs. This could, in turn, lead to marginalisation and institutionalisation.

Therefore, this section aims to examine clients with deafness (loss of hearing) and blindness (loss of vision), and the ways in which their needs could be met. We start with the basic anatomy of the organs of the ear and eye.

## Hearing loss

### The ear

The ear is the organ of hearing, and contains tiny bones and membranes which are sensitive to sound and vibration. It is divided into three parts:

1. External ear — this consists of pinna (auricle) and the external acoustic meatus or auditory canal.
2. Middle ear — an irregularly shaped and air-filled cavity in the skull. It is linked with the back of the nasal cavity by the auditory tube (eustachian tube). Three small bones in the middle ear malleus, incus and stapes link the ear drum to a small opening in the skull which leads to the inner ear.
   The eustachian tube is an air passage in which pressure is usually the same as atmospheric pressure. It is normally closed, and only opens when swallowing or yawning. If changes take place in the pressure outside the ear drum, eg. in an aircraft, the pressure is equalised by the opening of the eustachian tube to admit more air or release air from the middle ear.
3. Inner ear — this is filled with a fluid (perilymph) and contains a coiled tube, the cochlea. This is where we find the nerve endings. It is here that the sound vibrations are changed to nervous impulses.

**Functions of the ear** — to maintain normal posture and balance.

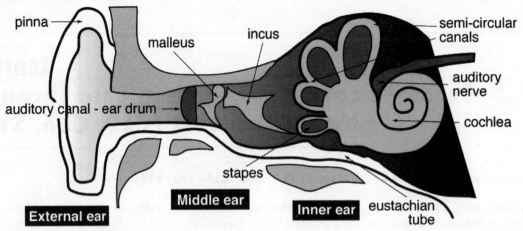

A simple diagram of the ear

# Deafness

Deafness is the inability to hear, due to sound waves failing to reach the part of the ear (cochlea) responsible for receiving and conducting messages to the brain. People with hearing difficulties are predisposed to stress and anxiety, especially if they are in hospital or a nursing home which is not their usual and familiar environment.

## Causes of deafness

These vary widely from conditions existing before or at birth (congenital) to psychological causes such as hysteria, illness or trauma.

## Forms of deafness

There are many forms. A person may be entirely without hearing, or partially deaf, or simply hard of hearing, but the common forms are:

### Pre-lingually deaf
This relates to people who have been deaf since birth, or early childhood, before the progress of normal speech and language. They communicate by lip reading or sign language.

### Post-lingually deaf
The problem occurs after normal speech and language have developed. Hearing aids and lip reading are the means of communication.

### Hard of hearing people
Clients are partially deaf but they are still able to communicate verbally to a certain extent with the help of hearing aids and lip reading. Communication with them will be based on their individual care plan.

> *Guidance*
> - develop and maintain a good relationship with the individual, based on a knowledge and understanding of the problems of deafness
> - follow guidelines towards promoting effective communication (*Unit 2*)

- know the means of communication or language that the person understands, eg. lip reading, symbols, written or sign language
- ensure that the environment is free from distractions — switch off noisy fans and turn off the radio or television
- look directly at the person with a warm welcoming facial expression – try to use gestures
- communicate with the person frequently through his or her own system of communication, eg. lip reading and sign language. Use the following approach:
  - face the light and let the person see your facial expressions. Do not smoke or eat
  - let the person understand you and do not put your hand over your mouth
  - speak at face level, so that the client can see movements of your lips and facial expression
  - touch the individual's hand to gain his or her attention if necessary
  - listen attentively to what he/she is saying and allow time to think and reply
  - speak slowly and distinctly; do not shout or raise your voice because those who are hard of hearing cannot hear high-pitched voices
  - check if the person uses a hearing aid; make sure that it is switched on and is working properly. Make sure he or she knows how to switch it off when not in use, and when and how to change the batteries
  - use non-verbal gestures in order to be more expressive in your communication
  - help the person to learn sign language and to lip read if attending a class
  - provide him or her with writing materials in order to assist communication if necessary
  - ensure that special picture cards depicting, for example, a toilet, drink, TV, bed or radio are available for the person's use, should the need arise
  - thank the person for his or her time at the end of the conversation.

## *Profoundly deaf*

These people have difficulty in coping with the written language and spoken words. They communicate through finger spelling where various positions of the fingers indicate the letters of the alphabet, and by signing which is a system of gestures and mime. They have specially trained dogs to attract their attention if the door bell rings.

## Management of problem

### *1. Assessment*

The purpose is to identify specific problems that the person may present, such as his or her lifestyle, pattern, and degree of deafness. A client may present any or all of the following problems at any stage and in any combination:
- language limitation and difficulty in understanding unfamiliar voices
- limited or no knowledge of communication aids, and difficulty in learning how to use a hearing aid or lip read
- isolation, because of lack of a means of communication
- suspicious attitude; believing that others are talking about him/her
- changes in normal speaking voice — he/she may shout without realising it
- restlessness and confusion.

### *2. Implementation of care*

Individual care plans will provide information on the management of the specific problems identified.

#### *Guidance*
- develop and maintain good relationships with patients, based on a knowledge and understanding of the problems of deafness

- know the means of communication or the language the patient understands and follow guidance on how to promote effective communication
- ensure that the hearing aid is in good working order and worn in the correct ear
- wax should be softened and removed
- encourage the person to use his or her own initiative and ability, however limited, to do things, to express ideas, opinions and take an interest in new experiences, such as in recreational and social activities: art work, drawing, sketches, bus-trips into the countryside
- ensure that the environment is free from distractions; during communication a special hearing and speech amplifier may be used
- give the patient time to answer and repeat what is said when necessary to ensure understanding
- participate in any training classes for communication with the deaf and blind.

It is important to get patients to do something no matter how small, as it gives them a sense of achievement and satisfaction. Always praise their effort.

## Evaluation of care

Evaluate the client's care when he or she is able to communicate effectively with others, taking into account the degree of disability. It must be remembered that deafness can be worse for people living in isolation.

## Hearing aids

There are many types of aids on the market; the NHS has about 15. As a result of technological advancement, some hearing aids can bring hearing by remote control; and most people use special 'environmental aids' to help them hear some sounds, eg. radio, telephone, television. This equipment is designed with special devices to amplify the sound in association with the hearing aids.

### *Care of the hearing aid*

The general principle of care is to be familiar with the hearing aid your clients uses and always follow the manufacturer's recommendations for use and care.

### *Guidance*

#### 1. *Always keep the hearing aid dry*
- remove before bathing, showering or swimming
- dry it with a soft cloth if it accidentally gets wet: NEVER use heat to dry it or allow it to come in contact with water
- help the individual to turn it off when not in use
- check that the battery is working before connecting the hearing aid to the client's correct ear
- remove the battery if the hearing aid will not be used for more than 24 hours.

#### 2. *Keep the hearing aid clean:*
- never use water, alcohol or a cleaning solvent
- detach ear mould from the aid
- wash the ear mould in warm soapy water
- remove any wax with a pin
- rinse in clean water, shake or blow through the tubing to remove drops of water
- make sure that the ear mould is always free from ear wax.

#### 3. *Storing the hearing aid:*
- ensure that it is marked with the owner's name
- store in its special case.

## Troubleshooting

| Problem | Possible cause | Action |
|---|---|---|
| Does not work | Not properly worn<br>Faulty amplifier or battery<br>Ear mould is plugged with ear wax<br>Not switched on or being worn in the wrong ear | Check off and on switch<br>Check or replace battery<br>Clean ear mould<br>Ensure that it is correctly worn and in the right ear |
| Faint or inaudible sound | Battery is low<br>Ear mould plugged with ear wax<br>Change in degree of hearing<br>The cord cracks or splits or twists<br>Volume is incorrectly adjusted | Check volume control<br>Teach client to turn off aid when not in use<br>Replace battery<br>Clean ear mould<br>Report for degree of hearing to be checked |
| Hearing aid 'whistles' and reverberates | Volume is set to high<br>Poor fitting<br>Obstruction by ear wax<br>Holes in the tube | Replace battery<br>Check obstruction<br>Report and send for repair or replacement |
| Complaint of pain and discomfort | Ear mould incorrectly fitted<br>Friction with spectacles if client wears both hearing aid and spectacles at the same time | Gently remove, check and reinsert the ear mold<br>Advise client to put the hearing aid on first<br>Report to supplier if problem persists |

## References

Flack M, Johnston M (1986) *Handbook for Care: Patients with Impaired Senses*. Beaconsfield Publishers Ltd, Bucks: 23–25

Nieuwenhuis R (1986) Breaking the speech barrier. *Nurs Times* **85**(15): 34–36

Robertson B (1992) *Study Guide for Health and Social Care Support Workers. NVQ in Care Level 2*. First Class Books Inc, USA

Robertson I (1986) Learned helplessness. *Nurs Times* **82**(51): 28–30

Roper N *et al* (1987) *The Elements of Nursing: Communication, Hearing and Seeing Problem*. Churchill Livingstone, Edinburgh:130

Tolson D (1991) Hearing aids. *Nurs Times* **87**(18): 36–38

## Audio visual aids

### Format: VHS video
Ref: CNE 4294: *Communication Strategies for Alzheimer's Patients*

Ref: CNE WA22: *Caring for the Hearing Impaired People*

Ref: 367C: *Hearing Loss in Residential Care*

Ref: CEAU237: *Communication Problems in the Elderly*

Oxford Educational Resources Ltd

# Assignment

The purpose of this homework is to assist you in preparing for your Workbased Assessment of Competence. As there is no pressure on you, feel free to work at your own pace, but avoid the temptation to procrastinate. After you have read your notes and suggested references, submit your work for correction. The completed work becomes part of your Personal Portfolio.

## Hearing loss (CL2: 1–2, CL6.1, S11: 1–3)

1. What do you understand by 'partially deaf and profoundly deaf'?
2. Draw and label a simple diagram of the ear, and list its functions.
3. Discuss how you would promote effective communication with a client who is profoundly deaf.
4. Describe what actions you would take to make the care environment safe for the people who are profoundly deaf and blind.

## Visually impaired people (CL2: 1–2, CL6.1, S11: 1–3)

People who lose their sense of sight move from a world of light and colour to a world of perpetual darkness. They usually feel isolated as they cannot see their surroundings or the person to whom they are speaking, and all visual means of communication are lost. Although losing the sense of sight, other senses such as smell, touch and hearing may be enhanced which may contribute to their ability to communicate.

Blind people are inclined to feel anxiety, stress and isolation in unfamiliar surroundings. They communicate by speech and touch, and feel their way around. Therefore, it is essential that their surroundings should not be changed so that they may feel safe, comfortable and reassured. People with visual handicap communicate by using the following methods:

- braille and moon type, which is a system of raised dots or lines, representing the letters of the alphabet, read by passing the tips of the fingers over them
- talking books, newspapers and magazines
- cassette tapes recording letters from relatives and friends.

### *Guidance*

- use basic caring skills to develop and maintain good interpersonal relationships. Act as the person's advocate
- follow guidelines on how to promote effective communication, and encourage the use of speech
- treat the person normally and never be patronising in your questions and answers
- avoid startling him or her, and always speak before reaching the individual
- introduce yourself to the person so that he or she learns to recognise your voice. Tell the person his or her whereabouts and the whereabouts of others present, if necessary:
  - always explain fully anything you want to do, and seek the person's co-operation
  - take care of his or her spectacles, making sure that they are:
  - worn as prescribed, clean and in good repair
  - stored in their case when not in use to avoid damage
  - they are reviewed by an optician every two years, or whenever necessary
  - mark the spectacles with the individual's name to prevent loss

- make sure that you understand the method of communication the person uses, such as braille, moon, talking books, cassette tape recording messages
- thank the person for his or her time at the end of conversation.

## Blindness

Blindness is defined as the deprivation of sight in one or both eyes, and may be temporary or permanent.

## Causes of blindness

There are many causes of blindness, varying from conditions that exist before birth (congenital), illness, injury to psychological causes such as hysterical blindness.

## The eye

The eye is the organ of sight situated in the eye socket in the skull, and is supplied by the optic nerve. It is almost spherical in shape, well-protected by bony walls except for the anterior aspect and at the back by fat to help protect the eye from injury.

Structurally, there are three layers of tissue in the walls of the eye. They are:

1. **Sclera** — a tough outer fibrous layer which maintains the shape of the eye.
2. **Choroid** — a layer of tissue lining the inside of the sclera, containing a network of blood vessels supplying food to the eye, particularly, retina cells.
3. **Retina** — a sensitive layer of cells which respond to light. It is the 'film' in the camera of the eye. Similar to the lens in a camera.

    **Lens** — an elastic circular biconvex transparent film which lies behind the pupil. It tends to change its shape, becoming thicker in the centre. Cataract is opacity of the lens.

    **Aqueous humour** — the fluid which fills the inside chamber and keeps the shape of the eye. An increase in the pressure of this fluid causes a condition known as glaucoma.

### Accessory organs of the eye:
- the eyelids are covers of skin above and below each eye which close freely or by a reflex action when we blink to protect the eyeballs from injury
- the conjunctiva is a fine transparent membrane which covers the eyeball
- the lachrymal glands produce tears which lubricate the eye.

### Functions of the eye

These are complex as different parts of the eye carry out different duties aimed at bringing about and protecting the mechanism of vision, for example:
- tears keep the eyes moist because moisture exudes from the lachrymal glands in the corner of the eye socket and the eyelids disperse the moisture around the eye
- the lens allows light rays to enter the eye from an object, focusing them on the retina
- the retina receives light rays from the lens and sends them through the optic nerve to the brain.

## Types of blindness

### Partial sight

There is no legal definition for partial sight. Guidelines state that the person is substantially and permanently handicapped by defective vision but has enough vision to read large print and move around without additional aids.

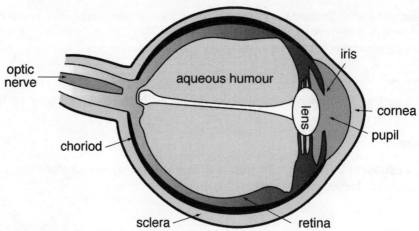

A simple diagram of the eye

### Remedy

Low vision aids, eg. binoculars for watching TV, spectacles for reading large print books, various aids to daily living, eg. speaking clock or watch, enlarged telephone dials, mobility aids, enlarged games and puzzles.

### Retraining

People whose visual acuity has deteriorated and can no longer continue in their employment may benefit from retraining. Training in a more appropriate occupation can be offered to suitable candidates by the Royal National Institute for the Blind at their training centre in Torquay.

The RNIB provides various services to support the education of visually-impaired children and young people, such as closed circuit TV.

### Blind

The person has no vision at all in either eye.

### Remedy

- teach the use of braille and moon type, which is a system of raised dots or lines, representing the letters of the alphabet, read by passing the tips of the fingers over them
- use talking books, newspapers and magazines
- listen to cassette tapes recording letters from relatives and friends
- provide guide dogs.

## Registration of a blind person

People with visual impairment will be assessed and certified by a consultant ophthalmologist who may recommend full registration as blind, or as partially sighted with the social services department. Registration entitles blind people to financial benefits, such as tax relief and aids to daily living supplied by social services.

For registration purposes, blindness is judged by the degree of visual acuity on the Snellen scale. Visual acuity is the best direct vision that can be obtained with appropriate spectacle correction as necessary, according to the Snellen scale. A person does not have to be totally without vision, but may be able to distinguish light from darkness, and to count fingers.

## Deaf and blind people

A few unfortunate people are both deaf and blind; a double barrier to communication. They may become isolated and their life can become a silent, dark world. They have no means of communication until someone takes their hands and makes contact with them by touch.

It is important to encourage the deaf-blind to use his or her own initiative in seeking and developing interests and new experience. Finger spelling may be the only method by which they can communicate.

Individuals often develop enhanced memory and other senses to compensate for loss of vision and hearing. They learn to find their way around and identify objects by touch. One of the most important duties of a carer is to take all reasonable steps to prevent clients from coming to any harm, ensuring that the environment is safe. Never leave the deaf-blind person in unfamiliar surroundings and make sure he/she knows you are leaving the room, even if it is only for a short period.

## Management of care

### *Assessment*

This is the collection of relevant information to establish what is the normal pattern of the person's life and to identify specific care needs. The assessment should address all aspects of care including risk-taking and the procedures it is necessary to follow. These should include:

- promoting self-confidence and encouraging mobility
- providing a safe environment with good lighting and keeping corridors free of obstacles
- making sure that doorways are free from potential hazards
- maintaining contact with the environment
- risk-taking and encouraging the independence of the individual.

## Implementation of care

Management is based on an individual client's care plan.

### *General guidance*
- explain the daily routine to the individual and his or her family and visitors, providing constant updates on what is taking place
- make sure that the person knows the times of meals and set his or her tray or place at the dining table in the same way for each meal
- leave drinks near the client, but warn him or her that you are doing so
- lay the person's clothes out in the same order every time he or she dresses
- ensure that the individual knows where all his or her personal possessions are and never move them
- escort the person by letting him or her take your arm and walk together
- arrange simple signals to indicate steps, stairs, pavements, obstacles
- indicate seating by placing the individual's hand on the back of the chair
- provide a walking aid if the person is unsteady on his or her feet
- always seek the client's permission to open and read his or her mail or put it on a tape cassette
- ensure that the person can always locate and use the emergency call bell system; quite often a portable one on a neck chain is used
- encourage individuals to participate in special card games, which are available for visually-impaired people
- assist the person to maintain contact with his or her environment through sound, eg. radio, tape cassettes

- the most important aspects of care include the promotion and maintenance of a safe environment, independence, self-respect and dignity of individual clients, and the prevention of loneliness which may be the result of the client feeling isolated
- encourage the individual to use speech and to express his or her wishes, ideas, feelings and lessen the likelihood of his/her speech becoming unintelligible.

## Evaluation of care

Evaluation can take place when a client is able to live independently with his or her disability, with little need for intervention and prompting by caring staff and relatives.

## Care of spectacles and prosthesis (artificial eyes)

### Spectacles

These are often mislaid and easily broken. Clients should be encouraged to wear their spectacles when they need them. They should be:
- engraved with the owner's name on the inside of the frame
- stored in the case when not in use
- cleaned with a soft cloth rather than with tissue paper
- checked for loose screws or broken frames.

### Artificial eyes

These are usually cared for by qualified nurses, but health care assistants may be instructed and supervised. The following procedures should be observed:
- follow the manufacturer's guidance and recommendations
- wash hands before handling the eye
- handle carefully to prevent scratching
- clean the eye over a sink or basin of warm water
- wet the eye under warm running water
- rub the eye gently with clean, sterile gauze
- rinse the eye under warm running water.

## Staff training

The RNIB can arrange courses for deaf-blind people to communicate with others. Workshops can be arranged for staff who work with visually-impaired children

# References

BBC (1995) *A Word of Difference. Straight Talk on Disability from BBC Radio.* Benefits agency, London.

Department of Health and Social Security (1990) *Social Security Benefits: A Guide for Blind and Partially Sighted People.* DHSS, London

Flack M, Johnston M (1986) *Handbook for Care. Patients with Impaired Senses.* Beaconsfield Publishers Ltd, Bucks

Roper N et al (1987) *The Elements of Nursing Communication:. Hearing and Seeing Problems.* Churchill Livingstone, Edinburgh.

Royal National Institute for the Blind (1994) *Education Support Services.* RNIB, London.

Royal National Institute for the Blind (1993) *Getting in Touch with Blind People.* RNIB, London

Royal National Institute for the Blind (1993) *Your Guide to RNIB for Visually Impaired People.* RNIB, London

## Audio visual aids

*Format: VHS video*

Ref: 344/2CT: *The Visually Handicapped : Part 2 — The Advancing Years*
Oxford Educational Resources Ltd
Ref: PR 10186: *Hearing is Seeing (audio description for visually impaired theatre-goers)*
Ref: CINEXSA: *Sight by Touch*
Ref: PR 10208 *Anna's Story*
Ref: PR 10590 *Taking the Plunge*
Royal National Institute for the Blind, London

## Assignment

The purpose of this homework is to assist you in preparing for your Workbased Assessment of Competence. As there is no pressure on you, feel free to work at your own pace, but avoid the temptation to procrastinate. After you have read your notes and suggested references, submit your work for correction. The completed work becomes part of your Personal Portfolio.

## Visually-impaired people (blindness) (CL2: 1–2, CL6.1, S11: 1–3)

1. Define the terms blindness and differentiate between 'partially sighted and blind people'.
2. Draw and label a simple diagram of the eye and list three of its functions.
3. Discuss how you would promote the independence of a visually-impaired elderly lady in your area of work, in relation to:
   a) personal cleanliness and grooming
   b) nutritional intake of nourishment
   c) recreational and social activity.
4. Discuss how you would promote effective communication with someone who is deaf and blind.

## People with dysarthria, aphasia and mental problems (CL1.1)

There may be some residents with speech difficulties, although they understand and know what they want to say. There is no disruption of reading and writing skills and they may have good eyesight. This condition is known as dysarthria.

### Guidance
- develop and maintain good interpersonal relationships
- ensure that the environment is free from distractions, eg. noise from radio, television
- ensure that the person is comfortable
- introduce the topic by 'breaking the ice', ie. talk about the weather
- speak slowly by using short sentences and smile occasionally
- do not rush or ramble as this could be confusing for the listener
- be a good listener; avoid criticising and using jargon
- be aware of your body language. Show interest, use a friendly tone and be positive
- be patient and introduce a sense of humour, occasionally
- use touch and eye contact but do not stare at the person, pace your talk

- ask questions, allow time to speak and listen attentively for **feedback**
- watch for gesture and facial expression
- clarify and check for understanding and show respect
- conclude the conversation by thanking the person for his or her time.

## Aphasia

This is a loss of the ability to speak or understand words.

### *Guidance*
- be patient with people suffering from this condition
- use communication aids, eg. pictures, pen and paper
- eliminate unnecessary noises, eg. television, radio
- speak slowly and allow time for the person to respond
- be supportive and talk normally, do not 'talk down' or shout
- ask the person to repeat if necessary rather than pretend that you understood what he/she said
- thank the person for his or her time at the end of the conversation.

## Mental health problems

Conversation with people suffering from depression, confusion or Alzheimer's disease can be very difficult and frustrating, especially if the patient is suffering from delusions, hallucinations and behavioural problems. The person may not at times be able to make reasonable responses and, if he or she does, they may be incoherent. It does not mean that the person does not hear or understand what you are saying.

### *Guidance*
Follow the guidance given in *Unit 19*, the 'Care and treatment of delusion and hallucinations'.

# References

BBC (1995) *A Word of Difference. Straight Talk on Disability from BBC Radio*. Benefits Agency, London

Hewitt FS (1981) The nurse and the patient, communication skills. Part 1 — getting it across. *Nurs Times*, Occasional paper: 25–28

Kershaw B et al (1989) *Helping to Care. A Handbook for Carers at Home and in Hospital*. Bailliere Tindall, London

Royal National Institute for the Blind (1993) *Your Guide to RNIB for Visually Impaired People*. RNIB, London

Royal National Institute for the Blind (1985) *Getting in Touch with Blind People*. RNIB, London

## Audio visual aids

### *Format: VHS video*
Ref: CINEXSA: *Sight by Touch*
Royal National Institute for the Blind
Ref: CNEUA 22: *Caring for the Hearing Impaired Patient*
Ref: CEAU 237: *Communication Problems in the Elderly 222*
Ref: CNE 4294: *Communication Strategies for Alzheimer's Patients*
Ref: 344/2CT: *Communication: Visually Handicapped* (tape cassette slides)
Oxford Educational Resources Ltd

# Assignment

The purpose of this homework is to assist you in preparing for your Workbased Assessment of Competence. As there is no pressure on you, feel free to work at your own pace, but avoid the temptation to procrastinate. After you have read your notes and suggested references, submit your work for correction. The completed work becomes part of your Personal Portfolio.

## Communication: clients with sensory deprivation (CL2, CL6.1, S11: 1–3)

1. Explain a range of techniques which could be used to communicate with:
   a) partially sighted people
   b) people who are hard of hearing
   c) people without sight and hearing (deaf/blind)
   d) a distressed person.
2. Conduct a small survey of clients with sensory impairment (registered or not) in your care area and discuss the outcome with the matron or person-in-charge.

# Unit 7
# Enable clients to achieve physical comfort (Z19)

## Nature and purpose of breathing (Z19: 1–2)

Breathing is one of the activities of daily living which takes place in the lungs. The respiratory system allows oxygen (O) to be taken into the blood and carbon dioxide ($CO_2$) to be removed. When we breath (inspiration), oxygen is taken in from the atmosphere through the nose, pharynx, larynx, trachea, bronchi, bronchioles and alveoli into the blood, and when we breath out (expiration), carbon dioxide is expelled from the lungs into outside air. The heart pumps the blood carrying the oxygen oxygen to tissues of the body, providing energy and helping the body to work properly. The organs of the respiratory system are:

### 1. The nose
The organ of smell and the first of the respiratory passages through which the incoming air passes. It is made up of cavities which are separated into right and left portions by the septum. The cavities are lined with numerous cilia-hair-like projections that flick to and fro. The main function of the nose is to warm, moisten and filter dust from the air before it reaches the lungs.

### 2. The pharynx
This is about 12 cm long and extends from the base of the skull to the sixth cervical vertebrae, and lies behind the nose, larynx and mouth. On its walls are the openings of the auditory tubes by which it is connected to the middle ear.

### 3. The larynx
This is situated in the front of the neck above the trachea. It grows larger in the male and is known as the 'Adam's apple', and has the special function of voice production. Two vocal cords lie across the larynx, and when air is passed over them in a certain way, they vibrate, and produce sound.

### 4. The trachea
A muscular tube about 10 to 11 cm long, generally known as the 'windpipe', this lies mainly in front of the oesophagus, and conveys air to and from the lungs. It is kept open by about 16 to 20 'C' shaped incomplete rings of cartilage at the back, and allows the tube to dilate during swallowing. It starts from the neck and divides into two — the left and the right bronchi, one for each lung.

### 5. The bronchi
The bronchi subdivide into smaller air passages, known as bronchioles. The bronchioles progressively divide and finally end as alveoli — a bunch of grapes. The walls of alveoli consist of a single layer of flattened cells where the exchange of gases for internal respiration takes place.

### 6. The lungs
These are inflatable thin-walled elastic sacs, pinkish in colour lying in the thorax. They are wrapped by a serous membrane called the pleura.

### 7. Diaphragm

This is a dome-shaped organ which separates the chest wall from the abdominal cavity. It forms the floor of the thoracic cavity and the roof of the abdominal cavity, and is attached to the lower ribs and the sternum.

### 8. Intercostal muscles

There are 11 pairs of intercostal muscles occupying the spaces between the 12 pairs of ribs. Because the first rib is fixed, when intercostal muscles contract, they pull all other ribs towards them, and they all move outwards when pulled upwards. In this way the chest cavity is enlarged.

### The act of respiration

The process relates to expansion and contraction of the lungs, and involves the main muscles of respiration which are intercostal muscles and the diaphragm. When at rest, the diaphragm is dome-shaped. During inspiration or breathing in, the chest walls expand by upward movement of the ribs, the intercostal muscles contract, and the diaphragm becomes flattened, to ensure the expansion of the chest. Air is then sucked into the lungs.

During breathing out or expiration, the diaphragm and intercostal muscles relax, and so expel the air, and the chest wall returns to its resting position. After expiration there is a pause before the next cycle begins. Deep breathing involves using the muscles of the neck, shoulders and abdomen.

### Respiratory rate

The lungs and air passages are never empty, and the exchange of gases continuously takes place. In normal breathing there are about 16 complete respiratory cycles per minute. These consist of three phases: inspiration, expiration and pause.

The respiration rate is counted after the cycle of inspiration and expiration is complete, ie. one breath in and one breath out equals one respiration. Respiration can be counted by observing the rise and fall of the chest wall over a given period of time (see measuring TPR).

### *Factors influencing respiratory rate*

The average adult respiration rate is between 16 and 20 breaths per minute and this may be influenced by:
- age (faster in an infant, up to 44 reparations per minute)
- exercise, because the muscles require more oxygen
- eating, speaking, laughing and coughing may cause minor variations
- diseases of the respiratory tract, eg. bronchitis, pneumonia, asthma, tuberculosis and allergic conditions
- smoking and chemical agents, eg. drugs
- obstruction of respiratory passages eg. foreign bodies, growth
- psychological reactions, eg. anxiety, fear, changes in mood.

### Discomforts associated with breathing

Breathing takes place instinctively unless an abnormality interferes with the process. This may be a blocked nose or a slight chest pain which becomes progressively uncomfortable so that eventually we seek help. Elderly people may experience problems and should be assessed. The assessment may identify some of the following problems:

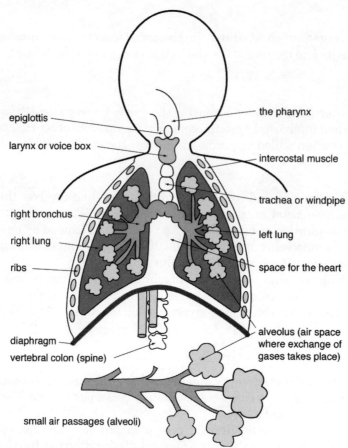

**A simple diagram showing the anatomy of the respiratory system**

## Cough

This is a voluntary expulsion of air from the lungs with the intention of expelling a foreign body or excessive mucus from the air passages. A cough may be productive with phlegm, mucus or sputum, or unproductive; dry and at times irritating.

**Intervention:** This will be based on the individual client's care plan.

### Guidance
- develop and maintain a good interpersonal relationship with the person
- observe and report chest pains, their frequency, the length and time a cough may last, nature of the cough, eg. dry and irritating at first and later with sputum
- find out the time when coughing is severe, eg. early in the morning
- encourage the client to sit up with a back rest and pillows. Observe and report on shortness of breath
- encourage the client to express his or her feelings and reassure any anxiety
- offer water or other refreshing fluid to sip in order to prevent dehydration
- provide a sputum mug and disposable tissues, and encourage him or her to cough and expectorate into the sputum mug
- support the client by the side of the chest and encourage him or her to cough and expectorate
- examine the sputum for any abnormalities, such as blood (haemoptysis)

- encourage good personal hygiene by offering handwashing facilities
- maintain a four-hourly temperature, pulse and respiration chart; manage care of pressure areas if the person is being cared for in bed or sitting up in a chair for a long time.

**Other treatments:**
- productive cough may need the help of a physiotherapist and a specimen should be sent to laboratory for investigations
- suggest that the client cuts down or stops smoking if he or she is a smoker and give health education information
- a drug may be prescribed to liquefy sputum if there is a respiratory infection.

## Sore throat

This is inflammation of the larynx or pharynx. A cough may also be present and troublesome.

*Intervention:* This will be based on the individual client's care plan.

### Guidance
- provide the client with help (*see Coughing*)
- provide a sputum mug, tissues and a disposable bag, if a cough is present
- offer a mouthwash, gargle and soothing drinks
- follow the care plan and intervention for cough.

## Nasal congestion (catarrh)

This is a simple inflammation of the mucus membrane accompanied by excessive secretion of mucus. It is usually a chronic condition of the nasopharynx or nose and may be caused by blocked sinuses.

*Intervention:* This will be based on the individual client's care plan.

### Guidance
- make the client comfortable in an upright position, either sitting up in a chair or in bed, with extra pillows
- provide a sputum mug in case a cough is present together with adequate disposable tissues and bags. Persuade the person to cough and spit out into the sputum mug
- offer liberal drinks and allow the person to rest
- be aware of the need for good personal hygiene.

## Dyspnoea

This is laboured breathing accompanied by pain and difficulty in inhaling and expelling air.

*Intervention:* This will be based on the individual client's care plan.

### Guidance
- promote good rapport with the client
- nurse the client in the most comfortable position for him/her, either upright in bed or sitting in a chair
- place a pillow on the bed table; ask the person to lean forward and use it as a support
- offer and encourage the client to eat small amounts of light nourishing meals.

## Chest pain

This is the body's way of indicating that something is wrong. It is a warning sign and may be accompanied by:
- shallow respiration, slow and difficult movement, restlessness

- adoption of an abnormal position, eg. gripping the painful area.

*Intervention:* This will be based on the individual client's care plan.

### Guidance
- talk to the person and encourage him or her to locate the pain and report your observations to the person-in-charge
- assist the client to change position and provide something to divert his or her attention, eg. music
- remain with the client and gently rub the area of pain. Encourage relaxation
- follow guidance on the coughing care plan.

### Choking and cessation of breathing

This situation may be the result of a foreign body obstructing the air passages. It is a medical emergency situation which requires immediate attention (see *Health, safety and security in the workplace: other emergencies* [CU1: 1–3]).

*Intervention:* This involves following an immediate action plan.

### Guidance
- stay calm; reassure and encourage the person to relax
- summon help immediately by calling loudly or ask someone to ring the alarm bell
- be aware of procedures relating to cardiac arrest and resuscitation
- encourage the client to lean forward and try to remove any visible obstruction from the back of the mouth
- remain with and reassure the casualty until further help arrives.

### Smoking

There is little doubt that smoking has harmful effects on health. It is reported that about 100,000 people die every year in England and Wales from smoking-related diseases, such as lung cancer and heart disease.

*Aim:* To encourage and enable the client to stop or reduce smoking.

### Guidance
- demonstrate understanding of the organisation's policy on smoking in authorised areas
- set a good example by refraining from smoking
- never permit smoking where oxygen is in use
- give health education information pointing out the adverse effects of smoking on health.

### Respiratory infection

This may include diseases of the lungs such as pneumonia, emphysema, tuberculosis, and lung abscess. The care and management of problems will be directed by the qualified person in charge (the team leader).

*Aim:* To treat the infection.

*Intervention:* This is based on the individual client's care plan.

### Guidance
- demonstrate an understanding of the organisational policy on infection control, such as isolation, good handwashing technique (see *Unit 3(b), Assist in the control of infection*)
- investigations, such as chest X-ray and examination of sputum specimens may be carried out.

## Administration of inhalations

Inhalations are gases, vapours and fumes of drugs used to produce an effect on the upper respiratory passages. Certain drugs, eg. eucalyptus oil, menthol, Friars Balsam (tincture of benzion) are sometimes administered in inhalation. There are various types of inhalations but the most commonly used are:

### 1. Oxygen

When oxygen therapy is prescribed, it will be administered and monitored by qualified staff. It may be administered by masks, such as ventimask or nasal cannula, tents and ventilators. The mouth and nose can become dry and drinking fluids is encouraged. Mouth care is maintained and ice may be given to suck. It is important to remember that there is increased fire risk when oxygen is being administered to clients. The following precautions should be taken:
- there should be no smoking or naked flame permitted
- no mechanical toys should be permitted
- no electric bells, razor or heating pads should be used.

### 2. Steam inhalations

Some drugs may be used for the relief of nasal congestion and purulent bronchitis. These are usually combined with hot water and the vapour inhaled by the client. Those which vaporise easily should be put into water not exceeding 50° C (120°F). Those which vaporise less readily may be placed in the receptacle first and have hot water poured over them

*Intervention:* This will be based on the individual clients' care plan.

### *Guidance*
- use the recommended inhaler. If earthenware Nelson's inhaler is used, half fill it with boiling water
- add the prescribed amount of menthol or Friars Balsam
- cover the mouthpiece with a gauze swab
- place the inhaler in a bowl covered over with a flannel and sit the client upright
- help the client to put his or her lips to the mouthpiece and advise to breath in through the mouth and out through the nose
- remain with the person to ensure safety and a proper use of the inhaler
- report any observations and the client's evaluation to the nurse-in-charge.

## References

Andrews C, Smith J (1992) *Medical Nursing*. NAS. Bailliere Tindall, London

Lim D (1982) Clearing the air. *Nurs Times* **78**(10): 256–257

Roberts A, Gardiner P (1991) Systems of life. The respiratory system Part 1. *Nurs Times* **87**(2): 53–56

Knepi J (1983) The control of breathing. *Nurs Mirror* May 11: 44–45

Wilson JW (1987) *Anatomy and Physiology in Health and Illness,* 6th edn. Churchill Livingstone, Edinburgh

## Audio visual aids

### *Format: VHS video*

Ref: CEAUA797: *EMS Vitals: Respiratory Problems* (VHS video)

Ref: CEAUA799: *EMS Vitals: Breathing Aids* (VHS video)

Oxford Educational Resources Ltd

## Assignment

The purpose of this homework is to assist you in preparing for your Workbased Assessment of Competence. As there is no pressure on you, feel free to work at your own pace, but avoid the temptation to procrastinate. After you have read your notes and suggested references, submit your work for correction. The completed work becomes part of your Personal Portfolio.

## Enable clients to breathe (Unit Z19: 1–2)

1. An elderly gentleman is in bed with a chest pain, temperature and cough. He normally smokes a pipe which he would not give up. Describe your role in helping to design his care plan in relation to:
   a) Physical welfare:
      - chest pain
      - cough, diets
      - personal cleanliness
      - pressure areas.
   b) Social welfare
      - smoking
      - recreational and social therapy
      - occupational therapy.
   c) Psychological welfare
      - understanding the aim of care and what will happen to him
      - anxiety, frustration.
   d) Observations that will be maintained.
2. Discuss how you would encourage the client to participate in his care.

## Help clients to rest, relax and sleep (Z19.2)

Everyone has periods of activity alternating with periods of inactivity, generally known as a *wakefulness cycle*. These activities are important in promoting clients' health by reducing tension and stress.

### Rest

This is a period when a person ceases mental or physical activity in order to recover strength or refresh him/herself. Other names for rest periods include 'siesta' in which the person may decide to lie down, doze, read or even maintain a period of silence in a relaxed state of well-being. In the care setting, residents are encouraged to rest, especially after the mid-day meal. Some clients may tend to 'rest' for longer periods than is necessary during the day, probably due to boredom, and they remain awake at night. During the rest periods, clients should not be disturbed unless absolutely necessary.

### Relaxation

This is a way of helping a person to be less rigid or tense. The aim is to identify the person's interests and plan ways of relaxing and amusing him or her, in order to reduce stress and tension.

## Helping clients to relax

Encouraging clients to develop self-control of the mind and relaxation of the body can be very beneficial. Undertaking simple relaxation exercises or yoga may help. Yoga involves a series of movements, positions and meditation. The needs of individual clients should be assessed before embarking on these exercises because contorting the body into any yoga position and holding it there for a long time can be difficult for most elderly people. However, under the supervision of skilful, trained professional, yoga can be a useful way to relax. Clients should change into comfortable clothing and lie down on a mat on the floor. Encourage them to concentrate on deep breathing exercises and listen to meditation tapes. A few simple yoga excercies can then be introduced. The carer should make sure that clients do not strain or try to do exercises that are unsuitable. If a client is unable to lie on the floor, a comfortable chair could be provided. Aromatherapy — the use of aromatic oils to massage different parts of the body — can be very refreshing and relaxing. Some care establishments provide this service.

Simple activities such as jigsaw puzzles, reading books, magazines, poetry and playing board games may be helpful in releasing tension and amusing residents. These are available in most care environments. Some clients may enjoy trying their hand at writing, drawing, painting or knitting. A gentle walk in the garden or sitting out under a sun umbrella is always appreciated. These activities may help to ensure that clients are reasonably and moderately occupied during the day and will promote adequate sleep at night.

## Sleep

This is a natural and repeated condition of the body and mind in which the eyes are closed, the person is relaxed and consciousness is temporarily suspended. A good sleep at night should enable the person to carry out his or her normal daily activities effectively the next day. In sleep, consciousness is suspended to the extent that the person fails to respond to outside stimuli. However, during this phase, it is possible for a loud noise or violent shaking to arouse the person.

It is claimed that adults spend up to a third of their lives sleeping, and the amount varies from one person to another. The average is about seven to eight hours a night. Some researchers believe that we do not need sleep at all and argue that, in principle, man is capable of living without it. Sieveking (1996) reported that a 54-year-old woman called Nguyen Thi Le Hang stopped sleeping suddenly in 1965 when her first child was born, and has not slept for the last 31 years. There is no report of any adverse effects.

## Purpose of sleep

It is a natural experience which is common to nearly all animate life. As people grow older, they may need less sleep. It is said that research has been unable to prove conclusively any essential function or purpose of sleep. Some believe that sleep:
- renews and maintains the growth of brain cells by repairing worn out tissues of the body, eg. healing wounds
- promotes, restores and conserves both mental and physical energy
- refreshes the individual and prepares the sleeper for the next period of wakefulness
- 'makes a person healthy, wealthy and wise'.

Traditionally, we retire to bed when we are tired or to rest when we feel ill. We lie still for part of the night and may move at intervals throughout the period of sleep. It starts when the muscles are relaxed, the person breathes slowly and deeply, and falls asleep within seven minutes of turning off the light.

## Lack of sleep

The experience associated with lack of or deprivation of sleep is usually very disconcerting, especially if one remains awake for long periods. Many factors may be responsible for this condition, but the outcome could be:
- irritability, depression, frustration, tiredness, anti-social behaviour and lethargy
- lack of concentration, lateness and poor job performance. If the condition is not arrested, it may lead to a chronic lack of sleep known as insomnia.

## The process of sleep

Sleep is straightforward, normal and uncomplicated. Most people go to bed because they are tired or to rest when they feel ill, close their eyes and fall asleep remaining in this state until they have had sufficient rest. In an adult the normal sleep pattern begins with a pre-sleep routine usually lasting for about 20 minutes. Once asleep, the person passes through various stages. The evidence for this is based on studies of electroencephalogram (EEG) readings. It is believed that during this period, we will spend about 25% of the time dreaming, 25% in deep sleep and 50% in a light sleep. When we wake in the morning, we are usually rousing during or towards the end of a dream episode.

## Stages of sleep

Recent research shows that sleep is divided into two parts — the *sleep cycle* and the *rapid eye movement (REM)* sleep of dreams. Each cycle starts with a light sleep, goes to a deeper sleep, then back to a lighter sleep and ends with a dream.

The four sleep cycles (Non REM) are as follows:

### Stage 1:
This is the passing from being awake, although drowsy, to a feeling of general relaxation followed by a loss of consciousness. During the initial stage, fleeting thoughts pass through the individual's mind and he/she can be awakened by any slight sound. In this stage the body relaxes and the heart rate, temperature and blood pressure appear normal. If undisturbed and after about 15 minutes, the person goes into the next stage which is actual sleep. Should the person lie awake 45 minutes or more, he or she may be experiencing *insomnia*.

### Stage 2:
This is the first true sleep where there is greater relaxation and thoughts have a dream-like quality. The individual is soundly asleep and will not respond to noise but, if awakened, may deny that he or she was asleep.

### Stage 3:
This stage occurs after 30 minutes of sleep where there is complete relaxation of bodily activities and the person is in a fairly deep sleep. Familiar noises do not usually wake the person and, if not disturbed, the next stage follows.

### Stage 4:
The sleeper is completely relaxed, rarely moves and is often difficult to waken being in a very deep sleep. If forcibly wakened, he or she may be disorientated. Quite often sleepwalking and incontinence of urine occur at this stage.

### Rapid eye movement

This is a period of light sleep in which dreams occur. The eyeballs move rapidly back and forth, hence the name rapid eye movement. There is increased muscular relaxation and some hormones are released affecting vitality, fatigue, metabolism and the ability to resist infection.

## References

Closs J (1988) Patients' sleep — wake rhythms in hospital. Part I. *Nurs Times* **84**(1): 48–50

Closs J (1988) Patients' sleep — rhythms in hospital. Part II. *Nurs Times* **84**( 2): 54–55

Adams K (1980) A time for rest and a time for play. *Nurs Mirror* **150**(10)6: 17–18

Getliffe K (1988) Clinical feature — sleep of the just. *Nurs Standard* **2**(11): 18–19

### Audio visual aids

#### Format: VHS video
Ref: 172CT: *Exercises for the Over 60s* (still frame VHS video or slide tape)
PAT 0609: *Nutrition and Exercise for the Elderly: Creating a Healthstyle*
Oxford Educational Resources Ltd

## Helping clients to sleep (Z19: 1–2)

Traditionally, sleep is looked upon as a time of restoration and preparation for the next period of wakefulness in order to enable the individual to function effectively. In the care setting some clients may find it difficult to have a good night's sleep, due to numerous problems, real or imaginary.

### Factors interfering with sleep

Insomnia is believed to occur when a client experiences difficulty in falling asleep, and may take as long as 90 minutes to fall asleep. In this case the person needs help to ensure that he or she is physically comfortable. Counselling skills may help to identify the cause and need for support. Interfering factors may be classified as:

#### *1. Physical factors*
These may include:
- hunger, eating and drinking certain food or beverages, eg. cheese and coffee, thirst or going to bed with a full stomach
- lack of fulfilment of pre-sleep routine and length of sleeping period
- effects of exercise due to over-stimulation, hypnotic drugs and stimulants, alcohol
- the time of going to bed and movement during sleep
- discomfort, such as pain, a coughing bout, illness
- a full bladder and the need to use the toilet.

#### *2. Psychological*
- anxiety, confusion, depression, irritability associated with sleep difficulties
- fear of sleeplessness or even going off to sleep
- bad dreams, nightmares and interrupted pre-sleep routine
- personal attitudes relating to change of independence to dependence status.

### 3. Social
- admission, especially for the first time bringing about changes in environment, routine and lifestyle
- stressful life events relating to long-term care
- sleeping with strangers, disturbance, eg. snoring
- sleeping space due to lack of single rooms, own bed or shared bed, pillows
- boredom, level of tiredness, marital or financial difficulties.

### 4. Environment
- noise of traffic outside the care environment, quietness, hot or cold atmosphere
- light, darkness, position of the bed
- familiar objects, security
- caring activities and routine procedures.

## Management of problems

Sleep is a sensitive and highly individualised activity and discomfort of any kind may interfere with the person's ability to rest or sleep. The process of caring involves an assessment of a client's sleeping pattern and asking questions about whether the person sleeps during the day, whether he or she prefers to sleep in a bed or chair at night, whether the person has any previous problems with sleep and, if so, how these were resolved.

The approach to care is based on maintaining good interpersonal relationships in an attempt to tackle an individual client's problems.

### *Pre-sleep routine*

Pre-sleep routine refers to those activities which people carry out routinely before retiring to bed at night. Most elderly people repeat a series of personal habits which are necessary for comfort and help to bring about relaxation and sleep. These activities may include:
- a bedtime drink, combing or brushing hair
- saying prayers
- talking to a particular person, eg. a fellow resident
- being tucked into bed by someone, preferably a member of staff.

Many clients continue to carry out their routine in the care environment and should be encouraged to do so. Information on the pre-sleep routine of individual residents is important and should be recorded in the individual care plan and made available to all night staff in order to provide care to meet the client's individual needs.

Those who cannot or do not practise pre-sleep routines, should have their needs assessed, and a care plan designed to help them develop good sleeping habit. Such an approach may identify the need for them to:
- go to bed when sleepy and not try to get more sleep by going to bed early
- when in bed, try to get all muscles as relaxed as possible. Those who are not able to do so, should be encouraged to think of something pleasant or listen to sounds outside, eg. birds, people, or traffic
- get up and do something if not asleep in ten minutes. Only return when they feel sleepy.

### *Hunger or thirst*
**Action**:
- check what is available in the care environment
- offer the person a choice of light refreshments
- ensure the client's satisfaction
- offer toilet facilities and leave the person comfortable.

## Pain

This is a symptom of something that is wrong and produces the discomfort. However, one type of pain which is sometimes associated with sleep is cramp. If a client wakes from sleep and complains of intense pain in the foot or calf with an inability to move, usually the big toe, the following action should be taken.

**Action:**
- find out if the person has had a cramp before, and if so, how did he or she cope with it
- raise the leg gently above the bed and massage it
- confirm effectiveness of the treatment
- offer a warm drink of his or her choice and make the person comfortable.

## Anxiety

Clients may be anxious or worried about nightmares, bad dreams or pending operations.

**Action:**
- use counselling skills and help to identify the problem
- sit down, hold his or her hands, and talk with the person. Encourage the person to express him/herself and listen attentively to what is being said
- reassure and offer the person a refreshing hot drink of choice. Supervised smoking may be allowed in a non-smoking area
- use a relaxation technique, eg. offer an opportunity for the client to listen to radio, music
- offer a warm drink of his or her choice, ensure satisfaction and reinforce the reassurance
- leave an alarm call bell or buzzer within easy reach and wish the person goodnight.

## Incontinence

**Action:**
- attend to the client's personal needs
- offer a refreshing drink after the procedure and wish him or her goodnight.

## Routine care procedures

The practice of carrying out routine caring procedures, eg. dealing with incontinence may disturb the night's sleep of both the person receiving the attention and any other clients' sharing the same room or in adjacent beds. The effects of deprivation of sleep have previously been discussed.

**Action:**
- prepare the equipment and trolley for routine care prior to settling clients for the night
- carry out the routine procedures as quietly as possible, ensuring that nothing is dropped
- ensure that clients who may be affected and the person receiving attention are reassured; offered a choice of warm drinks and adequately resettle.

## Temperature of the room

**Action:**
- check the ventilation and heating system of the room
- ensure that appropriate night attire is worn, and bedclothes are adequate for the time of year. Remove or re-adjust bedclothes as necessary
- offer a cold or warm drink of client's choice and make the person comfortable.

## Making it easier for clients to sleep

This involves management of problems as they are identified:
- ensure that the bed is comfortable with firm but not too hard a mattress and pillows. Place soft pillow on top for client's head to rest upon

- encourage client to use the toilet or commode before retiring to bed. Offer a warm bath or shower before bedtime
- offer bedtime beverage, eg. warm milky drink. Some clients may enjoy a small whisky or brandy added to a hot drink if allowed. Some may prefer a small sherry
- facilitate reading in bed to induce sleep for those who are able to read until they become drowsy
- encourage client to avoid daytime naps by providing age-related activities during the day
- manage problems as they are identified, eg. noise, hunger or thirst, temperature of the room
- inform the person-in-charge because if these remedial measures fail it may be necessary for the doctor to be informed. Medication may need to be prescribed as a last resort to help the client to relax and sleep
- consult clients before any lights are turned off or dimmed, because some derive security and sleep soundly in the presence of some form of light.

**The use of complementary therapies**

The following measures have been successfully used to assist people to relax and sleep.

*Massage*
This is popularly known as 'hands on therapy'. The therapist uses oil and systematically massages the body — the neck, upper back and shoulder, scalp, hands, arms, feet and legs. The treatment induces warmth and relaxation which can help to ease tension and pain. It is also said to bring about a feeling of security and well-being.

*Aromatherapy*
A form of treatment which extends the effects of massage and in which the therapist uses scented oil to massage a small part of the body. The aim is to increase the circulation of blood and lymph, soothe aches and pains, reduce muscular tension and promote a state of general well-being. It is claimed to stimulate the immune system.

**Observation and reporting**

Clients should be frequently observed at night and reported upon especially if they are taking night sedation. Take notice of the length of time the person has slept and make a report on the effectiveness, or lack of it, of any interventions given. It is also important to be aware that some clients may pretend to be asleep at night when carers do their rounds, as they feel that they must not 'bother anyone'.

*Guidance*
- demonstrate knowledge of individual sleeping habits
- spend some time watching the rise and fall of a client's chest
- if the person is awake, ask if there is anything you can do and offer a hot drink of his or her choice.

*Evaluation*
Report when a client is able to sleep naturally throughout the night without any disturbance.

# References

Carpenter R (1997) The sleep solution. *The Express*, February 8: 31–33
Manian R (1988) Clinical feature — can I sleep now, nurse? *Nurs Standard* **2**(12): 22–23
Sieveking P (ed) (1996) She couldn't sleep a wink – for 31 years. *The Sunday Telegraph*, October 6

Warner J (1997) Bedtime rituals of nursing home residents: A study. *Nurs Standard* **11**(20): 34–35
Whitfield W (1982) Breaking the habit. *Nurs Mirror* **155**(10): 59–60

# Assignment

The purpose of this homework is to assist you in preparing for your Workbased Assessment of Competence. As there is no pressure on you, feel free to work at your pace, but avoid the temptation to procrastinate. After you have read your notes and suggested references, submit your work for correction. The completed work becomes part of your Personal Portfolio.

## Help clients rest, relax and sleep (Z19: 1–2)

1. Discuss the importance of sleep and list the effects of lack of sleep.
2. It is over a week since Mrs Jones, a 75-year-old lady, was admitted, but since then she has lost her sleep cycle:
   a) give an account of this problem and discuss the reasons for her problem
   b) discuss what you would do to help her restore her sleep cycle.

# Unit 8
# Enable clients to eat and drink (NC12, NC13)

## Eating (NC12: 1-2, NC13: 1-2)

Eating and drinking are essential activities of daily living, and without it human life cannot exist. The body is made up of millions of complex cells which require a constant supply of energy — the source of which is food and water. Preferences are based on obtaining, preparing and consuming food in accordance with culture, lifestyle, likes and dislikes.

### Purpose of eating

Food and drink provide the nutrients and fluids necessary for growth until maturity is reached. After that, fluids and nourishment are required to replace worn out tissues. As we grow older, our bodies slow down and use less fuel (energy or calories). Extra care is needed in choosing foods which are the most nutritious and contain sufficient vitamins and minerals. In some cases, doctors may recommend therapeutic diets which are planned by dieticians.

In hospitals and health care homes, eating and drinking can be one of the most enjoyable parts of the day for as well as maintaining bodily health and function, it is a time for socialising. Enjoyment can be enhanced by varying the diet to provide all the energy and nutrients that are required for good health.

The nutritional needs of the elderly do not change a great deal. But with age and illness the body processes slow down, reducing the amount of energy required for the adequate functioning of the body. However, research suggests that, beyond the age of 70, declining health and a number of social and economic factors can contribute to reducing the intake of nourishment. It is important, when providing meals for elderly people, to consider how the diet will affect their weight. Carers should also check for signs of malnutrition, such as weakness, drowsiness, skin lesions, or the inability to combat infection.

To encourage clients to eat properly attention should be paid to varying the diet and taking cultural influences into account. Research shows that many health problems do not become evident until middle age, and can arise from the inadequate nutrient content of food, and from difficulties in persuading elderly clients to eat and drink, especially in their own homes in the community. These problems can result in poor responses to treatments prescribed for existing illness.

### Nutrition

This is the science of studying the process by which food is ingested by the body to supply nourishment. Good nutrition is essential for maintaining an optimum state of health. In other words, to remain in good health the person needs to eat a nutritionally well-balanced diet. This should be based on the Department of Health (1992) guidelines for a healthy diet, *The Balance of Good Health*.

## The Balance of Good Health

This is a new national food guide which aims to enlighten people and make it easier for them to understand and enjoy the benefits of healthy eating. It applies to most people, apart from children under two years of age, and suggests food nutrients that help the body to function. The five main categories of foods are:
- bread, cereals and potatoes
- fruit and vegetables
- milk and dairy products
- fatty and sugary foods
- meat, fish and alternatives.

|  | Bread, cereals and potatoes | Fruit and vegetables | Milk and dairy products | Meat, fish and alternatives | Fatty and sugar foods |
| --- | --- | --- | --- | --- | --- |
| Sources | Wholemeal bread, pasta, brown rice, cereals, baked or boiled potatoes in their skin, pulses, beans | Fresh, frozen, canned fruit and vegetables, dried fruit, oranges, grapefruits, salads, fruit juices | Yoghourt, milk, cheese, fromage frais, skimmed milk | Meat, poultry, fish, eggs, nuts, pulses, yeast extract, liver | Margarine, low fat spread, butter, salad oil, crisps, biscuits, cream cake, ice cream, puddings |
| Main nutritional value | Carbohydrate (starch) and fibre, calcium and iron, B vitamins | Vitamin C, minerals, fibre, carotene | Calcium, protein, vitamins B12, A and D | Protein, iron, Vitamin B (B12), magnesium, zinc | Vitamin D, high in salt, sugar and fat |
| Quantity | Eat plenty of whole grain or high fibre types. Avoid frying, rich sauces or dressings | Eat as much as you like and choose a wide variety. Avoid adding dressings, butter or sugar | Eat moderate amounts where possible. Choose lower fat options | Eat moderate amounts of these foods, selecting lower fat options | Eat these foods infrequently or in minimal amounts |

## The concept of a balance of good health

It is based on eating the right amount of a variety of foods which is necessary to maintain a healthy weight. Recommendations include eating plenty of foods rich in starch and fibre, and five or more portions of fruit and vegetables daily. There is, as yet, no specific information on the actual size of portions. Fatty and sugary foods are discouraged and certain food stuffs are to be avoided, eg. thickly spread butter, frequent fried foods (eg. chips), poultry with skin not removed. Use of salt should be reduced and only use the amount of herbs and spices that is recommended. Alcohol should be kept to reasonable amounts, ie. 1 or 2 units a day.

## Nutrition for elderly people

The majority of people over 65 years of age need to remain fit and well and maintain physical activity. They need food intakes that will provide them with higher energy requirements, and age-related exercise is recommended. Although they may appear to eat an appropriate amount of nutrients, it should be remembered that no single food contains all the nutrients required; a mixture of these in the right proportion can be classified into the essential constituents of *a healthy diet*. Carers should ensure that they have a sound knowledge of the essential foods that need to be included in a well-balanced diet for elderly pepole. This should include knowledge about sources of vitamin and mineral supplements.

### Dietary constituents

### Carbohydrates
Sources:     Meat, fish, fruit and root vegetables, pasta.
Function:    Provide the body with heat and energy.

### Proteins
These are made up of amino acids which are broken down by the digestive system and absorbed through the intestinal wall. There are two types — first class from animal and second class derived from vegetable origin.

Sources:     First class:    Meat, fish, eggs, milk, cheese
             Second class:   Peas, beans, nuts and lentils, soya beans.
Function:    Growth and repair of body tissues and cells; provide energy.

### Fats
Sources:     Animal fats (saturated fat): milk, butter, eggs, meat, oily fish, such as herring, cod, vegetable fats (unsaturated): vegetable oils, margarine, nuts.
Function:    Provide heat and energy; support certain organs of the body such as eyes and the kidneys. Excess fat is stored in the body and saturated fats are linked with increased cholesterol levels.

### Dietary fibre
Indigestible part of the diet:
Sources:     Cereals, wholemeal bread and pasta, vegetables, fruit.
Function:    Gives bulk to the diet and satisfies the appetite, stimulates movement of the bowels. Should be accompanied by exercise and plenty of fluid.

### Vitamins
These are chemical compounds necessary to health. There are two types:
Sources:     Fat soluble:    Vitamins A, D, E and K
             Water soluble:  Vitamins B, C and P.
Function:    Regulate energy and the process of metabolism for general health of tissues. Deficiency can lead to specific conditions.

### Mineral salts
Organic compounds necessary for all body processes. They are required in minute quantities. The main sources are:
Sources:     Meat, fish, dairy products, green vegetables, rice, seafood (sardines, shellfish) liver, spinach and pulses, nuts, wholemeal bread, cereals, eggs.
Function:
- calcium for healthy teeth, nails and bones
- phosphorous for healthy teeth, bones and energy

- sodium (salt) important for blood, bones and body fluid. Too much can cause problems
- magnesium essential for bone, muscle function and nerve
- iron necessary for red blood cell formation
- copper vital for healthy blood vessels and ligaments
- iodine needed for proper functioning of the thyroid gland
- zinc needed for growth, clear skin and hair.

## Water

This is a liquid comprising of two parts of hydrogen and one part of oxygen ($H_2O$). It is essential for life and makes up about 70% of body weight in men and 60% in women. It is the main constituent of body fluids — we need about 2500 mls (5½ pints) per day, and death will follow extreme dehydration.

Function: It provides the moist environment required by all living cells of the body. Water dilutes and moistens food, assists in the regulation of body temperature, dilutes waste products and toxins in the body. It contributes to formation of urine and faeces.

## The digestive system

A basic knowledge of human physiology and how the food is used by the body is important in the care of clients. Some residents may have difficulty in swallowing their food, and knowledge of this will be useful when feeding helpless clients. The term *digestive system* is a collective name used to describe the alimentary tract and the process in which foodstuffs are altered by chemical substances called enzymes (chemical messengers) for absorption. The activities of the system are classified as:

- Ingestion — taking of food into the alimentary system
- Digestion — breaking food down into small particles by chewing and swallowing for action by the enzymes
- Absorption — the process by which digested foodstuffs enter the bloodstream through the small intestine
- Elimination — disposing of the waste products of the breakdown process.

## Organs of digestion

The alimentary tract is a tube about 10 metres long which stretches from the mouth to the anus. As food passes through this tube, it is broken down by enzymes, which are chemical messengers, into a form suitable for absorption. The digestive system comprises:

### Mouth

This is where digestion begins. It receives the food, chews and swallows it. Various structures in the mouth are sensitive to stimuli, such as temperature, but the tongue is the main organ of taste. The taste buds pick up the sensation which the brain interprets as flavour, helping to make food palatable.

### Salivary glands

The six pairs of glands secrete saliva to lubricate food and start digestion in response to the sight, smell and thought of food.

### Oesophagus

This is a muscular tube which passes from the pharynx, through the diaphragm into the stomach. It produces mucus which lubricates food as it goes down into the stomach by peristalsis.

### Stomach

A large pouch-like muscular organ which acts as a temporary reservoir for food which remains here long enough to allow gastric juices time to act on the foodstuffs.

### Liver

A large wedged-shaped organ; described as the largest organ in the body. It lies beneath the diaphragm and produces bile and eliminates toxic substances.

### Small intestine

After the food leaves the stomach, it passes through the small intestine which lies coiled up in the abdominal cavity surrounded by the large intestine. It is about seven metres in length and the first part is called the duodenum. Its 'C' shape houses the head of the pancreas, into which flows pancreatic juice and bile from the liver. Most nutrients are absorbed into the body in the small intestine.

### Large intestine

This is about 1.5 metres long, begins at the caecum and terminates at the rectum in the pelvic cavity. It is divided into the caecum, ascending, transverse colon, descending colon, sigmoid or pelvic colon, rectum and anal canal. Indigestible fibre and semi-solid waste pass into the large intestine where it forms large, soft stools. Water is reabsorbed from here into the body.

### Rectum

This is a slightly dilated part of the colon which is about 13 cm long. It stores stools until they can be excreted.

## The act of swallowing

The process occurs in three stages. When the food has been sufficiently moistened by saliva it is formed into a soft mass called bolus, and swallowed by the action of the tongue:

- the mouth is closed and the tongue and cheeks push the bolus backwards into pharynx
- the muscles of the pharynx propel the bolus down into the oesophagus. The soft palate rises up and blocks the nasal part of the pharynx and the tongue closes the route back to the mouth
- the larynx is lifted up and forward so that its opening is closed by the epiglottis coming into contact with the base of the tongue to prevent the food from being inhaled
- the presence of the bolus in the pharynx stimulates a wave of peristalsis which propels the bolus through the oesophagus to the stomach.

Peristaltic waves of contraction only pass along the oesophagus after swallowing, otherwise the walls are relaxed.

### Factors influencing swallowing

Swallowing can be affected by a number of difficulties (dysphagia), such as:

- **Physical**: appetite, sight, type and consistency of food, condition of the mouth, smell of food or drink, illness such as Huntington's Chorea, Parkinson's disease, choking, dependency status such as being fed, infection, position in care
- **Social**: cultural, religious beliefs, eg. fasting
- **Psychological**: depression, anxiety, thought of food, sight of blood and accident

The management of these difficulties will depend upon the cause of the problem.

*Enable clients to eat and drink*

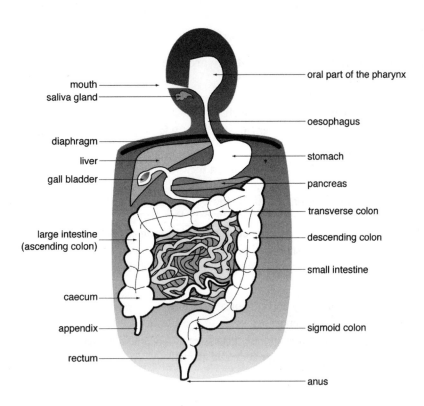

**A simple diagram of the alimentary system**

### Guidance
- maintain a good interpersonal relationship with the client
- demonstrate an in-depth knowledge of the client and of first aid, eg. in choking
- maintain records of what food is likely to cause the problem
- ensure that meat and other products such as sausages or segments of oranges are finely cut to meet the client's need
- ensure that the client is satisfied with the texture of the food
- allow the person time to swallow
- ensure that the person maintains a comfortable position
- observe and report on clients with ill-fitting dentures. Sometimes the gums shrink, and clients may have difficulty in keeping their dentures in place.

## Helping clients to eat (NC12: 1–2, N13.1)

Meal times should be looked forward to as a social occasion. The dining room should be tastefully decorated with good ventilation. Clients should be encouraged, if possible, to use the dining room for their meals. If clients do not wish to eat their meals in the dining room, arrange for them to have meals in their rooms.

## Mobile patients/clients

1. The **dining table** or **tray** should be suitably prepared:
   - clean table/table cloth or tray cloth
   - cutlery, condiments, serviette, drink
   - flowers on the table can add a special touch
   - special cutlery, non slip mat and other aids if necessary for a disabled patient/client.

2. **Personal cleanliness:**
   - check that mobile patients/clients have washed their hands and made themselves presentable before a meal
   - offer the use of a commode or bedpan to those who are confined to bed, followed by handwashing facilities. Wear a clean protective apron and tie back long hair
   - ensure that patients/clients are wearing dentures and hearing aids where appropriate
   - keep fingernails clean and fingers out of the food
   - protect any cuts or abrasions with a waterproof plaster and do not smoke.

3. **Serving of meals:**
   - be sure that people are properly and comfortably seated
   - check that any special diet is served
   - offer a choice of menu if possible and ask if they would like small or large portions
   - serve hot/cold food and drink appropriately and attractively. Also, ask if they would like sauce or gravy poured over their vegetables or meat.

4. **During meals:**
   - allow enough time to eat and enjoy the meal
   - serve one course at a time. Do not serve the next course until everyone has finished and dishes have been removed
   - encourage patients/clients to eat the food served at mealtimes rather than to eat between meals. Offer second helpings as may be required by individual clients
   - assist in cutting up food and pouring out drinks as necessary
   - observe and report on the amount of food eaten and drink taken, and if clients refuse food or have difficulty in chewing or swallowing, report this to the person-in-charge.

5. **After meals:**
   - clear away dishes/trays promptly after the meal is finished. Stack crockery and cutlery in the kitchen ready for washing
   - report any complaints made by patients/clients to the person-in-charge
   - offer tea or coffee, or a drink of the person's choice
   - encourage patients/clients to clean their teeth or dentures, or offer a mouthwash, in accordance with their individual personal hygiene regimen
   - offer fresh fruit as a means of cleaning teeth and mouth after a meal.

## Helpless patients

Some people feel embarrassed and humiliated by having to be fed. When feeding helpless patients, emphasis should be placed on encouraging independence, re-education and allowing an individual to feed and drink him/herself as far as is possible.
- prepare a tray with cutlery, condiments
- maintain a good interpersonal relationship, offer toilet and handwashing facilities before a meal. Check that dentures and hearing aid where appropriate are in use

- make the person comfortable supported by pillows; explain the content of the meal
- place yourself in a position — sitting or standing, so that the person can see you clearly
- protect the client's clothing with a serviette tucked under his/her chin
- offer a choice of eating utensils, ie. spoon or fork
- establish a means of communication, eg. ask the person to nod when the mouth is empty if he or she is unable to speak
- assist the person to feed him/herself by placing a spoon loaded with food in the client's hand and directing it to his or her mouth
- allow time to breath and swallow between mouthfuls. Give a longer rest at intervals, if swallowing is difficult
- promote conversation, although this may be difficult while eating, but there should be no need for absolute silence throughout the meal
- observe and report the amount of food eaten, including refusal of food, and any untoward incident during the meal to the person-in-charge
- remove the tray, offer a mouthwash and make the person comfortable after the meal.

## Factors which may affect adequate nutritional intake

The desire to eat and drink is often suppressed because of the following, and could lead to malnutrition and dehydration if untreated:

- general malaise and feelings of nausea, frailty, lethargy, drowsiness
- anorexia (loss of appetite, not to be confused with the medical condition known as anorexia nervosa), immobility, direct influence of injury and illness)
- pain, abdominal discomfort which may be due to constipation
- difficulty in swallowing (dysphasia); may also be a side-effect of drug therapy
- psychological conditions, eg. depression, stress, anxiety, confusion, over-activity
- environmental conditions, eg. unpleasant sights or smells, lack of choice, staff attitudes
- ill fitting dentures or lack of dentures, sore mouth, tongue or gums, poor eyesight
- religious beliefs about food, or special diets, poverty, alcohol
- unfamiliar food and/or routine, together with interrupted or rushed meals.

## Guidance on promoting adequate nutritional intake

- identify and report on specific problems such as poor fitting dentures, constipation, poor eye sight, or someone smoking in the immediate vicinity
- maintain a good interpersonal relationship at all times
- ensure a clean and comfortable environment with attention to utensils and presentation
- give the client a choice of menu at the time of serving the meal, together with an opportunity to see and smell the food available
- ensure facilities for light snacks or alternative nourishment, eg. Build-Up, Complan
- maintain a monthly record of client's weight.

## Tube feeding

This procedure involves passing a nasogastric tube directly into the patient's stomach. A gastric tube may also be inserted through the abdominal wall into the stomach. The tube is prescribed by the doctor and a nutritionally balanced liquid diet is fed through it.

### Guidance on care plan

- take care when moving, bathing or dressing the person to avoid pulling the tube out
- maintain a fluid balance chart
- report immediately any signs of discomfort and blockage of the tube

- watch for irritation around the nostril or abdominal site
- keep all food and beverages away from people whose orders indicate 'nil by mouth'.

# References

Brown K (1991) Improving intakes. *Nurs Times* **87**(20): 64–68
Dudek SG (1987) *Nutrition Handbook for Nurses.* J B Lippincott, Philadelphia
Farbrother M (1993) What can I eat? *Nurs Times* **89**(14): 63
Health Education Authority (1994) *The Balance of Good Health.* HEA, London
Moran D (1994) *Fit for Life.* Windsor Healthcare Ltd, Bracknell, Berkshire
Nursing Times (1995) *Pocket Guide to Nutrition. What is a Healthy Diet?* Macmillan Ltd, London
National Dairy Council (1993) *Keeping Fit in Retirement.* A National Dairy Council Publication, London
Robertson B (1992) *Study Guide for Health and Social Care Support Workers.* First Class Books Inc, USA
Wilson JW (1987) *Anatomy and Physiology in Health and Illness*, 6th edn. Churchill Livingstone, Edinburgh
Woolaway MC et al (1985) A study of the nutrition content of hospital meals. *Comm Med* **7**: 193–197
Wynn M, Wynn A (1993) A catering concern. Nutritional standards for older people. *Nurs Times* **89**(20): 61–64

## Audio visual aids

### Format: VHS video

Ref: 425CT: *Healthy Eating for Elderly People*
Ref: CEA8661: *Nutritional Assessment of the Elderly*
Ref: 128CT: *Food Hints for the Over 60s*
Ref: PAT0605: *Nutrition and Exercise for the Elderly: Eat Right, Feel Better*
Ref: PAT0606: *Nutrition and Exercise for the Elderly: Problems of Nutrition for the Elderly*
Oxford Educational Resources Ltd

# Assignment

The purpose of this homework is to assist you in preparing for your Workbased Assessment of Competence. As there is no pressure on you, feel free to work at your own pace, but avoid the temptation to procrastinate. After you have read your notes and suggested references, submit your work for correction. The completed work becomes part of your Personal Portfolio.

# Enabling clients to eat and drink

## Eating (NC12: 1–2, NC13:1–2)

1. State what you understand by the term 'healthy diet'.
2. Discuss the balance of good health and foods classified under its five categories.
3. Make a list of vitamins and mineral supplements and their sources.
4. List seven constituents of a healthy diet.
5. Discuss factors which may affect a client's dietary needs and choice.

6. Explain the importance of enabling clients to choose food and drink.
7. A newly admitted client refuses to eat or drink. What do you think could be the reasons for this behaviour?
8. A notice on a client's bed reads 'nil by mouth'. What do you understand by this?

## Assignment

The purpose of this homework is to assist you in preparing for your Workbased Assessment of Competence. As there is no pressure on you, feel free to work at your own pace, but avoid the temptation to procrastinate. After you have read your notes and suggested references, submit your work for correction. The completed work becomes part of your Personal Portfolio.

## Enabling clients to eat (N12: 1-2, N13: 1-2)

1. Describe how you would prepare and care for the following clients at meal times:
   (a) Mobile client:
       (i) action before meal
       (ii) action during meal
       (iii) action after meal.
   (b) Helpless client:
       (i) action before meal
       (ii) action during meal
       (iii) action after meal.
2. State briefly what action you would take if a mobile client:
   (i) refuses to eat
   (ii) refuses to drink.
3. State briefly what you would do if a helpless client:
   (i) refuses to eat
   (ii) refuses to drink.
4. What would lead you to believe that a client is not having an adequate diet?
5. Describe procedures for monitoring an individual's intake of nourishment.
6. Discuss how you would help a helpless person you are feeding to maintain his self respect and dignity.

## Helping clients to drink (NC12: 1-2, N13: 1-2)

### The nature and purpose of drinking

The daily intake of fluids is one of the important items in the diet and without it, the balance of water in the body cannot be maintained and dehydration sets in. Fluids are essential for life and although a starving man can survive without food for about a month, he can only live for a few days without water.

Water represents about 70% of the body weight and is available from many sources, such as fluids taken by mouth, solid food, and water content of fruits. It is claimed that the average daily intake of water is about 3 litres, and should the intake be insufficient, the person will experience a sensation of thirst. If this is not relieved, he/she may complain of dryness of the mouth, lack of energy and appear dull. During this condition small quantities of fluid of the individual's choice may be given by mouth.

## Dehydration

This is a condition in which the body is deprived of water for a considerable length of time. The condition is accompanied with a serious loss of weight. The person may have furring of the tongue, the skin loses its elasticity, the face appears pinched and drawn and eyes are sunken in the sockets. If the condition is not treated, the person may have kidney failure leading to unconsciousness and death. High concentrations of uric acid result from inadequate fluid intake or to fluid loss caused by excessive perspiration.

### *Loss of water*

The body may lose water if the client is suffering from vomiting, fevers, extreme diarrhoea, haemorrhage, incontinence, perspiration, severe burns or wounds. Elderly people with weak bladder control may withhold their intake of water in the hope that it will reduce the need to ask for a bedpan or urinal. Excessive use of some drugs, such as diuretics, may cause loss of water. Any gross loss of fluid is followed by a loss of body weight.

## Prevention of dehydration

The care plan should include the following approaches:
- liberal and oral intake of fluid
- introduction of fluids by intravenous/subcutaneous infusion or rectum
- maintenance of a fluid balance chart to facilitate a clear picture of body fluid balance.

### *Oral and liberal intake of fluids*

The fluids usually used include plain water. The amount will depend on whether the individual is capable of taking fluid by the mouth. In any case developing and maintaining a good interpersonal relationship with clients is very important.

> *Guidance*
> - ensure that fresh water is readily available. Drinks may be chilled, probably with ice
> - offer to pour a drink whenever you enter a client's room to ensure that he or she drinks it
> - offer foods such as jelly, ice cream, soup if the person's diet allows them
> - encourage intake of fruits with high water content, eg. grapes
> - maintain the fluid balance chart, including records of weight as any severe loss of body fluids is always accompanied by loss of weight.

### *Intravenous route*

Fluids are normally administered by mouth depending on the condition of the person. In certain severe cases fluid may be given by other routes such as per rectum, subcutaneous (under the skin) and by intravenous infusion. The fluids used may be normal saline, dextrose, glucose, transfusion of fresh blood, blood plasma and blood serum. The amount given depends on the need of the person in relation to the condition. The intravenous route is the responsibility of qualified nurses. Care assistants can observe and report on the flow meter and quantity of remaining fluid in the bottle.

## Fluid balance chart

The fluid balance chart is a daily record of body fluid intake and output maintained by the use of a special chart. It is a 24-hour record of a total intake of fluids less the total amount in urine, vomit or diarrhoea. The main purpose of this observation is to enable members of the health care team to keep a check on the physical condition of their clients to prevent dehydration. These measurements must be accurately and neatly recorded to provide a clear picture of the body fluid balance.

## Design of the chart

The chart is designed to show both input and output sections, together with time, types of fluid, volume and routes of intake and the amount of output within a 24-hour period.

## Measuring fluid intake

To accurately measure a person's intake, it is necessary to record all fluids taken. Measure fluids taken by mouth as soon as consumed. This may be a cup of tea, bowl of soup, water from bedside jugs, coffee or juice. Amounts taken are usually expressed in millilitres (ml). There are 30 mls in one fluid ounce. It is important to know how much the containers hold. In some cases, the amount and frequency of fluid may be ordered for the daily intake

## Measuring the output

In certain illnesses, eg. when fever is present, fluid may be lost in perspiration. This type of fluid loss cannot be accurately measured. It has been reported that loss by perspiration could be about 1000 mls in 24 hours. Urine is a reliable output measurement. On average, a person may void about 1200–1500 mls per day.

### Guidance

For a person who is mobile, a specimen pan is placed in the toilet seat. Ask him not to empty the pan. For people using a bedpan, urinal or commode, remove the specimen pan to the sluice and use the following procedures:

- wash and dry your hands thoroughly and put on disposable apron and gloves
- pour the urine into graduated specimen container or jug kept in the sluice for this purpose
- place the container on a level surface and note the amount of output
- look for abnormalities, eg. blood, colour, mucus, discharge
- empty the urine into toilet and flush
- clean and disinfect all equipment after use
- remove and dispose of the disposable apron and gloves; wash your hands thoroughly
- record the output and report any abnormalities.

## Special conditions

Fluid balance charts may be maintained for clients with a variety of conditions such as:

## Oedema

This is a condition in which fluid is retained in the body tissue. It may cause painful swelling and weight gain. Heart and kidney disease and the use of too much salt can cause the condition.

## Care plan for oedema

Aim of the care plan is to:
- maintain a good interpersonal relationship with the person
- encourage him or her to wear loose-fitting clothing

- raise the extremity (limb) with a foot stool or pillow
- maintain the fluid balance chart and offer a pleasant tasting mouthwash
- help the person to keep to a special diet which may be ordered, eg. low fluid or low salt diet.

## *Evaluation*
When the person improves and is able to assume his or her independence.

## *Dehydration*
The condition means too little fluid or a loss of fluid in the body and may be due to:
- excessive vomiting
- severe bleeding or burns
- high fevers; untreated diabetes resulting in excessive micturition (passing of urine)
- weak bladder control and incontinence
- other causes such as wounds.

### *Signs and symptoms*
- dull and apathetic appearance
- dry mouth and cracked lips
- wrinkling of the skin
- excessive urinary output
- sore, furred or inflamed tongue.

### *Care plan*
The aim is to:
- ensure that fresh water is readily available for the person to drink. Always offer to pour a drink for the person whenever you enter his or her room because the person will not feel able to do so independently
- offer foods such as jelly, ice cream, soup if the person's condition allows
- encourage intake of fruits with high water content, eg. grapes
- maintain fluid balance chart.

### *Evaluation*
When the person recovers and is able to assume his or her independence and normal drinking habit.

*Enable clients to eat and drink*

**24-hour fluid balance chart**

Surname:............................... Forenames:...................................

Hospital/Nursing home...................................................................

Address:........................................................................................

Tel.no............................... Age/Dob........................ Sex....................

Ward/dept........................... GP...............................................

Consultant:.....................................................................................

| | Fluid intake | | | | | | Fluid output | | | | |
|---|---|---|---|---|---|---|---|---|---|---|---|
| | Intravenous | | Oral | | Intravenous | | Other | Urine | Gastric content | Other | Remarks |
| Time | Type of fluid | ml | Fluid | ml | Type of fluid | ml | ml | ml | ml | Type | ml |
| | | | | | | | | | | | |
| | | | | | | | | | | | |
| | | | | | | | | | | | |
| | | | | | | | | | | | |
| | | | | | | | | | | | |
| | | | | | | | | | | | |
| | | | | | | | | | | | |
| | | | | | | | | | | | |
| | | | | | | | | | | | |
| | | | | | | | | | | | |
| **Totals** | | | | | | | | | | | |
| | | | Total intake= ml | | | | | Total output= | | | ml |
| | | | Blood/ ml | | infusion | | | Insensible loss= | | | ml |
| | | | | | Balance +/- | | | | | | ml |

# Assignment

The purpose of this homework is to assist you in preparing for your Workbased Assessment of Competence. As there is no pressure on you, feel free to work at your own pace, but avoid the temptation to procrastinate. After you have read your notes and suggested references, submit your work for correction. The completed work becomes part of your Personal Portfolio.

## Enable client to drink (NC12: 1-2, NC13: 1-2)

1. Discuss the act of swallowing and list 12 factors which may influence a client's ability to swallow.
2. Describe a situation in which a resident may have difficulty in swallowing. What help would you give to the person?
3. A client is reported to be suffering from dehydration.
   a) What do you think could be the cause(s) of this condition?
   b) What are the signs and symptoms of this problem?
   c) Discuss ways in which the person could be helped to take adequate fluid intake.
   d) Describe your role and the observations and report you would make to the person-in-charge which may indicate that the person is responding to care.
4. Discuss the importance of maintaining a fluid balance chart, and your role in maintaining this document.

## Therapeutic and special diets

Caring for people, whether sick or well, involves the use of a variety of approaches to treat and help them to survive and maintain good health. Among the commonly used methods are the use of natural substances (naturopathy), such as sunlight, fresh air, pure foodstuffs and herbs without resorting to the use of drugs or surgery to treat and prevent diseases. This is based on the belief that symptoms of disease are seen as the body's attempt to get rid of collected waste. The treatment, therefore, aims to help the body to return to, and maintain normal good health.

Other methods include psychotherapy for mental health problems, aromatherapy based on the use of aromatic oils, hydrotherapy which is the use of water, massage — a method of rubbing the body to stimulate circulation, and dietetics which is concerned with the use of specific diets.

### Diets

The term refers to the food we eat and the choices of meals we regularly make according to the needs of the body in order to maintain good health. As people grow older, their nutritional requirements change, because of changes in their body relative to absorption, excretion and use of nutrients. A diet is what is eaten, and dietetics is the science of regulating diets in order to keep the body healthy. Diets are used to treat certain conditions and will require a dietician to assess the person, and prescribe suitable dietary treatment. During the 1940s, treatment for tuberculosis was based mainly on a well-balanced diet and fresh air.

### Therapeutic diets

This diet is basically *The Balance of Good Health* which is usually modified by a dietician and prepared by trained cooks in the residential care homes or hospitals. This is necessary in order to manage, treat or prevent disease by altering the consistency and adapting the content of the food or both. Therapeutic diets are medically prescribed and involve:

- assessment of an individual's food intake and essential substances such as proteins, vitamins and fats to see if it falls below a certain level of recommended daily intake
- appraisal of how the person tolerates certain food, eg. if he or she feels ill after eating a certain food, then it has to be excluded from the diet, eg. coeliac disease, intolerance to gluten where all wheat products must be excluded from the person's diet
- identification of deficiencies in minerals and vitamins which can be remedied with supplements readily available, eg. iron in somebody suffering from anaemia
- treatment of illnesses in some highly specialised situations, with a combination of drugs and diets, eg. AIDS, diabetes
- prescribe specialised diets for diagnostic purposes and treatment, eg. exclusion diet for food allergies, irritable bowel syndrome.

## Special diets

Over the centuries, different foodstuffs were valued for their medicinal properties. For example, garlic was known to cure many disorders and cabbage used as a wound dressing. In the eighteenth century, lime juice was administered to British sailors to prevent scurvy (scorbutus) which led to the slang term 'limey'. In the present care environment, most diets are regarded as normal, ordinary and well-balanced. A well-balanced diet is one which contains sufficient amounts of nutrients — proteins, fats, carbohydrates, vitamins and minerals — in the right proportion to ensure good health. A special diet is where a normal diet is modified to help in the treatment of a medical condition, eg. diabetes, Crohn's disease or ulcerative colitis, and the person is required to follow this diet as part of his medical treatment.

A diet to reduce weight (ie. a slimming diet) may be termed a special diet if the person concerned has been advised to lose weight for medical reasons. Vegetarian or vegan diets are a matter of choice for individuals who refuse to eat meat, fish or any kind of dairy products and are not usually termed special diet.

### Types of special diets
These diets include:
- light or convalescent diet. This is nutritious but easily digested high calorie foodstuffs
- fluid or milk diet. May mean only milk or may include other fluids
- high protein/high energy diet for those who are underweight. This replaces lost protein, helps to alleviate bedsores and severe burns and generally builds up a person
- low protein diet for liver and kidney complaints, hypertension, uraemia
- low fat diet used in the conditions of the gall bladder, jaundice and in lowering cholesterol levels
- high fibre diet prevents constipation and stimulates a lazy bowel
- high fibre/low irritant diet rests the gut and reduces inflammation of intestinal tract
- low salt or no added salt diet reduces sodium content in the body; used particularly where there is tissue oedema and aids against hypertension
- weight reduction diet to aid against physical strain, eg. back pain, heart disease, varicose veins
- metabolic diet used in disorders in children, eg. phenalketonuria
- ethnic diets, where religious laws govern the choice, eg. Sikhs, Muslims, Hindus, Orthodox Jews.

## Management of a special dietary programme

When a client is put on a diet a number of changes are likely to occur which may affect him or her for the first few days. It is likely that he or she may have difficulty in adjusting to or tolerating the new diet. This problem should be reported to the person-in-charge who may subsequently consult the dietician. Relatives and other visitors should be advised of the foods which are suitable and those which are unsuitable for the person receiving therapeutic diet.

### Guidance
- develop and maintain a good relationship with the client by explaining the purpose of the diet and helping him or her to cope
- monitor his or her progress regularly and report accurately in accordance with the care plan
- report to the person-in-charge if the person has difficulty in tolerating the diet
- check the person's bedside locker regularly to make sure that no unsuitable foods are either bought or brought in by visitors or relatives
- record certain aspects of the person's dietary requirement regularly, eg. weight
- ensure that the therapeutic diet is given only to the person for whom it has been specifically prescribed. It should never be used for anyone else.

## Serving the special diet

At meal times, the person-in-charge must make sure that every member of the care team know which clients or patients are on special diets. They should be persuaded to eat if necessary, and the staff should be asked to report if anyone does not. Food should be attractively served, and really hot or cold according to what it is. The staff should also know the patients or clients for whom fluid balance charts have to be recorded.

## Diabetic diet

The aim of a diabetic diet is to prevent excessive changes in blood sugar levels. It involves a controlled carbohydrate diet which is low in fat content and high in dietary fibre. Each client will have a diet specifically designed for his/her needs by a dietician. This will be an essential part of the treatment controlling the diabetes and clients/patients maintain this diet for life.

Careful control of the carbohydrate content which is necessary for normal daily activities should be maintained, and should:
- exclude simple sugars (glucose, sucrose) from the diet wherever possible
- reduce salt intake and moderate alcohol intake
- help client to lose weight if he/she is obese as weight reduction plays a crucial part in the control of diabetes. It appears to increase a diabetic's lifespan and may be valuable for helping the other conditions, such as hypertension that often go hand in hand with diabetes
- use artificial sweeteners in moderation and only as a part of a calorie-controlled reducing diet.

### Exercise and diabetes
Regular exercise should form part of everyone's daily routine. It can help to control this condition, by achieving an ideal body weight and reducing blood pressure and mental stress. The type of exercise advised for the elderly should be age-related and preferably prescribed by a physiotherapist.

## Guidelines for good health

In recent years, medical science has recognised the importance of manipulating the body chemistry to maintain good health, and to treat and prevent diseases. In 1983, the National Advisory Committee on Health Education in Britain highlighted the relationship between diet and health. It recommended a change in our national diet to ensure a more balanced approach to nutrients, in order to ensure a decrease in the number of diet-related illnesses.

The main recommendations include cutting down the fat intake from both animal and vegetables sources, and reducing high intakes of salt and alcohol. In order to maintain energy levels, it is important to increase the amount of carbohydrate in the diet from cereal-based products rather than from sugar or sugary foods. By following these guidelines, nutrients which are not beneficial are reduced but adequate supplies of protein, vitamins and minerals are maintained.

## Basic guidelines for a healthy diet

The following suggestions will help provide a balanced diet to maintain good health. We should:
- ensure a good daily intake of vegetables, especially green leafy vegetables, such as cabbage, broccoli
- ensure a good intake of fibre
- eat a varied and interesting diet
- take alcohol in moderation
- limit salt intake in cooking
- eat fresh foods and, whenever possible, avoid foods containing additives
- ensure a good but not excessive intake of protein-rich foods
- avoid being or becoming obese by eating excessively, especially of fatty foods
- take regular exercise
- do not smoke.

It is obvious that the role of diet is not simply limited to those who have diabetes or those with other medical diseases; we are all at risk from poor eating habits to some extent and benefit from using nutritional treatments in one way or another. Dietary treatments can be used in many common diseases and ailments, such as skin conditions — eczema, dermatitis, acne — to improve hair and nails and in pre-menstrual problems.

## References

Balmforth H (1992) *A Chef's Guide to Nutrition*. Cambridge University Press, Cambridge

Booth B (1990) Nutritional therapies. *Nurs Times* **89**(37): 44–46

Davidson S , Passmore R (1979) *Human Nutrition and Dietetics*. Churchill Livingstone, Edinburgh

Davies S , Stewart A (1989) *Nutritional Medicine*. Pan Books, London

Department of Health and Social Services Report (1979) *Eating for Health*. HMSO, London

Department of Health and Social Services Report (1969) *Report on Public Health and Medical Subjects*. No. 120. HMSO, London

Department of Health and Social Services (1979) *Report on Dietary Amounts of Food and Nutrients for Groups of People in the United Kingdom*. No. 15, HMSO, London

Maryon-Davies A ,Thomas J (1984) *Diet 2000*. Pan Books, London

McLaren DS (1981) *Nutrition and Its Disorders*. Churchill Livingstone, London

# Assignment

The purpose of this homework is to assist you in preparing for your Workbased Assessment of Competence. As there is no pressure on you, feel free to work at your own pace, but avoid the temptation to procrastinate. After you have read your notes and suggested references, submit your work for correction. The completed work becomes part of your Personal Portfolio.

## Therapeutic and special diets

1. Define the terms, and differentiate between therapeutic and special diets.
2. There are numerous reasons why people are prescribed special diets. List six of these diets and give possible reasons.
3. Describe your duty in making sure that these diets are correctly served.
4. What do you understand by 'special diet'? Give an example in which a special diet may be ordered, and your role in ensuring that the individual takes his/her diet as prescribed.

## Food Hygiene Act 1990

During 1989, there was a series of outbreaks of food poisoning linked with salmonella, listeria and botulism discovered in yoghurt, especially in the north west of England. The incidence was so alarming that the government set up the Richmond Committee to find out the cause of the outbreak. The mandate was very wide and covered the way food was produced, distributed, retailed, catered for, and handled in the home. The committee completed its task and in January 1991 the report became law.

The main aim of the Act is particularly concerned with the safety and quality of food people eat from the farm to the point at which it is served in restaurants. It makes it an offence to sell food that is unfit for human use or carry out business in unhygienic premises or in an environment where food is exposed to the risk of contamination. The main target area is restaurants and cafes because it is believed that caterers have more influence than most on the quality and safety of the food we eat. Under the Act, local authorities are given the responsibility for enforcing the law through their food examiners, and in England and Wales, food examiners include environmental health officers or trading standard officers. The main regulations featured in the Act are:

- registration of premises
- rights of appeal and compensation
- food hygiene training for food handlers.

### Registration

All premises used for food, including vehicles used for hot dogs and ice cream, are required to register. This also includes nursing and residential care homes. In order for local authorities to have an overview of food premises in the areas, registration is free and applications cannot be refused.

### Duties of food examiners

They have the power to enter any food premises to inspect the safety and quality of food being served. They are authorised to:

- inspect food to see whether it is safe for human consumption
- obtain specimens for bacteriological examination

- require improvements to be made to unhygienic premises
- ask a justice of the peace to condemn and close down any premises in extreme cases.

## Rights of appeal

The people affected by the action(s) of food examiners have the right to appeal and to seek compensation.

## Handling of food

### Food

This is defined under the Act as every item of food and drink, including milk or water or ingredients of food, such as gravy.

### Storage

It is believed that the risk of contracting food poisoning is increased if the process is not handled as recommended, especially in the area of care. The basic handling of food includes:

#### Cleanliness of environment
The kitchen must be kept clean including storage spaces, especially the refrigerator. All utensils that are used in the preparation of food should be capable of being cleaned, prevent absorption of liquid and the risk of contamination.

#### Cool
It is important that food should be stored below 5°C in the refrigerator. No food should be stored for more than 24 hours from the time it is brought into the area. In residential care homes, it is customary for residents to have a personal stock of food. They should be advised to keep food dated. Raw and cooked food must be kept in separate areas, and under no circumstances should raw meat, fish, poultry or eggs be stored in clients' rooms. Food should be kept covered and either refrigerated or served piping hot.

#### Wrapping
All food already prepared for eating must remain in its original wrapper and should be stored until the sell by or use by date. Once the food has been unwrapped and served, it must be consumed or disposed of if not used. Waste bins must be covered at all times with a well-fitted lid.

#### Covering
All food must be covered. Any food for individual use must be sealed and placed in a clean plastic box, and properly labelled with the person's name and date of preparation. Again, once the food is uncovered, it must be eaten or thrown away in a proper container.

#### Personal cleanliness
It is important to always maintain good personal hygiene. When serving food, hands should be washed and dried thoroughly both before and after the procedure. Cuts and sores should be covered with waterproof dressings, and clean disposable plastic aprons should be worn when handling open food. Hands should never come in contact with the food. There should be no smoking wherever food is served, and sneezing over food should be avoided. Ensure that wasted food is disposed of in appropriate containers with properly fitted lids.

#### First aid
It is a requirement that first aid materials should be readily available to food handlers.

#### Training
Everyone involved is required to attend a practical basic food hygiene course appropriate to their role. Some local authorities provide this training and issue certificates.

# References

Foodsense (1991) *A Guide for Carers and Employers. The Food Safety Act 1990.* Foodsense, London

Foodsense (1991) *The Food Safety Act and You: A Guide from HM Government.* Foodsense, London

## Audio visual aids

*Format: VHS video*

Ref: 259CT: *Food Free from Germs*
Ref: 301CT: *Clean Food*
Oxford Educational Resources Ltd

# Assignment

The purpose of this homework is to assist you in preparing for your Workbased Assessment of Competence. As there is no pressure on you, feel free to work at your own pace, but avoid the temptation to procrastinate. After you have read your notes and suggested references, submit your work for correction. The completed work becomes part of your Personal Portfolio.

## Food Hygiene Act 1990

1. Explain what you understand by the Food Hygiene Act 1990. Discuss your role within the Act.
2. Where could you find guidance on food hygiene and storage?
3. List certain precautions you would take when serving food to residents in your place of work. Include information about your own personal hygiene precautions.

# Diabetes

Diabetes is a disorder of the carbohydrate metabolism in which there is a deficiency of insulin. The actual cause is uncertain but it is believed that the disease affects the islets of Langerhans in the pancreas. Normally, sugar is absorbed from food in the intestine into the bloodstream and stored in the liver, where it can be used as energy. For the body to use this sugar, insulin converts it so that it can pass from the blood into the tissues of the body. In diabetes, the level of sugar in the blood is too high or too low, depending on the type of diabetes. Unless treated, it can become unstable and lead to sugar in the urine. This can cause:

- sugar to draw water into the urine, making the diabetic person want to urinate frequently throughout the day and night, as this extra water is lost, the body becomes dehydrated, causing the person to become extremely thirsty
- sugar in the urine increases the risk of high levels of bacteria and can lead to urinary infections.

## Types of diabetes

1. Diabetes mellitus — due to deficiency of insulin resulting in high blood sugar (hyperglycaemia) and altered fat and protein metabolism.
2. Diabetes insipidus — is marked by an increased flow of urine accompanied by extreme thirst.

*Signs and symptoms*

Clients may complain of:

- thirst, fatigue, itching skin (pruritus) and muscle cramp
- frequent micturation (polyuria) with sugar present and very often dialectic acid and acetone in the comatose stage
- lowered resistance to infection, serious especially in the young
- blurred vision, weight loss and the lowering of spirits (depression).

## Management of diabetes

The problem can be managed by any of the following ways and in various combinations:
- diet alone
- diet with insulin
- diet and tablets
- diet and weight control.

Whatever the form of treatment, it is important to remember that clients will always need a diabetic diet. Clients should have their own personal diet supplied by a dietician.

## Principles of care

The carer should:
- monitor client's intake and report any food not consumed
- encourage client to eat regular meals containing starchy foods, eg. bread, potato, pasta, rice and make sure that the client does not miss meals
- encourage intake of snacks between meals if recommended by the doctor, dietician or diabetes nurse; include age-related exercises
- cover client's cuts and scratches as diabetics heal slowly and are prone to infection
- give clients the opportunity to discuss and seek clarification on treatment and respect their views, wishes and rights
- advise the client on health issues regarding sweet and sugary food or drink
- report any change in activity or food intake, especially as insulin dosages may need to be altered to compensate for changes
- encourage clients to lose the extra weight and give appropriate information
- encourage clients to eat a wholemeal or high fibre food with each meal
- ensure that clothing and bed clothes do not impede blood circulation
- advise against diabetic products as they are expensive, not low calorie and some contain a sweetener called sorbitol which can cause diarrhoea. Diabetic squash and jams or marmalade may be taken
- provide good personal hygiene and good skin care
- persuade clients to avoid fat and fatty food, especially if overweight
- report any changes in the colour of the skin or temperature, or urinalysis
- provide clients with appropriate information to encourage independence
- encourage moderation in the intake of alcohol. Alcohol should never be taken on an empty stomach
- test urine for sugar (glucose), acetone and acetic acid as directed.

## Complications of diabetes

Complications may occur and the most common are:
- cataract and diabetic retinitis, boils and carbuncles
- painful neuritis, gangrene, diseases of the lungs with accompanying breathing difficulties.

## Hyperglycaemia (diabetic coma)

This is the result of too little insulin or too much sugar in the blood. It occurs when blood sugar levels are high and acidosis (inability of the body to excrete toxins) is present. Although the onset is gradual, this is a life threatening condition requiring immediate care.

*Early signs*
- increased micturation of urine
- abdominal pain, nausea, drowsiness.

*Later signs*
- heavy breathing, flushed face, breath smells of pear drops (acetone), dry skin
- loss of consciousness followed by death.

*Management*
- insulin is injected by a qualified nurse
- stay with the client and offer support
- observe and report any signs of abnormal symptoms immediately, eg. restlessness, struggling to breathe, excessive hunger.

## Hypoglycaemia

This is a condition in which blood sugar becomes too low resulting from too much insulin or too little sugar, especially if clients take insulin or diabetic tablets. There is a danger of insulin shock when clients:

- take more insulin than is needed
- miss or delay a meal or snack
- take strenuous exercise over and above their usual exercise
- do not eat enough starchy food
- take too much alcohol.

*Early signs*
The onset is very sudden and client may show signs of:
- shaking, trembling, confusion, tingling sensations, palpitations
- absent-mindedness or being argumentative
- lethargy, weakness, dizziness
- sweating, unconsciousness, leading to death.

*Management*
Observe and report any attacks of hypoglycaemia to the person-in-charge who should manage the problem in accordance with agreed prescribed treatment in the person's care plan. This should make the person feel better within a few minutes, after which he/she should either have:
- I cup of milk and a biscuit **or**
- 2 digestive biscuits **or**
- 2 slices of bread as a sandwich.

Alternatively, if it is time for the next meal, they should eat it straight away. If your clients frequently suffer from hypoglycaemia, their doctors should be notified. If a diabetic client taking insulin or diabetic tablets becomes ill, it is very important that they should not stop taking their medication. This is because illness, eg. influenza, diarrhoea, colds will cause a natural rise in blood sugar. Non-diabetic people can cope with this, but people with diabetes must continue with their medication.

# References

Faulkner A (1996) *Nursing: The Reflective Approach to Adult Nursing*. Chapman and Hall, London

McMaMahon C, Harding J (Eds.) (1993) *Knowledge to Care: A Handbook for Care Assistants*. Blackwell Scientific Publications, London

Robertson B (1992) *Study Guide for Health & Social Care Support Workers, NVQ in Care Level 2: Model 10*. First Class Books Inc, USA

## Audio visual aids

### Format: VHS video

Ref: CNE 7815: *Nursing Management of Diabetes in Adults*

Ref: CEAU802: *EMS Vitals: Diabetic Emergencies*

Oxford Educational Resources Ltd

# Assignment

The purpose of this homework is to assist you in preparing for your Workbased Assessment of Competence. As there is no pressure on you, feel free to work at your own pace, but avoid the temptation to procrastinate. After you have read your notes and suggested references, submit your work for correction. The completed work becomes part of your Personal Portfolio.

# Diabetes

1. What is 'diabetes'?
2. List four signs and symptoms of this disease.
3. Differentiate between diabetes mellitus and diabetes insipidus.
4. How would you know that an elderly person with diabetes is suffering from:
    a) hyperglycaemic coma?
    b) hypoglycaemic coma?
    c) discuss your role in the immediate management of these conditions.
5. Discuss how you would ensure that the client takes his or her diet.
6. What is the significance of testing a urine specimen from a person suffering from this condition?

# Unit 9
# Assist clients to access and use toilet facilities (Z11)

## Principles of elimination (Z11: 1-2)

Elimination is one of the activities of daily living which all individuals perform regularly throughout life. The process involves getting rid of body wastes for the body to function properly. During illness, the daily pattern of elimination changes and the person who is ill must seek help. For example, if a stroke causes paralysis of the left side of the body, some cultures, such as Muslims who only use the left hand to clean themselves, would need additional help. It is important to understand the process of elimination in order to provide effective care. We begin by looking at the characteristics of normal and abnormal body wastes known collectively as stools or faeces, and the basic anatomy of the alimentary system.

### Stools or faeces

These are waste matter excreted by the bowel and consisting mainly of food which has escaped digestion, bacteria (living or dead), water and indigestible cellulose.

### *Characteristics*
Stool varies in colour according to the diet. In starchy foods or a milk diet, it is light brown in colour, while stools from meat are usually a dark brown colour. Its consistency should be well-formed, firm, soft and cylindrical in shape to correspond with the intestine.

### *Amount*
The amount also varies with the diet but could be at least 150 grams to 250 grams (4ozs) daily. It could be as low as 50 grams daily in some elderly people with an unpleasant but not highly offensive odour under normal circumstances.

### Common abnormalities

### *Fluid motions*
Diarrhoea which varies in colour from light brown to green. The greenish colour is due to rapid passage of the faeces through the intestine so that bile has no time to act upon it.

### *Parasites*
Round worms, thread worms and segments of tape worms are found in infected cases.

### *Blood*
This may present as streaks or larger amounts which is, at times, bright red due to bleeding in the lower intestinal tract (colon and rectum). If bleeding is high up, eg. gastric ulcer, the blood is altered and becomes dark brown or black in appearance and is known as Melaena. At times, a similar appearance may be caused by excess fruit in the diet or if the client is taking an iron supplement.

### Pus
It is not commonly found in faeces but may be recognised as yellowish-white material, eg. in ruptured abscesses in the alimentary tract and some types of dysentery.

### Mucus
This may appear as a slimy jelly-like substance which mixes with stool, commonly seen in cases of constipation. At times, it may occur separately in the form of small masses.

### Hard
Hard and even dry motions are common if the client suffers from constipation. It has a lumpy appearance and is no longer cylindrical in shape.

## Mechanism of elimination

Defecation is the act of emptying faeces which accumulate in the rectum in sufficient bulk. In an infant, emptying the bowels happens automatically through the process known as *reflex action* when the rectum is distended. As the child grows older, he/she learns to control this process.

When the upper part of the rectum is distended, a conscious sensation is produced, and the person becomes aware of a desire to open the bowels. On reaching the lavatory, faeces in the rectum cause further distension and sets off another set of impulses and defecation begins voluntarily.

### The process is as follows:
- muscular walls of the rectum contract to form a moving contraction canal, and the muscles of the pelvic floor contract as well
- abdominal pressure is raised by holding the breath and contracting the diaphragm. The abdominal wall muscles contract, and the pressure inside the chest pushes down on the diaphragm
- the anal sphincter muscle relaxes and faeces are squeezed along the length of the rectum and out through the anus.

## Helping a client to eliminate

For some residents, the process does not occur voluntarily. Normally, the muscles in the walls of the rectum relax at the call to empty the rectum. If this is ignored, then the impulse ceases and the desire to defecate passes off. Persistent failure to respond to this natural process may result in the collection of faeces in the rectum and constipation.

When the person is taken to the lavatory, he or she may experience difficulty in emptying the rectum and will need help. Knowledge of how the act of elimination takes place could be useful in this instance.

### Guidance
- ensure that the client sits comfortably on the lavatory seat and explain the process
- provide privacy but discretely be available should your assistance be needed
- make sure that toilet roll and handwashing facilities are at hand
- instruct the person to breathe in, hold his or her breath for a few minutes, then push hard and, at the same time, breathe out silently
- ascertain and report on the outcome.

Hopefully, both the bowel and the bladder will open simultaneously in response to the psychological effect of turning on the cold water tap.

## Constipation

This is caused by an incomplete or infrequent action of the bowels and may result in the rectum filling with hard faeces.

### Characteristics

Most people consider themselves constipated if bowels are not opened at least once, twice or three times a day. Others may only have their bowels opened every third or fourth day, without any ill effects.

### Causes

- lack of absorbable fibre in the large bowel
- an intestinal obstruction
- absence of peristalsis as a result of weakness of intestinal muscles
- neglect of normal eliminating habit
- lack of exercise
- injury to the part of the brain that controls defecation.

### Signs and symptoms

- headache, nausea, vomiting, fatigue, lack of appetite (anorexia)
- indigestion, abdominal pain, distension, distress and rectal pain
- confusion, restlessness, wandering.

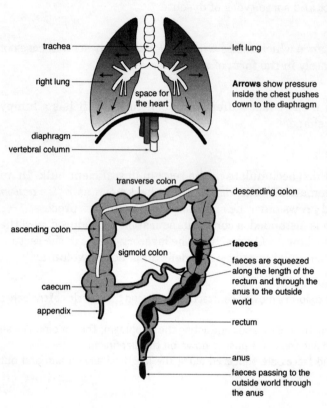

Diagram showing the act of defecation

### Management of the problem

*Intervention:*
This is based on a prior assessment of the person and a care plan should be designed to restore his or her normal eliminating habit, eg. enema, laxa- tives, suppositories, manual evacuation, habit training, exercise.

*Guidance*
- establish and maintain good interpersonal relationship skills
- assist in preparing and supporting the person during the procedure
- provide privacy, self-respect and dignity
- assist the person to walk to the toilet or transport them in a wheelchair or sani-chair. Help them from chair to toilet if necessary.

## Assist client to use facilities

Offer a bedpan or sani-chair if the person is in bed by adopting the following procedures:
- wash your hands, put on disposable apron and gloves and warm the bedpan
- explain the procedures to the client, arrange the bedclothes and ask the person to bend his or her knees by raising the hips. Assist if need be
- place the bedpan in position. If the person is unable to raise hips, roll him or her away from you, place and roll him or her onto the pan
- raise the person to a sitting position if possible, and cover him or her with a blanket
- place toilet roll and call bell within easy reach, and ask the person to signal when he or she finishes
- never leave a person on a bedpan for more than 10 minutes — observe unobtrusively as far as possible and ask if he or she needs help
- when the person has finished, remove and cover the bedpan immediately. Assist with wiping the anus if he or she is unable to perform this activity unaided
- provide the person with handwashing facilities as may be necessary
- examine the content of the bedpan for any abnormalities
- dispose of the waste matter by putting the bedpan in the washer, remove and dispose of any gloves and disposable aprons
- wash and dry your hands thoroughly.

### Bedpan
It is very difficult and embarrassing for people to use a bedpan in bed. The procedure should be carried out with sensitivity and in private to maintain client's self-respect and dignity.

### Bedside commode
Some people have the ability to get out of bed but cannot walk to the toilet. They may be offered a bedside commode, which is a chair with a hole in the seat and a bedpan below. It is used as a toilet, but the pan is removed and emptied after use.

## Evaluation of care

A successful outcome is when the person's normal bowel action returns. Continue to observe and report results and any abnormalities to the person-in-charge.

## Prevention of constipation

### Guidance
- ensure that the client eats a healthy diet as prescribed which includes dietary fibre, fruits and an adequate fluid intake
- assist in educating the individual to respond to the sensation of a full bowel and to do gentle exercises as often as possible
- respond in a sensitive way to the needs of clients when they call
- observe, record and report on the bowel function of clients
- staff should update their knowledge on current research findings on constipation.

# Diarrhoea

Changes from the normal bowel function may be caused by illness rather than the ageing process. Normally, the stool is soft and of a firm shape, of medium colour with a distinguishable odour. But at times some elderly people cannot control their bowel action because of the frequency with which semi-solid or liquid faecal matter is passed from the bowels. This condition is known as faecal incontinence or diarrhoea.

## Characteristic

Diarrohea is a frequent discharge of liquid stools from the bowels leading to the loss of a considerable amount of water, causing marked loss of potassium and weakness of the muscle. In severe cases, it may be accompanied by dehydration and the person suffers from exhaustion, embarrassment and needs skin cleansing and special protection. Sounds and odour of defecation may cause extreme embarrassment as will the frequency of asking for a bedpan or help to use the lavatory. The condition may also cause pain and severe wind from the large amount of gas suddenly produced. This may further embarrass the client.

## Causes

- food poisoning, eating indigestible food, a sudden change to high fibre diet
- psychological factors, eg. anxiety, fear, extreme nervousness
- some drugs, eg. antibiotics, excessive use of purgatives or laxatives
- alternating constipation and diarrhoea (faecal impaction with overflow).

## Management of the problem

This will be based on prior assessment of the problem, and designing a care plan to restore the person's normal bowel action. Methods may include fluid replacement, dietary supplements, maintenance of good personal hygiene and isolation with separate washing facilities.

### *Guidance*

- establish good interpersonal relationship with the person
- help to collect data, eg. frequency of the bowel action, vomiting, dry and cracked lips, formation of sores in a dirty mouth and dehydration, which may support the care plan
- provide privacy, self-respect and dignity. The client may be isolated in a room with his/her own washing facilities
- keep constant observation to ensure that isolation techniques are carried out and that the room is well ventilated and draught-free
- reassure the client; explain all the procedures of this type of care and seek his/her co-operation
- ensure that any diet supplements are taken as ordered by the dietician
- offer fruit drinks as prescribed, eg. four-hourly to keep the mouth clean, moist and fresh and to help the flow of saliva
- assist in maintaining a fluid balance chart with special attention to the frequency of stools
- give the client an opportunity to express personal views such as choice, and report any complaint of pain to the person-in-charge
- maintain good personal hygiene by following the same procedures as those in the use of bedpan
- wet soft toilet tissue and use it to clean the perianal area followed by application of a suitable soothing cream to alleviate any sores around the anal area
- treat pressure areas four-hourly if the client is nursed in bed
- encourage and promote gentle exercise according to his/her ability
- keep the skin clean and dry with particular attention given to skin creases
- encourage the client to change position as often as possible
- help to prevent the spread of infection by following procedures for disposal of contents of bedpans
- wear disposable gloves, gowns or protective aprons when in contact with client or faeces

- use and maintain a meticulous handwashing technique
- observe procedures for collecting specimens of faeces for laboratory examination
- be aware of procedures for control of cross-infection, eg. dealing with soiled linen, client's clothes.

**Diarrhoea** is a very distressing and embarrassing condition. It is, therefore, important to respond to the client's needs for personal care with sensitivity and great urgency.

## References

Flack M, Johnston M (1986) *Handbook for Care*. Beaconsfield Publishers Ltd, Bucks

Gidley C (1987) Now wash your hands. *Nurs Times* **83**(29): 41–42

Irvine ER (1986) *The Older patient. An Introduction to Geriatric Nursing*. Hodder and Stoughton, London

Roberts A (1991) Systems of life. The digestive system — Part 4. *Nurs Times* **87**(24): 61–64

Young P (1984) *Nursing the Aged*. Woodhead Faulkner Ltd, Cambridge

**Audio visual aid**

*Format: VHS video*
Ref: 73/5CT Part 5: *Anatomy and Physiology of Digestive System*
Oxford Educational Resources Ltd

## Assignment

The purpose of this homework is to assist you in preparing for your Workbased Assessment of Competence. As there is no pressure on you, feel free to work at your own pace, but avoid the temptation to procrastinate. After you have read your notes and suggested references, submit your work for correction. The completed work becomes part of your Personal Portfolio.

## Enable client to eliminate (Z11: 1–2)

1. Constipation is a problem which everyone, especially, the elderly experience.
    a) Discuss how you suspect that an elderly lady in your care is having a problem?
    b) List approaches which may be used to overcome this problem.
    c) State how you personally will help to prevent this problem, listing a variety of foods you know can help in resolving it.
2. Describe how you would assist a client who has difficulty in emptying his or her rectum while he/she is still sitting on the toilet.
3. Identify and list some causes of diarrhoea.
4. Discuss the precautions you would take, and observations you would make when removing a bedpan from a client with diarrhoea.

## Care of the bowels (Z11: 1–2)

When constipation occurs, the aim of treatment is to convert hard dry faecal matter into soft and easily evacuated stoolsl by introducing liquefying agents into the rectum. Various remedies may be used in the form of aperients and laxatives such as Fybogel, Isogel, lactitol, lactulose. The aim is to soften stools, add bulk or stimulate the bowel into action. But strong purgatives should be avoided.

Enemas and suppositories are well-known remedies which are initially prescribed by the doctor for the management of constipation. Thereafter, management of the problem becomes the responsibility of the nursing or caring staff.

## Enemas

This is an injection of fluid into the rectum to empty the bowels of faeces. The aim is to stimulate the bowel to empty.

### *Types of enema*

#### *Retention enema*

This enema which contains drugs in the fluid is aimed to have local effect on the bowel, eg.
- olive oil or arachis oil given to soften impacted or hard faeces
- barium enema: is an injection of barium sulphate into the rectum for X-ray examination
- cortisone enema for ulcerative colitis
- opiate, phosphate and other preparations.

#### *Evacuant enema*

This is an enema given to empty the rectum and relieve constipation, eg. disposable enema. An evacuant enema consists of either water or soap and water.

### *Purpose of enemas*

Enemas may be given to:
- empty the rectum of faeces and relieve abdominal distension due to flatus
- introduce drugs for local treatment, establish diagnosis and relieve retention of urine
- prepare the individual for an operation of the bowel.

### *Administration*

Normally the procedure is carried out by a professionally qualified person but care asisstants may be asked to help. The person carrying out the procedure should:
- warm the disposable enema pack in water of a temperature of 38°C for about 10 minutes
- check the temperature because if it is too hot it may scald or if too cold it may cause shock
- put on a disposable apron and/or gloves
- lubricate the nozzle of the disposable enema and insert into the anus for about three to four inches
- squeeze the solution slowly into the rectum by rolling the bag until it is empty
- remove the nozzle and discard the entire pack into a disposable bag. Wipe clean the anal region.

### *Equipment*

A tray or trolley may be used containing:
- desired pack, eg. disposable enema
- receiver or disposable bag, swabs, incontinence pad to protect the bed
- lubricant, eg. K-Y jelly
- bedpan and cover or sani-chair nearby
- a bowl of warm water at a temperature of 38°C.

### *Procedure*

#### *Guidance*
- prepare the client by forming a rapport with him or her

- explain the procedure and encourage the client to relax
- screen the bed and close windows as necessary
- place the client in the left lateral position with the buttocks close to the edge of bed
- make the client comfortable but do not expose him or her unnecessarily. Cover with a treatment blanket
- offer the client the use of an urinal as may be necessary
- take the tray or trolley to the client's room or bedside
- support and reassure the client during administration.

## After the administration

### Guidance

- encourage or allow the client to rest quietly in bed for about 15 minutes, and retain the enema as long as possible
- support the client, offer the use of a bedpan, sani-chair or accompany him or her to the lavatory
- observe and report on the result in relation to the presence of any abnormalities, eg. blood
- offer handwashing and drying facilities
- assist in clearing and putting away the equipment.

When an enema is given to relieve retention of urine, it is important to note the return and discover whether urine has been passed. For this purpose, the returned enema must be measured and compared with the quantity of enema given; unless evidence from another source is obtained, eg. confirmation by client that he or she has passed urine.

### Frequency of administration of enema

In some cases enemas may be repeated daily or on alternate days as may be necessary, until the rectum is empty — discovered by examination — and the client's normal bowel action is restored.

### Retention enema

Sometimes if the constipation is particularly stubborn, hard faeces may be softened by arachis oil, with an enema being given before the client retires to bed at night. This is followed with an evacuant enema in the morning.

### Special procedure

Before administration of an enema an attempt should be made to empty the rectum so that the enema will be retained. Oily enemas should be warmed before use.

## Suppositories

These are solid, cone-shaped substances inserted into the rectum to dissolve the hard faeces at body temperature. Common types are glycerine, Anusol, aminophylline and bisacodyl.

### Purpose

Suppositories are given to:
- relieve constipation
- soften hard, impacted faecal matter
- relieve broncho-spasm and chronic bronchitis
- provide soothing effects, such as local anaesthetic, astringent.

## Administration

In order to obtain maximum effect, suppositories should be inserted into one side of the faecal mass in contact with the rectal membrane.

## Equipment

- suppositories
- lubricant — K-Y jelly with swabs
- disposable finger stalls or right or left hand disposable gloves
- disposable apron
- a bowl with warm water, an incontinence pad and a disposable bag.

## Procedure

### Guidance

The client should be prepared as for the procedure for the administration of an enema. The person carrying out the procedure should:

- use a disposable apron, finger stall or left or right hand glove
- hold up the suppositories between the thumb and forefingers, smear with K-Y jelly or dip them in warm water to facilitate easy introduction into the rectum
- help the client to bear down in order to relax the anal sphincter
- insert the suppositories one at a time into the rectum, and as far up as possible into one side of the hard faeces, and in contact with mucous membrane of the bowel
- allow the client to rest quietly for about 15 minutes for the suppositories to dissolve
- accompany the client to the lavatory or offer the use of a bedside sani-chair or commode
- clear away, wash and return the equipment
- remove disposable apron, gloves or finger stall, wash and dry hands thoroughly
- report the result to the person-in-charge or record in the appropriate record.

## Observation

Following administration of enema and suppositories, the content of bedpan should be inspected and a report made on the characteristics of the result, eg. whether it was merely coloured fluid, contains particle of faeces or a 'good result'. The stool should be observed for any abnormalities of shape, colour, smell, blood or mucus. Care should be taken in emptying the bedpan to prevent the risk of infection.

## Reference

Irvine RE (ed) (1986) *The Older Patient — An Introduction to Geriatric Nursing.* Hodder and Stoughton, London: ch 19

### Audio visual aid

**Format: VHS video**
Ref: NT 18: *Giving Enema or Suppositories*
Oxford Educational Resources Ltd

## Assignment

The purpose of this homework is to assist you in preparing for your Workbased Assessment of competence. As there is no pressure on you, feel free to work at your own pace, but avoid the temptation to procrastinate. After you have read your notes and suggested references, submit your work for correction. The completed work becomes part of your Personal Portfolio.

## Care of the bowels (Z11: 1–2)

1. Discuss the role of care assistants in the care of a client with constipation before, during and after the administration of:
   a) an enema
   b) suppositories.
2. What equipment should the care assistant prepare before carrying out an enema?
3. Go through the report you would make to the person-in-charge on the outcome of the treatment.

## Promotion of continence (Z12: 1–2)

Many elderly people in care suffer from urinary incontinence, and it is estimated that the number of elderly people aged over 65 with regular urinary incontinence in an average health district of 250,000 population is 1040 (male) and 2640 (female) (Thomas *et al*, 1980). Generally, it is believed that it affects over three million people in the United Kingdom, and costs the National Health Service considerable sums of money each year trying to control the problem.

Incontinence, whenever one voids urine or faeces without control, is not a disease but a symptom that there is a problem that needs treatment: a problem that can only undermine dignity. It is a distressing condition which is sometimes known as 'the secret disability', because many sufferers are too ashamed and miserable to seek help or to talk about it.

### Effects of incontinence on the person

For some elderly people, their incontinence is not a new or recent occurrence; some have hidden it for years, and it is only revealed when they have required care for something else. For many elderly people, the loss of urinary control causes great embarrassment which results in:
- avoiding visiting friends for fear of leaving wet patches on chairs
- wearing dark clothes which makes dampness less noticeable
- stopping all sporting activities for fear of leakage
- avoiding outings for fear of a lack of public lavatories. Clients isolate themselves to avoid taking part in social activities because of the smell
- feeling ashamed about discussing the elimination of body wastes with other people
- denying that they are incontinent. In some cases soiled garments may be found hidden away in cupboards and drawers.

### Normal urinary system

In infancy, micturition is controlled by a spinal reflex and as the child grows older he or she acquires conscious control of the bladder. For most of the time good **bladder** control is an acceptable norm, and urine is passed four to six times a day.

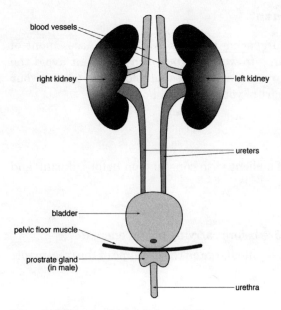

**A simple diagram of the urinary system**

If a person is continent, he/she will be able to store and pass urine at will in suitable places, and at convenient times. The bladder, being a muscular bag, acts as a reservoir of urine over a period of time, and as a pump during voiding to overcome the resistance in the urethra. It holds about two to three pints of urine, and while filling, the muscles around the urethra remain tightly closed. There are two shut off valves leading from the bladder that are helped by the surrounding pelvic floor muscles to keep the urine in the bladder. As a result, a person can comfortably manage without emptying the bladder for several hours.

When the bladder is full, nerve impulses from the stretched bladder travel to the brain. If the brain is satisfied that the person is in a suitable place to pass urine, the bladder muscles relax and release the urine down the urethra. At this stage the person voluntarily tightens up the pelvic floor muscles. In some people the normal control of the bladder is lost, and they become incontinent.

## Types of incontinence

There are many types of incontinence but the most common are:
- **Stress**: more common in women aged 45–60 than in men, as a result of childbirth. A slight leakage of urine on laughing, crying, sneezing, or similar exertion.

Causes: weakness of the sphincter pressure, putting pressure on the bladder. The valves fail to close and urine leaks out.

Management: pelvic floor exercises, electrical stimulation of the bladder muscles by a physiotherapist.

- **Overflow**: common in men aged 55 and over, due to an enlarged prostate gland. The pressure in the bladder exceeds the urethral resistance causing a small, regular escape of urine with incomplete micturation.

Causes: pressure on the sphincter, urethra obstruction, fibrosis of the bladder neck in women, spinal injury or damage, impacted faeces, infection, illness accompanied by dementia, diabetes.

Management: surgery, catheterisation and a check may be made for diabetes.

## Other contributing factors:

Other factors which may contribute to incontinence are:

### Physical:
- injury to the urinary tract
- obstruction of the urethra in either sex
- brain damage such as cerebrovascular accident (CVA), tumour, dementia

- acute urinary tract infections causing irritation of the walls of the bladder (cystitis). Also bladder stones (calculi)
- acute illness such as pneumonia, fevers, cardiac failure, diabetes
- constipation, obesity, impacted faeces
- reduced mobility due to arthritis, haemiplegia, painful feet, bunions
- drugs, especially night sedation, major tranquillisers, diuretics and those causing constipation, eg. analgesics.

*Psychological:*
- anxiety, depression, fear, stress, confusion.

*Social:*
- due to the effects of ageing, control of the bladder muscle decreases, resulting in a wasting of the lining of the urethra in both men and women. However, the ageing process alone, does not cause incontinence
- the need to pass urine more frequently, made worse by cold weather
- clothes, due to difficulty in adjusting or removing them, eg. trousers
- excessive use of alcohol.

*Environmental:*
- sudden change in environment, such as admission to hospital or a home
- unfamiliar routine
- lavatories: difficult to use because of unpleasant smells, cold, dirty, difficult to find, inconsistent supply of soft toilet paper
- institutional: helpers' attitudes may exacerbate incontinence

## Promoting continence

### 1. Assessment

The assessment process involves the collection and analysis of information to identify client's specific care needs by members of the care team, who will subsequently formulate a care plan. Direct questions should be asked about: the type and severity of urinary symptoms, how often the client passes urine during the day and night and whether there is any warning or accidents on the way to the toilet. Although doctors will frequently carry out medical examination in support of these observations, the whole team should acquire the skills to make basic observations and assessment.

### 2. Planning of care

The care plan should consider methods for managing the problem which include the following, dependent on the ability of the person to participate in his or her care:
- pelvic floor exercises usually supervised and recommended by the physiotherapist
- bladder training regime
- catherisation (intermittent or continuous).

It should also establish:
- good rapport with sensitivity to client's needs
- care of any underlying problem, eg. constipation, impacted faeces
- availability of adequate toilet facilities, eg. urinals, bed pans, commodes, extra handrails, walking aids, raised toilet seats
- education and training of the clients in a settled way of behaviour by constant prompting (habit training and behaviour modification)
- needs of newly admitted clients
- prevention of constipation with the provision of a high fibre diet with adequate fluid intake of about three–five pints (1.5–3 litres, or 8 cups) per day.

## 3. Implementation of care

Bladder training is the most popular method and relates to the use of a specified and established regime. The home should provide a local policy for management of care.

### *Guidance*
- maintain good interpersonal relationships with clients showing sensitivity to their needs for privacy, self-respect and dignity. Be familiar with local policy for management of care
- provide a relaxed environment without unnecessary intrusion
- encourage clients to use normal toilet facilities as far as possible rather than bedpans or commodes except perhaps at night
- encourage regular routine lavatory visits or provision of facilities, eg. two–three hourly during the day. At night make sure that facilities are easily accessible and encourage four-hourly visits to the lavatory despite the state of 'dryness' or 'wetness' of those who wet the bed
- provide regular skin care, wash and pat dry. Check skin regularly for redness, evidence of sores or weeping areas
- clean the client carefully and supply fresh nightwear or clothes whenever necessary
- encourage sufficient fluid intake according to the care plan. Offer a last drink two–three hours before bedtime. Maintain a fluid balance chart
- encourage recommended high fibre diet to prevent constipation
- provide ladies with a fuller skirt rather than trousers, and stockings instead of tights. For men, trousers with a long velcro fastening
- change soiled beds or clothing immediately, taking precautions to prevent the spread of infection
- observe and report on signs of clients' discomfort when they are wearing special sheaths
- be aware of the routine care of indwelling catheters for drainage.

### *The use of special clothing, waterproof pads and pants*
- loose and easily accessible waterproof dresses; stockings for ladies, trousers with velcro instead of a zip or buttons for men
- sanitary pads and waterproof pants, eg. marsupial pants with a pouch. Pants, eg. Pampers® standard incontinence pads (Incopads®) are difficult to place under the client and may leak from the unsealed edges. 'Kyle®' washable drawsheets are comfortable and can absorb volumes of water
- sheaths should be fitted over the penis, held on by an adhesive strap and drained into a bag — observe for any discomfort
- long-term or intermittent catheterisation using the smallest possible diameter (16 or 18FG — French Gauge®) or 'Foley's®' catheter
- laundry facilities with provision for changing and rinsing wet clothes, and a linen store, in accordance with organisational policy
- social and recreational activities to prevent boredom
- smell: neutralising deodorant (Nilodor) can be used in appliances
- colour coding, if any, to identify the doors of toilets as part of reality-orientation programme.

## 4. Evaluation of care

This is the final stage of individualised client care plans and involves continuous monitoring of care, to assess the progress or lack of it. It must be remembered that one of the most important factors influencing the promotion of continence is staff attitude and promptness in responding to the needs of clients.

A good individualised care programme can substantially reduce the incidence of incontinence which becomes more common if staff expect it. The current practice in some care establishments is to place the standard incontinence pad under the person in an attempt to protect the bed or chair. This is not generally accepted because of the effects on a person's appearance, ability to move, and self-esteem. The environment should receive special attention and must be free from the unpleasant odour of stale urine. A high standard of personal hygiene and prevention of infection is of paramount importance.

# References

Cheater F (1991) Continence training programme. *Nurs Stand* **6**(8): 24–27

Coloplast Limited (1992): *Objective Continence: A Model for the Promotion of Continence.* Coloplast Ltd, Cambridge

Coloplast Limited (1992): *A Pharmacist's Guide to Continence Care.* Coloplast Ltd, Cambridge

Department of Health (1991) *An Agenda for Action on Continence Services.* HMSO, London

Flack M, Johnson M (1986) *Handbook for Care.* Beaconsfield Publishers Ltd, Bucks

Irvine RE (1986) *Continence and Bladder Problems.* Hodder and Stoughton, London: chs 17, 18

Nursing Times (1996) *The NT Guide to Urinary Continence Assessment.* Macmillan Magazines, London

Norton C (ed) (1996) *Nursing for Continence,* 2nd edn. Beaconsfield Publishers Ltd, Bucks

Roberts A (1989) Systems of life: urinary incontinence 1–2: *Nurs Times Systems of Life* 170, 171: *Senior Systems* 35, 36(85), 15, 19. April 12 and May 10, 1989 (respectively)

Thomas TM *et al* (1980) Prevalence of urinary incontinence. *Br Med J* **281**: 1243–1245

Tobin GW (1992) *Incontinence in the Elderly.* Edward Arnold, London

### Audio visual aids

*Format: VHS video*

Ref: 400/1-2 CT: *The Management of Incontinence* (and in cassette tape)

Ref: 198/1CT: *Prevention of Urinary Infection*

Ref: 406: *Incontinence — It Doesn't Have to be a Problem*

Ref: CME 9102: *Approach to Urinary Incontinence in the Elderly*

Oxford Educational Resources Ltd

# Assignment

The purpose of this homework is to assist you in preparing for your Workbased Assessment of Competence. As there is no pressure on you, feel free to work at your own pace, but avoid the temptation to procrastinate. After you have read your notes and suggested references, submit your work for correction. The completed work becomes part of your Personal Portfolio.

## Promotion of continence (Z12: 1–2)

1. What is incontinence?
2. What factors could contribute to this condition?
3. Discuss the procedure for managing this problem in your area of work.
4. What do you think could be the effects of this problem on the individual and his or her family?

## Care of catheter and drainage bags (Z12.2)

It is recognised that all clients with catheters are at risk of urinary tract infection. The organisms causing the infection may spread from the infected urinary tract into the blood, producing serious blood poisoning (septicaemia). The care of the catheter and the drainage bag is a crucial part of total care of people with incontinence. The course of standards and practice for care of the drainage system must be based on informed evidence, supported by the local policy. As a rule, professionally qualified practitioners are responsible for total client care, assisted by care assistants.

### Catheter

A catheter is a hollow, soft tube which is passed up the urethra into the bladder. The balloon end of the indwelling urethral catheter is filled with sterile water through the valve, to keep it in position in order to drain urine continuously from the bladder into a collecting drainage bag.

#### Changing the catheter

The need to change indwelling catheters depends on individual clients, as quite often the inside of catheters become packed with deposits which may affect the flow of urine. It is, therefore, necessary for a care plan to indicate the frequency with which a catheter needs to be changed. The procedure should be carried out with great sensitivity in order to maintain the client's privacy, self-respect and dignity, and in accordance with local policy for care of catheters.

#### Procedure

The staff carrying out the procedure should:
- be familiar with local policy for changing the catheter
- wash and dry their hands before and after handling the drainage system
- clean the urethral meatus (area where the catheter enters the body) daily using a warm soapy flannel and then dry the thigh thoroughly
- wash and wipe dry thoroughly the length of the catheter, away from the body down to the tube and connection bag
- remove any dried secretions that have collected on the catheter
- empty the urinary bag before bathing or showering, but leave the bag attached to the catheter
- arrange the catheter in such a way that the client does not sit on it.

### The drainage bag

There are a wide variety of urine drainage bags to choose from. The most commonly used are the body-worn appliances which drain the urine into a collecting bag. Their suitability depends upon size, urine output and where the clients want to wear them, eg. thigh for women and calf for men. Bags may be worn on the thigh or calf using:
- leg straps
- a holster suspended from a waist-belt
- a waist-belt
- knickers with a pocket to hold the bag.

#### Emptying the drainage bag

The bag is changed when it is full and becomes uncomfortable, pulling on the catheter. It must be constantly observed to prevent an overflow which may siphon the urine back into the bladder, causing great pain and discomfort. Its weight should not be pulling down on the urethral area. The process requires the use of a special aseptic technique in order to avoid introduction of infection. Be aware of local policy for changing of urinary drainage bag. In most cases, this is the responsibility of professionally qualified staff.

## Procedure
The staff carrying out the procedure should:
- be familiar with local policy for changing the urinary drainage bag
- wash and dry their hands thoroughly
- open the tap and empty all the urine into the toilet. Note the amount
- close the tap and wipe it dry with a clean tissue or toilet paper to remove excess urine, and dispose of this in the toilet
- avoid touching the tap with hands or other objects or items of clothing.

If the client cannot go to the toilet, a container (bedpan, urinal, a measuring jug etc) may be used. But ensure that the urine is disposed of in the toilet and the container is treated in accordance with routine practice and policy.

## Changing the drainage bag
This is carried out arbitrarily. Some people leave the bag connected to the catheter for seven days, and others change it after three days because it is wearing out or starting to smell. In either case, the procedure should be carried out under aseptic conditions, in accordance with local policy.

## Procedure
The staff carrying out the procedure should:
- wash and dry their hands thoroughly
- put on a disposable plastic apron and a pair of sterile gloves
- avoid touching the ends of any connecting tubing
- pinch or clamp the ends of the catheter using the thumb and forefingers
- remove the protective cap from the new bag and immediately insert the new drainage bag tube into the catheter
- replace the protective cap onto the old bag
- secure the new bag using the chosen method of support
- empty urine from the used drainage bag into the toilet
- dispose of the used empty drainage bag according to local arrangement for the collection of soiled dressings, catheters and drainage bags
- never put used drainage bags down the toilet
- remove disposable apron and gloves
- wash and dry hands thoroughly.

## Attachment of a night drainage bag

A two-litre bag may be attached to the tap on the leg bag using a connector. This practice maintains a closed system and prevents interruption of sleep during emptying of a leg bag.

## Procedure
The staff carrying out the procedure should:
- be familiar with local policy for handling the night drainage bag
- wash and dry their hands thoroughly
- insert the tap of the leg bag into the clean connector and the two-litre bag for night use
- open the tap on the leg bag and drain the urine into the larger bag to ensure that the system is working efficiently

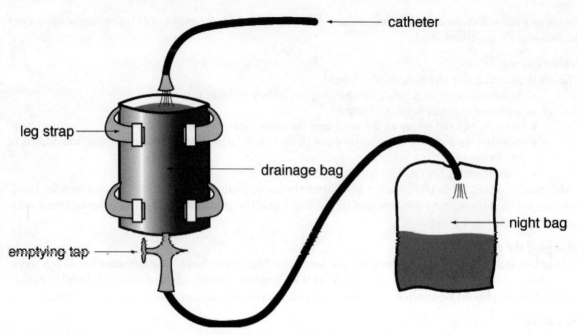

**A simple diagram showing a urine drainage system**

- attach the two-litre bag to the frame or stand of individual choice
- wash and dry hands thoroughly.

### Removal of the night drainage bag

*Procedure*

On getting out of bed the client should:
- wash and dry hands thoroughly
- close the tap of the leg bag
- disconnect the connector and the two-litre night drainage bag
- note the amount and empty urine into the toilet
- wash and dry hands thoroughly.

## Management of specific problems

### *Guidance*
- observe and report to the person-in-charge who may undertake the following measures.

| Problems | Action |
|---|---|
| Blockage of catheter | 1. Encourage client to change position or walk around |
| | 2. Encourage liberal fluid intake |
| Urine leaks | 1. Ensure that the catheter is not kinked or being sat on |
| | 2. Ensure that the catheter is not blocked and urine is draining into the bag |
| | 3. Check for a gap between the catheter and the body |
| Client complains of pain and discomfort | 1. Talk to the client and try to establish the cause |
| | 2. Check that the catheter is in position and draining well |
| | 3. Encourage the client to change position or walk about or do a gentle exercise according to his/her ability |

## Role of care assistants

The care of catheter and drainage bag is the responsibility of the person-in-charge, and may be delegated to experienced and competent staff. If this is so, they should demonstrate knowledge of local policy and information contained in the care plan. The following suggestions may be helpful.

### *Guidance*
- promote and maintain good interpersonal relationships
- maintain and assist clients to good standards of basic personal hygiene
- ensure that there are no kinks in the tubing
- keep the drainage bag below the level of the bladder
- ensure optimum drainage by maintaining the catheter in the correct upright position either on a stand or supported on the thigh or calf
- report to the person-in-charge if any of the following is observed:
  - *catcher falls out*
  - *urine is not being drained*
  - *client complains of persistent pain*
  - *a rise in temperature (fever)*
  - *blood in urine (haematuria)*
- encourage the client to perform pelvic floor exercises regularly
- encourage the client to take regular exercise
- ensure that the client takes adequate nourishment and recommended fibre in his/her diet
- encourage a liberal intake of fluid
- protect the client from unnecessary embarrassment when carrying out the procedure
- observe and report on any redness or broken skin and unpleasant body odour
- try and reassure the client at all times.

## References

Clifford C (1982) *Bacteriuria — A Possible Consequence of Urinary Tract Infection*. Proceedings of the Conference organised by the Nursing Practice Research Unit at Northwick Park Hospital, London

Glenister H (1987) The passage of infection. *Nurs Times* **83**(22): 68–73

Gould D (1994) Keeping on tract: infection control, urinary tract. *Nurs Times* **90**(5): 58–64

Roe B (1990) *Catheter Care: A Guide for Users and Their Carers*. HG Wallace Ltd, Essex

### Audio visual aids

*Format: VHS video*
*Beware of the Urinary Catheter*
Ref: PYR77: *Clean Intermittent Catheterization*
Oxford Educational Resources Ltd

## Assignment

The purpose of this homework is to assist you in preparing for your Workbased Assessment of Competence. As there is no pressure on you, feel free to work at your own pace, but avoid the temptation to procrastinate. After you have read your notes and suggested references, submit your work for correction. The completed work becomes part of your Personal Portfolio.

### Care of catheter and drainage bags (Z12.2)

A 78-year-old gentleman has an indwelling catheter and a drainage bag *in situ*. Discuss the role of care assistants in relation to:

a) Keeping the urinary catheter clean.
b) Care of the drainage bag.
c) Personal cleanliness; bathing or showering of the client.
d) General mobility of the person.
e) Maintaining self-respect and dignity of the person.
f) Encouraging the client to help with the care of the equipment.

# Unit 10
# Assist clients with personal hygiene and appearance (Z9)

## Personal grooming and dressing (Z9: 1–2)

One of the most important aspects of individualised client care, is a knowledge of the grooming and dressing habits that form part of an individual's lifestyle. The aim of personal cleanliness is to promote good health, refresh the individual and contribute to his or her overall comfort and morale. Over the years, substances for cleansing the skin, hair, mouth and teeth have been refined and as a result people spend large sums of money to maintain their personal appearance, ie. creams which claim to rejuvenate ageing skin. *The Express,* January 14, 1997 reported, 'A fresh complexion on ageing for £5' an 'intelligent anti-ageing cream which is set to shake up the cosmetics industry'. Even clothes have undergone changes in style and fashion, and some people will only wear expensive designer clothes.

### Grooming

This is the habit of ensuring a tidy, smart and fresh appearance. The mouth and nose have a natural flora of bacteria which may cause infections. The skin perspires and produces oily substances called sebum. To avoid unpleasant body odour clinging to clothes, especially underwear and socks these should be changed and washed frequently. Encouraging clients in habits of cleanliness helps them to express their individual rights for choice, self-respect and dignity. When illness causes declining physical and mental ability, some clients lose interest in their personal grooming and dress, and expect carers to maintain their hygiene routines. This may be carried out until the person is well enough to resume responsibility for his or her own appearance.

### Dressing

The way people dress is a means of non-verbal communication, and a powerful tool for expressing and preserving the individual's personality. Dress can signify the ethnic origin of the person, the organisation or professional groups to which they belong. It can also indicate the level of income, social status, personal preference, style and attitudes of a person. It is an important part of a general care plan. People take pride in being well-dressed, and clothes express their personality, especially when chosen for special occasions. Wearing their own clothes is a most powerful way for a client to preserve his or her individuality. Well-dressed clients and their relatives are more likely to be content.

### Factors influencing personal grooming and dressing

An assessment of the individual ability to carry out personal grooming and dressing on a daily basis needs to be made. This should include how the person prefers to look and his/her choice of clothes, ie. casual or formal. Some people like to maintain their appearance and lifestyle by wearing more

stylish clothes on special occasions, such as birthdays and visiting times. The following factors control and influence how individuals groom and dress themselves:
- personal beliefs, preferences, culture, custom and tradition
- choice — availability and cost of clothes, and how these are laundered
- style and fashion: these may be influenced by special occasions or suitability for weather conditions
- standard of cleanliness: the frequency with which clothes and footwear are changed. If a client suffers excessive body odour, he/she should be encouraged to change underwear, socks, stockings etc more frequently.

### Promotion of personal grooming
This is based on a holistic approach to care and the care plan should be designed to identify specific areas in which clients can be encouraged to assume responsibility for their personal grooming and dressing. The client will need support in the use of prostheses and dressing equipment.

#### *Guidance*
- maintain good interpersonal relationships with clients and others concerned
- encourage the client to wear personal clothes to boost his or her morale, self-respect and dignity
- offer clients an opportunity to see and choose from a variety of clothes to suit their personality in relation to style, colours and fashion
- complete toileting and washing before dressing and undressing
- allow the client sufficient time to dress in the privacy of his or her room without haste
- assist where necessary in fastening zips, buttons, belts and other fastenings
- encourage frequent change of clothes, especially those which are worn next to the skin, eg. pants, vests
- ensure that he or she has adequate storage space and laundry facilities
- provide matching clothes, eg. matching tops and bottoms of pyjamas at night
- ensure that he or she has the use of adapted clothing and dressing aids if these are necessary
- ensure that the client has suitable footwear and assist in putting them on if necessary. A footrest or stool and a shoehorn may be useful
- assist helpless clients to dress themselves by putting out their clothes in the proper order. They may need help with underwear, trousers, stockings and shoes
- encourage clients who like to wear their costume jewellery to do so, although expensive items may pose a security problem.

### Condition of the skin

**Washing** Personal cleansing should normally be carried out independently on a daily basis and in private, unless help is absolutely necessary. Most able clients care for their skin by washing with soap and water, rinsing and drying thoroughly, night and morning. This can be an 'all over' wash using a basin of water or immersion in a bath or shower. A care plan should identify individual clients who need to wash in bed, and a bowl of water should be placed within easy reach on a suitable bed table (cantilever), together with other washing aids.

#### *Guidance*
- examine and report on the condition of the skin its colour, any scars, blemishes or tattoos
- look for signs of dryness, chafing, soreness, redness, a break in the skin. Report if the client complains of extreme irritation, if there is burrowing under the skin, scratches which may lead to infection, acne, bruising, discoloration, moist or wrinkled skin and extreme perspiration. Also note any deformity or sores.

*Female*
The moist membrane in the perineal (genital) areas should receive special attention and so should the folds of skin under the breasts. These areas usually become tender, sore and red if not properly washed, rinsed and dried. Report any sign of soreness.

*Male*
Pay special care to the genital area. If he is not circumcised, gently retract the foreskin, wash with a soapy flannel, rinse and dry thoroughly before replacing the foreskin. Talcum powder, cream or deodorants may be used according to the personal preference of the client. Report any sign of redness.

**Handwashing** Regular washing of hands contributes to the comfort of the elderly person. Every client should be encouraged to wash and dry their hands thoroughly before meals and after visiting the toilet. If handwashing before a meal is not possible, the use of finger wipes should be encouraged. It should be remembered that frequent removal of the skin's natural oily secretion (sebum) may cause chafing and broken skin leading to infection. Emollient hand cream or a suitable hand cream may be applied after adequate drying.

**Hair** There are about 100,000 hairs on the scalp and a person may loose about 80–100 a month through combing. It grows about 1 mm in three days, loses its original colour and becomes grey or white. Hair becomes thinner and more brittle. Baldness and an increase of facial hair may occur in some women due to reduced oestrogen after the menopause. An attractive hairstyle is a morale booster at any age, and great care must be taken to help clients to always look their best. A professional hairdresser should visit the home regularly as some clients may wish to pay for the service. Male clients should be encouraged to shave themselves if possible in order to maintain their self-respect, dignity and independence.

### Guidance
- encourage the client to brush and comb his or her hair twice a day according to his or her lifestyle, and offer the use of a hand mirror during this procedure. Some people of African origins would like their hair combed carefully otherwise it could break
- some hair is particularly brittle so use oils or lotions to keep it in good condition
- wash and set the hair preferably once a week according to the client's personal preference, using an appropriate shampoo to keep the scalp free from dandruff
- report the client's needs for a hairdressing service. Never cut the client's hair but do examine its condition regularly and report on:
    - any extreme irritation or scratching
    - sores and infection of the scalp, any signs of matted hair, broken scalp, dandruff or lice
- shave male clients with an electric razor and apply either pre or after shaving lotions according to his wishes
- help those with beards and moustaches to wash and trim them regularly
- encourage female clients to have their hair set periodically, especially on special occasions, such as their birthdays
- ensure that female clients with facial hair receive regular attention. Suitable cream may also be used to remove unwanted hair
- keep individual combs and brushes clean and do not use them on other people
- encourage male clients to wash and shave themselves and clean their own teeth or dentures.

**Nails (hands and feet)** Keep clean and cut every week. The best time is after a bath when the nails have been softened by hot water.

### Guidance
- soak nails and remove any obvious dirt with a blunt instrument before using a nail brush
- wash and dry feet thoroughly and sprinkle talcum powder according to the client's wishes
- examine between the toes and report any sign of blisters, corns or verrucas
- apply cuticle cream after washing and drying to prevent ragged cuticles
- cut fingernails according to the shape of the fingers in a rounded fashion. Some female clients wear false fingernails and care should be taken in cutting these nails and applying nail vanish in accordance with the individual's wishes.
- trim toenails straight across with appropriate nail clippers and file to prevent in-growing toenails. This is best carried out after a bath. In most cases, especially with diabetes, toenails are best treated by the podiatrist (chiropodist)
- encourage clients to change their socks and stockings frequently, especially in hot weather.

**Shaving** This is an individual choice and many male clients do prefer a clean-shaven face. Many women like to shave their legs and armpits. Shave after bathing when the skin is soft, or use a warm face flannel to soften the skin.

### Guidance
- wash and dry your hands thoroughly
- explain the procedure and what you are going to do and seek the client's co-operation
- use the client's personal shaving equipment, eg. razor, towel and face flannel
- encourage the person to wash his face and apply shaving cream, hold the skin taut
- shave male clients with an electric razor and apply either pre or after shaving lotions according to the client's preference. Some people may prefer a wet shave; provide them with the appropriate equipment
- shave in the direction of the hair growth and wipe the face with a warm face flannel
- apply after-shave lotion as required and make the client comfortable
- clear, wash and put away the equipment
- wash and dry your hands thoroughly
- observe and report any skin rashes to the person-in-charge.

## References

Faulkner A (1996) *Nursing: The Reflective Approach to Adult Nursing Practice*. Chapman and Hall, London

Roper N, Logan WW, Tierney A (1985) *The Elements of Nursing*. Churchill Livingstone, Edinburgh

Flack M, Johnson M (1986) *Handbook for Care. Practical Guidelines for Care Assistants and Nursing Auxiliaries*. Beaconsfield Publishers Ltd, Bucks

**Audio visual aid**

***Format: VHS video***
Ref: NT6: *Personal Hygiene*
Oxford Educational Resources Ltd

# Care of face, ears, eyes and prosthesis (Z9: 1–2)

The face and eyes are called the mirror of the body and reflect a person's personality. As people grow older, subtle changes become evident, such as a sharpening of features. Eyes may lack their former sparkle due to the ageing process, and the altered shape of the jaws makes it harder to wear dentures comfortably. It is necessary to ensure that frequent attention is paid to clients' faces and eyes.

## The face

The wizened and shrunken appearance of the face is due partly to loss of subcutaneous fat and partly to the degeneration of facial bones.

### Guidance
- encourage clients to wash their faces with soap, water and a facecloth according to their individual cleansing regimes and to dry thoroughly
- assist them to wash behind their ears and in corners of their noses
- help female clients to use face creams and other cosmetic preparations according to individual preference and style. Also encourage the use of suitable cleansing creams and moisturisers
- observe and report any signs of chafing, spots or breaks in the skin
- encourage female clients to use their normal cosmetics. Some may benefit from beauty therapy and manicure services.

## The eyes

The eyes should be treated with care and attention. Any abnormalities, such as redness of the eyelids and irritation must be reported. At times there may be discharges which may cause the eyelids to stick together, an indication of the onset of infection. The person-in-charge may take and send a swab specimen for pathological investigation.

## Action plan

### Guidance
- encourage clients to wash their eyes daily with soapy flannel or towel, and to avoid excessive rubbing when drying the eyes
- observe and report any redness of the skin around the eye, or any swelling. If a discharge is present, a specimen swab will be taken and sent for laboratory examination
- report if the eyelids are stuck together. Gently dab the affected eye with a swab soaked in normal saline and leave to dissolve the dried sticky discharge. Clean the eye gently wiping from the bridge of the nose to the temple. Discard the swab. Repeat the process until the discharge is removed
- use a dry swab to dry the eye and wash and dry your hands thoroughly afterwards.

## The ears

These are organs of hearing and consist of the external ear — the pinna and auditory canal, the middle ear and the internal ear. Some clients may have problems with hearing, due to an excessive build up of wax. Some may also have discharging ears as a result of infection.

### Guidance
- encourage clients to wash the outer ear with their own face cloths or cotton wool swabs
- look into the outer ear for signs of wax and discharge and report your observation to the person-in-charge. Excessive build up of wax may need syringing out by a doctor or trained nurse

- advise the person to avoid rubbing the affected ear as a swab specimen may be taken for laboratory examination
- ensure that the affected ear is thoroughly mopped up if drops to soften the wax are inserted
- encourage clients to wear their hearing aids.

## Prosthesis

This is the fitting of artificial parts to the body, such as an arm, leg, dentures, eyes or breast. Those used as mobility or sensory devices require special care to ensure that they are well-looked after and are working properly. The care of specific prosthesis has been dealt with in other sections, see care of the dentures, artificial eyes.

### *Guidance*
- know the correct way to use a device before helping a client to use it
- make sure the person knows how to use the device. Mark it with the person's name in an obtrusive way
- inspect the device regularly, before and after use, making sure that it is in good condition
- keep the equipment within easy reach of the person
- check for any physical problems that might develop with use, such as pinching, swelling, rubbing, sore spots
- keep the device clean in accordance with the manufacturer's recommendations
- encourage other staff to help with care of devices if they are able and to report any fault.

## References

McMahon RCA, Harding J (1993) *Knowledge to Care: A Handbook for Care Assistants*. Blackwell Scientific Publications, London

Robertson B (1992) *Study Guide for Health and Social Care Support Workers: NVQ in Care Level 2*. First Class Books Inc, USA

## Audio visual aids

### *Format: VHS video*
Ref: 77C/059A: *Ingrowing Toe Nail* (live video action)
Ref: 251/1-2CT: *Rehabilitation of Bilateral Amputee* (cassette tape)
Oxford Educational Resources Ltd

# Assignment

The purpose of this homework is to assist you in preparing for your Workbased Assessment of Competence. As there is no pressure on you, feel free to work at your own pace, but avoid the temptation to procrastinate. After you have read your notes and suggested references, submit your work for correction. The completed work becomes part of your Personal Portfolio.

## Personal grooming and dressing (Z9: 1–2)

1. Discuss the nature and purpose of grooming and dressing, and how you would help elderly people to care for their general appearance and lifestyle.
2. How would you help elderly people to maintain their personal appearance with attention to their:
   (a) clothes?
   (b) face?
   (c) ears?
   (d) hair?
   (e) nails (hands and feet)?
   (f) What other areas would you pay particular attention to:
      (i) for a woman?
      (ii) for a man?
3. What report would you make to the person-in-charge regarding an individual's state of personal grooming?

## Care of the mouth, teeth and dentures (Z9: 1–2)

Care of the mouth is regarded as one of the most basic but essential activities of care, especially residents who are unconscious or seriously ill. They require special care of the mouth for comfort, maintenance of self-respect and dignity, and prevention of infection. Normally, the mouth is kept clean by saliva, eating and drinking, followed by regular cleaning of teeth and dentures. During illness or neglect, the mouth may become very dry and in some cases there is an offensive odour. If this state is allowed to continue, debris of food may collect, the person loses his/her appetite, and inflammation of the mouth may develop with ulceration (stomatitis). Gums may also become inflamed with a fungal infection (thrush). Eating and drinking and even talking may become difficult and uncomfortable, and the client may become prone to other types of infection.

In order to promote and maintain the health and well-being of the individual client, the mouth, teeth, gums and tongue must be routinely kept clean. The frequency with which this is done varies according to individual clients' abilities to care for themselves, but the person-in-charge will be able to direct and advise on the frequency of care, especially for those who are helpless.

### The mouth

The mouth is an external opening in the face. It is a common passage for both food and air. The upper and lower lips form the front opening and are lined with a mucous membrane which gives them the characteristic red colour. The floor of the mouth is occupied by the tongue and the roof is formed by the bony hard palate. Generally, the mouth is kept moist by saliva which is secreted constantly from the six salivary glands. The back of the mouth leads to the pharynx.

### Functions of the mouth
The mouth:
- takes in, masticates and prepares food for the act of swallowing
- secretes and mixes saliva with food; the food then passes into the pharynx
- communicates, eg. speech production
- breathes
- absorbs medication, eg. glycerinetrinitrate.

### Content of the mouth
The mouth contains the following:

#### 1. The tongue
This is a muscular organ covered by a special type of mucous membrane. Unlike the rest of the mouth which is smooth, the tongue is rough and contains special cells called taste buds (for distinguishing sweet, sour, bitter, and salt), and is attached to the back of the floor of the mouth.

### Functions of the tongue
- helps in the maintenance of speech
- helps in mastication and passes food back into the pharynx in the act of swallowing
- moves food about the mouth; and contains taste buds for distinguishing bitter, sweet, sour and salt.

#### 2. Uvula
Muscular projection from the back of the roof of the mouth used in swallowing.

#### 3. Tonsils
These are two patches of lymphoid tissue, each lying on either side of the back of the mouth between the pillar of fauces.

#### 4. Saliva
A watery fluid containing ptyalin (amylase) enzyme, which acts on cooked starches. It is believed that about 1000 ml is produced daily. Its production is influenced by the sight and smell of food. Some residents may show side-effects to specific drugs which may increase the flow of saliva (dribbling) or cause a dry mouth. It is important to have a knowledge of your residents and report your observations to the person-in-charge.

### Functions
- keeps the mouth moist and lubricates food
- aids in the act of swallowing by moistening food as it passes to the oesophagus and the stomach.

#### 5. Teeth
The main mass of the tooth consists of a substance called dentine, which is a very hard material resembling bone in composition but which has no canals.

### Types of teeth
Each individual has two sets of teeth during his/her lifetime. These are made up as follows:
- temporary or milk: a set of childhood teeth, consists of 20 in number
- permanent: a set of adult teeth, consists of 32 in number.

### Functions
- essential for cutting and mastication of food
- prevents food slipping while eating, grinding and pounding food for swallowing.

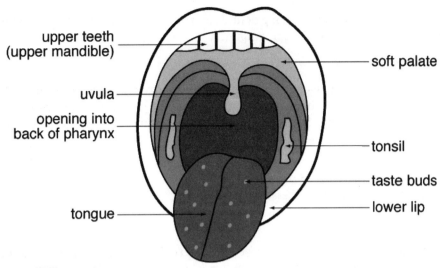

A simple diagram of the mouth

## Promoting a healthy, moist and fresh mouth

Most elderly people enjoy mealtimes. They have their own teeth or dentures and communicate and socialise without experiencing any problems. Others because of illness or mental disorders, for example, are not so fortunate. Ill fitting dentures and poor mouth hygiene can exacerbate existing illness or may even cause infections which can prevent eating and lead to emaciation, weight loss indigestion or malnutrition. During illness, clients may experience difficulty drinking and this may, in turn, cause a dry mouth, furred tongue, cracked lips, dehydration and infection.

### Action

- monitor and record fluid intake in accordance with the care plan
- encourage clients to drink plenty of citrus fruit juices to stimulate the flow of saliva
- report ill-fitting dentures to the person-in-charge who may refer the client to a dentist
- encourage clients with well-fitting dentures to wear them at meal times
- encourage clients to eat fresh fruits as they help to cleanse and keep the mouth moist
- provide a mouthwash to remove debris of food stuck to the gum and teeth after meals
- give the client ice cubes to suck in hot weather to keep the mouth moist.

## Dentures

These are sets of artificial teeth made specially for individual clients. There are different ways of cleaning dentures, eg. paste and toothbrush. Some clients prefer to have their dentures soaked in a solution of their own choosing, and then brushed and rinsed. Dentures should be scrubbed under clean, warm running water with a small denture brush using a special dentifrice, rinsed and soaked in sterident in a denture mug or a container labelled with the client's name, and stored overnight. Clients should be given a mouth wash after dentures have been cleaned and replaced.

## Care of teeth and mouth

Foods containing starches and sugars are usually acted upon by the saliva and bacteria present in the mouth. The bacteria cover the teeth and produce acids known as plaque which, if not removed, may attack the dentine of the teeth causing dental cavities (holes), and the gums in which the teeth are set can become inflamed, resulting in gingivitis.

## 1. Mobile patient/client

Most mobile clients are likely to clean their teeth twice or three times a day, preferably after each meal. A minority may need assistance and encouragement for personal mouth care in the morning and before retiring to bed at night. This is because bacteria tend to be more active during the night, building up plaque.

### Equipment
- toothbrush and toothpaste of choice
- chlorhexidine mouthwash in a beaker
- a bowl for used mouthwash.

### Procedure
Toothbrushes have been shown to be the most effective tool for removing plaque. Gums and teeth should be brushed regularly, after every meal followed by a chorhexidine mouthwash.

## 2. Seriously ill or unconscious patient/client

In acute illness, the mouth will require frequent and careful attention, as neglect may lead to serious complications. Whenever mouth care is given, the carer should develop a good relationship with the client, by explaining the procedures to him/her.

### Equipment: a tray containing:
- mouthwash, foam sticks, sponge mouth cleaner or small gauze swabs
- denture floss, white paraffin or lip salve. Wooden spatula for initial mouth inspection
- plastic sponge applicators — alternatively, a gauze swab may be wrapped securely round a finger. Care must be taken as some clients may bite
- a sterile mouth package containing: disposable forceps, cotton wool swabs, disposable receptacles for lotions (gallipots), disposable towels for protecting the client
- disposable bag for used swabs, cleaning lotions, eg. sodium bicarbonate, 1% solution to remove dried mucus and coating, glycerine of thymol mouthwash to rinse and freshen the mouth. Proprietary mouthwashes may be used, eg. sodium bicarbonate
- Vaseline may be used for soothing dry and sore lips
- a labelled denture bowl as necessary.

### Procedure
- wash and dry your hands prior to carrying out the procedure, and cover any cuts or grazes with waterproof dressing
- screen the bed, sit the client in a comfortable position and protect his/her clothing with a sterile towel
- inspect the mouth for cracks, swelling or thrush and report to the person-in-charge
- remove dentures, if present, and place them in a labelled denture mug containing water
- pour out cleansing lotions
- mount the swabs supplied onto the forceps ensuring that they are properly secured
- dip only the corners of the swab or plastic sponges in the cleaning lotion and squeeze off excess as this could cause client to choke or even drown
- clean methodically starting with the lips and work inside to the back and sides
- clean inside and outside of the gums and both sides of the teeth. Ensure that all surfaces of the teeth and the crevices between the teeth receive attention
- clean the tongue last — from back to front using firm strokes

- rinse the mouth by dipping the sponge in the mouthwash, working from the cheeks and the back of the mouth forwards, finishing with the lips
- give a conscious client a piece of lemon to suck to help stimulate saliva, replace dentures if worn and report the state of the mouth to the person-in-charge.

## Neglected care

The outcome of neglect may lead to the following complications:
- sores and crusts on the lips and teeth
- cracked lips, furring of the tongue, inflammation of the gums and tongue, dental cavities
- bad breath and the spread of infection to the chest and lungs, stomach, middle ear and other parts of the body.

Regular mouth care and dental inspection should be undertaken, especially on the frail and seriously ill. Report any abnormalities at once to the person-in-charge.

## References

Boyle S (1992) Assessing mouth care. *Nurs Times* **88**(15): 44–46
Campbell J (1993) The mechanics of eating and drinking. *Nurs Times* **89**(21): 32–33
Crosby C (1989) Method in mouth care. *Nurs Times* **85**(35): 38–41
Millinson K (1991) Taking care of John's mouth. *Nurs Times* **87**(21): 34–35
Parrot A (1991) Teaching mouth care. *Nurs Times* **87**(38): 48
Wilson KJW (1990) *Anatomy and Physiology*. Churchill Livingstone, Edinburgh

## Assignment

The purpose of this homework is to assist you in preparing for your Workbased Assessment of competence. As there is no pressure on you, feel free to work at your own pace, but avoid the temptation to procrastinate. After you have read your notes and suggested references, submit your work for correction. The completed work becomes part of your Personal Portfolio.

## Care of the mouth and dentures (Z9: 1–2)

1. Discuss the importance of mouth care in care of elderly residents.
2. Describe how you would care for the following residents and the report you would make to the person-in-charge about their mouths:
   a) the mobile
   b) the bedridden
   c) the seriously ill.
3. A client refuses to eat because he or she cannot taste the food and complains of pain when trying to chew, to the extent that even the sight of food makes him/her feel sick.
   a) What do you think could be the cause of these problems?
   b) What action would you take?
   c) How do you think the problems could be resolved?
4. Discuss how you would care for a frail elderly resident's dentures from the time he or she wakes up in the morning until he/she retires to bed at night.
5. Discuss how you would help a resident to maintain a healthy, moist and fresh mouth.

## Personal cleanliness (bathing) (Z9: 1-2)

Hygiene is the science of health which embraces individuals and how they maintain their personal cleanliness to ensure good health. When a person is ill, he or she may experience difficulty in maintaining adequate standards of personal hygiene, especially if the procedure is accompanied by pain or other discomfort. The outcome may be the onset of unpleasant problems, such as infection, with a lowering of spirits, self-esteem and dignity. Carers should assist with personal hygiene, and help maintain individual well-being, without subjecting the client to embarrassing procedures.

### The need for privacy

Personal hygiene is an individual's concern and is achieved by removing items of personal clothing and washing the body one part at a time. In the care setting a client is exposed to total strangers frequently of the opposite gender. In these circumstances the client should be approached in a sensitive way, in order to maintain individual privacy, dignity and self-respect. Modesty is valued by all, especially people of other religions and cultural groups.

### Principles of care

People vary in their habits. For some, a bath is a daily necessity while others see it as an unfamiliar ordeal requiring considerable encouragement. When it comes to changing poor personal hygienic practices, a balance should be struck between a client's condition, and a desire to promote health through cleanliness. Some care homes operate within a set system based on an established daily routine where clients have their baths on specific days. There is a need to consider modification of this system to meet the needs of clients, as the final outcome should be to maintain their individual lifestyle and habits within an acceptable limit. Quite often, upbringing and culture tend to influence the way some people clean themselves. Consequently, flexibility is required to meet these needs, based on an assessment of an individual's ability to carry out personal cleanliness routines independently, and on a daily basis as the need arises.

### Assessment

The decision to bathe a client should be based on analysis of information collected to determine his or her cleansing habits, such as how often a bath is taken — once or twice a week; the time — morning or evening; and preference — shower or bath. Some people never have a bath but always take a shower, while others prefer a bath.

### Bathing

Bathing stimulates general circulation and prevents infection. It encourages exercise, prevents the development of pressure sores, promotes relaxation and refreshment of the body after a day's work. It offers an opportunity to identify problems, eg. infection, rashes, oedema and the general condition of the body. A variety of baths are prescribed to bring about healing, eg. disinfectant baths, although the most common reason for a bath is cleanliness.

### Design of care plan

It should identify:
- which areas are to be cleaned by carers and why, eg. application of prescribed lotions
- which areas should not be washed or treated, eg. marking where a client is receiving radiotherapy

- the level of independence to be aimed for should work towards achieving the carers and clients goals. Some clients may continue to need help while others will regain their independence
- the need to use specific bathing aids, such as hoist or lifts.

**Implementation of care**

Clients should be encouraged to carry out the procedure independently and in private, unless help is necessary. If assistance is given, carers should use this opportunity to promote and improve their social interaction with clients by allowing them to express their views and choices. Clients' questions should always be answered truthfully.

### *Guidance*
- offer clients the use of toilet facilities before starting the procedure
- use extreme caution to prevent slips and falls, eg. the use of a non-slip or rubber mats
- test the temperature of the bath water before the client goes in the bathroom
- ensure that once the required temperature is reached, no more water is added, especially for those elderly who do not register hot or cold efficiently as they get older
- give consideration to individual clients' cultural customs
- assist the individual in and out of the bath or shower, use bathing aids such as hoists or lifts if necessary
- check with the person-in-charge before you leave a person alone to bathe
- provide warmth, privacy and dignity, and explain procedures to clients
- ensure that bath seats, handles, transfer boards, stools and hoists are available.

**Approaches to personal cleansing**

*Shower*

Clients who are able to use the shower on their own should have the means of summoning help, eg. they should be shown where the bell is situated and how it operates.

### *Guidance*
- assemble equipment, eg. towel, face cloths, soap, clean gown or clothes, a bath board with slats or perforations to allow water through
- encourage clients to use shower chairs and not to stand for long periods
- check the water temperature before the person enters the shower
- assist the client in the shower and steady him/her with your arms
- make sure that the wheelchair wheels are locked during transfer to the shower chair
- give assistance as needed in washing, rinsing, drying and dressing the client.

*Baths*

Clients who are mobile clients should be encouraged to use the bathroom. Some may need help to wash inaccessible areas, eg. back or feet. It is important that they have access to a means of summoning help and are shown how to operate any such devices, eg. nurse call alarm bells.

### *Guidance*
- offer the individual an opportunity to use toilet facilities before starting the procedure
- assemble the same equipment as for a shower
- fill the bath half full, running cold water into the bath first, then the hot

- mix the water well and test the temperature with a bath thermometer. This should not be more than 38° C. If there is no bath thermometer, check the water temperature with the back of your hand. Ask the client who is going to have the bath to check that the temperature is comfortable
- never allow residents into the bath unless both of you are satisfied with all aspects of the procedure, especially the temperature of the water
- make sure that there is a non-slip mat in the bath and assist as necessary
- help to wash, rinse, dry, talcum and dress the client as may be necessary
- use a bathing aid, eg. hoist or lift or seek help if there is a danger of the person falling or slipping
- wrap the person in a dry warm towel after the bath to prevent chilling, and ensure that he or she is thoroughly dried, dressed and escorted from the bathroom
- return to the bathroom, clean the bath and remove used towels
- leave the bath in as clean a state as you would like to find it.

## Bedbaths

### Guidance

- assemble equipment, eg. towels, soap, face cloths, bath blankets, bowl, disposable wipes, linen skip for dirty linen, nightdress, pyjamas, talcum powder, deodorant and any other requirements for the client, eg. cologne, cosmetics, toothbrush, toothpaste, disposable denture bowl (if required). Nail scissors and nail file, comb and hairbrush
- explain to the person what you are going to do and seek his or her cooperation
- close all the windows and doors to prevent drafts and offer toilet facilities
- strip the bed. Replace the top sheet with a bath blanket
- remove nightdress or pyjamas and any unnecessary pillows
- place a second bath blanket under the client and make him or her comfortable
- pour warm water (temperature not more than 38°C) into a bowl, two-thirds full
- wash client systematically from the face, neck and ears, rinse and dry thoroughly
- encourage the person to wash and dry his or her face. If the client is unable to do so, wash each eye from the inner to the outer corner, using water only. Change the water frequently
- rinse thoroughly and ask if he or she feels dry, to encourage communication
- attend to finger and toenails, hair and offer mouth care as necessary
- apply domestics — deodorant or talcum powder sparingly, as required by the client
- replace pyjamas trousers. Remove blankets, make up the bed and leave the client comfortable
- clear away the trolley and report the outcome of care to the person-in-charge
- observe and report on the client's satisfaction and any skin rashes, sores or bruises.

## Bathing specific areas

### Arms and hands

Start with the arm furthest away from you. Place a towel under the arm, then wash and rinse paying particular attention to the axilla. An assistant can dry the arms and hands while you prepare to wash the next area.

### Chest and upper abdomen

- wash and dry carefully, paying particular attention to under the breasts in women
- apply talcum powder sparingly and according to the client's personal preferences.

### Upper back

- encourage the client to sit up. If he/she finds it difficult to do so, then gently turn him or her on the side
- fold back the top sheet and protect it with a towel

- wash the buttocks and perineal area (ie. between the legs) with a disposable face cloth, using circular motions. Rinse and dry thoroughly
- observe and report any unusual marks, ie. redness as this is a sign of the onset of pressure sores.

## Legs and feet
- wash and dry well using the same principles as those used for the arms. Soak feet in a bowl of warm water if possible
- observe and report on any swelling or redness. These may indicate deep vein thrombosis
- encourage the client to exercise his/her legs and ankles. If he or she is unable to do so, carry out passive exercises.

## Toilet and perineal (genital) areas
- place a second towel between legs. Prepare and provide the client with a disposable wipe or appropriate cloth and towels
- encourage the client to carry out the procedure personally if possible, in order to promote and maintain his or her self-respect, dignity and independence
- assist the client, if he or she is unable to do so.

### Female clients
When assisting a female client, wash from front to back to avoid bacteria from the anal area contaminating the urethra and causing urinary infection.

### Male clients
When assisting an uncircumcised client, gently fold back the foreskin and dry the penis before replacing the foreskin.
- wash and dry the scrotum carefully
- follow the guidance given on care of clients with incontinence.

## After the bath
- dress the client in appropriate clothes
- remove and place any soiled personal clothing in an appropriate linen skip or a labelled plastic bag
- follow appropriate procedures for laundering soiled clothing
- remove, wash and put away equipment
- wash and leave the bath in the state you would like to find it
- report the outcome to the person-in-charge.

## Evaluation of Care

The aim of care is achieved when clients are able to carry out their own personal cleansing without help or with very little support. Their efforts should be praised no matter how limited and how long it takes them to accomplish specific tasks. In certain circumstances, it may be possible to leave them alone and return to help as required in order to promote independence. But equipment and an alarm call bell should be within easy reach should they need to summon help.

## References

Cochrane GM, Wilson AK (1990) *Hoists and Lifts*. Disability Information Trust, Oxford
Flack M, Johnston M (1986) *Handbook for Care*. Beaconsfield Publishers Ltd, Bucks
Greaves A (1985) We'll just freshen you up dear. *Nurs Times* **81** (10): 3–4
Gooch J (1989) Skin hygiene. *Prof Nurse* **5**(1):13–18

Mandelstam M (1993) *How to get Equipment for Disability.* Jessica Kingsley Publishers, London

McMahon R (1991) The prevalence of skin problems beneath the breasts of in-patients. *Nurs Times* **87**(39): 48–51

McMahon A, Harding J (1993) *Knowledge to Care.* Blackwell Scientific Publishers, London

Roper N *et al* (1987) *The Elements of Nursing.* Churchill Livingstone, Edinburgh

## Assignment

The purpose of this homework is to assist you in preparing for your Workbased Assessment of Competence. As there is no pressure on you, feel free to work at your own pace, but avoid the temptation to procrastinate. After you have read your notes and suggested references, submit your work for correction. The completed work becomes part of your Personal Portfolio.

## Personal cleanliness (bathing) (Z9: 1–2)

1. Define briefly what you understand by the term 'personal cleanliness'.
2. Give four reasons why people should maintain their personal cleanliness.
3. An elderly Asian gentleman aged 78 years, has been in the home for two weeks and during this time he has refused any attention to his personal hygiene:
   (a) What do you think could be the reasons for his behaviour?
   (b) How would you reconcile his need for a bath and at the same time respect his right and choice?
   (c) Assuming that he has agreed to have a bath, how would you go about it?
   (d) What precautions would you take regarding:
      i) his feet, hands, beard?
      ii) temperature of the water?
4. Discuss special precautions you would take to avoid causing embarrassment to a client during bathing.

# Unit 11
# Assist clients to move, exercise and maintain desirable posture (CU6, Z6, Z7)

## Positions used in care (Z7: 1–2)

People who are ill are usually cared for in bed, although some may prefer sitting up comfortably in chairs if their condition allows. Being in bed or sitting up in a chair for a considerable length of time can cause problems, such as pressure sores. Other complications may include thrombosis, loss of muscle tone, contracture leading to wasting of the muscles. Prevention of these problems will depend upon observation and the frequency with which their positions are changed. Special equipment is available for clients who are being cared for in bed or sitting up in chairs for prolonged periods (Dealey, 1997).

The positions used vary with the needs of the person, and the care plan must provide guidance on the best position. It is important to note that the use of these positions, and the best way of maintaining them can contribute to the overall care and comfort of the individual. They can be used for either short- or long-term care, but it is important to remember that they require equal and constant attention, in order to minimise the effects of complications, such as pressure sores. Positions commonly used are:

### Lying in bed

#### 1. Supine
The individual should lie flat on the back, face upwards. A pillow or two may be placed under the head for comfort, providing medical condition allows. A bedcradle is used to prevent the bedding causing pressure on the feet. A flat pillow may be placed along the length of the lower leg to relieve pressure of the heels. This position is not suitable for use with clients at high risk of developing deep vein thrombosis. The reasons for use are:
- gynaecological examinations, catheterisation
- administration of enema.

#### 2. Lateral positions (left or right)
The person lies on the side with the head supported by pillows. Care should be taken with the person's earlobe. The underneath shoulder should be brought slightly forward, and the upper arm comfortably supported on a pillow. The upper leg should be slightly flexed and also supported with a pillow, while the lower leg should be extended. The client's back may be supported by a pillow. This position is normally used when sleeping or resting. The reasons for use are:
- recovery from general anaesthesia, care of unconscious patients
- rectal and vaginal examinations, giving enemas, suppositories.

#### 3. Upright position (Fowler's position)
The individual sits upright in bed with the back supported by at least six pillows. The person may lean forward on the bedtable on which a soft pillow has been placed. The reasons for use are:

- in the case of severe asthma, dyspnoea (difficulty in breathing), heart failure
- to assist expansion of the lungs, and in chronic chest conditions
- to make it easier for the individual to clear his or her chest.

### 4. Prone position

In this position the person lies with the face down with one pillow under the head which is turned to one side. The ankles may be raised on a pillow or sponge rubber pad so that the toes are free of the bed surface. The reasons for use are:
- to prevent pressure sores occurring
- relief of flatulence and distension of the abdomen
- to help drainage from the front of the body (postural drainage of the chest)
- in the care of residents with spinal injuries, burns and other injuries.

### 5. Sitting position in bed

The individual should sit upright in bed with the body inclined slightly backwards. It is a modified form of the Fowler's position with the back supported by a bedrest and pillows. The feet should rest at right angles against a wedge or bolster to prevent the client from sliding down the bed. Care should be taken that the skin is not damaged as the person slides down.

Alternatively, if the condition allows, the foot of the bed may be raised by about three inches with a special wooden block. The bedding should be loose on the person's feet. A bedcradle may be used to relieve any pressure on the toes. The reasons for use are the same as with Fowler's position

## Sitting up in a chair

### *Guidance*

When a resident sits down, it is important to:
- make sure that he or she settles into a comfortable seat and sits in a comfortable position which enables the lumbar spine or small of the back to be well-supported
- check that the width of the seat allows for the full breadth of the hips. Also, that the depth of the seat allows for support to the full length of the thighs, the lumbar spine and the sacrum against the back of the chair
- place a hard object under the cushion to help if the seat is too soft to provide a firm base
- ensure that the chairs have arms on which the person can rest his or her arms
- encourage the person to sit upright with feet resting firmly and comfortably on the floor; if they do not, then provide a low foot rest
- discourage the person from sitting in a chair which allows the bottom to sink much lower than the knees. This is because the person may be forced to slump and have difficulty in getting up
- discourage the use of deck chairs and sagging armchairs. The reason is that they do not support the back properly, and usually cause the spine to curve and the person to assume an unnatural posture
- place a small table as close as possible to the chair for the person to rest his or her book, drinks
- ensure that the person is well-protected from any unfavourable weather condition with a small blanket or travelling rug.

## Using leg rests

It is important that the leg rests should be adjusted to allow for a slight flex of the knee. The heels should be kept clear of the rest, and the hips at a right angle. Consideration should be given where possible to elevating one leg at a time. It is necessary to ensure that pressure is removed from the sacral area, particularly for clients with pressure sores.

### Getting clients out of bed

*Guidance*

Some elderly people suffer from arthritis which makes it difficult for them to get out of bed in the morning. A small number suffer from hypertension in which a sudden change in position may cause giddiness. They may lose their balance or fall down if made to get up suddenly. They should be handled with extreme care as follows:

- sit the person up gradually and swing his or her legs gently over the edge of the bed. Feet may touch the floor
- ask the individual to rest for a while. After recovery, request him or her to place both arms on the bed and gently lift his or her body upwards keeping the back as straight as possible. A walking stick or a Zimmer frame may be helpful for this movement
- encourage him or her to gradually push him or herself up straight into a standing position
- provide a gentle support as necessary, and encourage the person to walk to a suitable arm chair, preferably unaided.

### 6. Lifting

Moving people is a major cause of accidents and injuries in the caring professions. Some people cannot or should not move themselves, and lifting properly involves the use of good lifting techniques; how you stand, move and position your body.

It is important to consider the client's disability, size and weight before any attempt is made to lift the person. Able clients should be assisted to help themselves as far as possible.

*Principles of lifting*

- wash and dry your hands thoroughly before and after the procedure
- never lift, carry or transfer anyone in a way that is likely to cause injury to the individual, yourself or to others
- arrange the room and furniture as necessary before lifting
- ensure that there is adequate space to perform the lift in safety
- all lifting should be carried out by at least two carers or nurses
- use the correct lifting technique and an appropriate aid, eg. hoist, Ambulift and accessories.

*Remember — every move can injure your back*

## References

Hollis M (1991) *Safer Lifting for Patients,* 3rd edn. Blackwell Scientific Publications, Oxford

Charlish A (1986) *The Damart Guide for Back Pain Sufferers.* Ward Lock Ltd, Slough

Dealey C (1997) *Managing Pressure Sore Prevention.* Quay Books, Mark Allen Group, Dinton

Flack M, Johnston M (1986) *Handbook for Care.* Beaconsfield Publishers Ltd, Bucks

## Moving and handling clients (Z7: 1–2)

Moving and handling people is a fundamental part of care and takes place when carrying out a wide range of clinical procedures in low beds, chairs or wheelchairs. The elderly or incapacitated may need help in using the toilet and, if bedridden because of painful joints, they will need to be moved from sitting to prone positions. They may not be able to get in and out of baths or showers without help, and if they are seriously ill and in need of continuous care, they will need to be moved to prevent bedsores. These tasks may be carried out in their homes in the community, and in care

establishments. Furthermore, with an increasing number of the elderly in the population, some of whom cannot and should not move themselves, there is a corresponding increase in the workload for carers and an increased risk of back injury. Research shows that some procedures carry specific risks, for example:
- prolonged stooping postures when attending to the patient/client
- awkward posture when moving the resident or patient in bed
- awkward posture when attending to a resident or patient in a double bed.

## Legislation

During the past decade, emphasis has been directed towards encouraging organisations and employers to produce policies, procedures and suitable equipment so that moving and handling people can be carried out safely, without injury to either the client or the staff doing the lifting.

## Health and Safety at Work Act 1974/92

This Act highlights the responsibilities of both the employers and employees to provide a safe place of work. It states that the employer has a duty 'to ensure, in so far as is reasonably practicable, the health, and safety and welfare at work of all his/her employees'. This duty includes providing suitable equipment and training, local policies, procedures and codes of practice in order to maintain a safe standard of care for all involved in handling.

## The EU regulations

These regulations which came into effect in January 1993, emphasised the need for training carers in manual handling. It also requires management to ensure that:
- all hazardous manual-handling tasks are avoided where possible
- if risky manual-handling tasks are unavoidable, they must be assessed in advance. Once assessment has been done, action should be taken to remove or reduce the risk of injury
- a safe manual-handling policy, incorporating training and assessment must be in place.

## Policy guidelines

There is currently a movement towards non-manual handling with an emphasis on the use of mechanical lifting aids. The approach is based on assessment of the needs and capabilities of individual clients, and ways of handling them. A care plan should provide guidance on each resident with handling problems based on:
- the weight of the person
- the extent of the person's ability to assist, bear weight and any other relevant information
- the technique to be employed to handle the particular client should be consistent.

## Lifting and handling aids

There are a wide variety of lifting and moving aids which should be used as frequently as possible and not left stored away in ward store rooms, passages, corridors or in corners of bathrooms. Some are simple to use and others require an orientation programme on how to use them. Those commonly in use are:

### *Hoists*

Hoists are designed to meet the needs of individuals who are heavy to lift. They are electrically, hydraulically or manually operated with a restriction on maximum weight. They are usually used with slings for lifting residents in and out of the bath, and from a car into a wheelchair or vice versa. There are other models for domestic use, such as a toilet combined commode and shower and transport aids. Be familiar with operating instruction on their use.

### Sliding board

A small board is placed between the bed and the chair or between the chair and the bath. The person sits on it and slides gently across to the desired position. The two surfaces must be of the same or similar height.

### Drawsheet

This sheet is usually placed under a resident to prevent soiling of the main sheet. But, a strong drawsheet may be used to move a resident in bed or transport people with back injuries from a trolley to bed. It is essential that the client's head is supported and the drawsheet firmly held.

### Transfer belt

This is used to transfer helpless people. It is put around the person's waist to provide a grip during transfer. It may be used to grasp people with painful joints and allergic skin conditions.

### Monkey pole

The 'pole' may be attached to the head of the bed, ceiling or fixed to the wall. The person grasps the pole with both hands and pulls him or herself off the bed. It has many uses, such as helping the person to change position, turn in bed, or for using toilet facilities, ie. bedpans. Some people use it as an exercise bar to strengthen their arm and leg muscles.

### Turning bed

The bed is designed to alter the person's position. The person may be suspended in a net to allow circulation of air around the person, and relieve pressure from areas which are predisposed to pressure sores. It may be operated manually or electrically, but requires regular attention.

### Turntable

The table is a circular disk which pivots when a person stands on it. It is useful for transferring people who are paralysed on one side (hemiplegic) and cannot walk.

### Handling and moving residents or patients

The *Nursing Times* (1996) guide to manual handling suggests that if such handling is unavoidable, you should protect your back and, before you start, ask yourself the following questions:

### 1. Is handling really necessary?
    **Action**: consider,
- *whether patients can move themselves*
- *equipment and or other staff needed and how you will carry out the task.*

### 2. Are you fit for the task?
    **Action**: consider whether you have had appropriate training, are anxious or tired and are wearing appropriate clothing and footwear.

### 3. Can the resident or patient cope with the procedure?
    **Action**: consider the patient's weight, diagnosis and ability to co-operate.

**4. Do you have the right equipment?**
   **Action:** consider using equipment whenever possible.

**5. Is the environment safe?**
   **Action:** consider the space and any obstacles.

### Handling and lifting techniques

#### Guidance
- always wash and dry your hands thoroughly before and after the procedure
- be familiar with and follow local policy, procedures and practices for lifting residents
- check with the person-in-charge on the agreed method of handling a particular client
- maintain a good interpersonal relationship with the person, and always explain the procedures you are going to use, prior to starting and seek his or her cooperation
- check whether you need to share the load or use a lifting aid, only after you have been trained on how to use the equipment
- remove all obstacles, check for wet floor, brakes on wheelchairs
- remove any jewellery to avoid injury to the resident and yourself
- explain and discuss the techniques with a colleague who may be assisting you
- move as close as possible to the resident
- promote the client's independence by encouraging maximum participation of the person
- position your feet carefully with a wide base of support
- tuck in chin, keep head stable: tighten the natural corset — stomach and buttock muscles
- bend knees, keep the back naturally straight and do not twist
- ensure that your grip is both safe and easy and breathe out when lifting or lowering
- do not lift while stretching, eg. lifting objects above your head
- do not drag client's heel or buttocks when moving him or her up and down the bed, as friction may occur resulting in the break down of the skin and formation of pressure sores.

#### Additional guidance
- be aware of the problem areas. Observe and report your findings to the person-in-charge
- demonstrate knowledge of all residents designated for manual handling and moving and their individual care plans
- assist in assessment of client's needs as may be delegated or directed by the team leader
- help to create a safe working environment by reporting and recording any accidents or incidents in appropriate documents in accordance with local policy
- ensure that you are fit for the job and do not exceed the level of your responsibility
- maintain an accurate record on instructions you received in manual handling operations.

*Remember — every move can injure your back*

### Evaluation

It is important to identify your own capacity and ability for moving residents when you are requested to assist in manual handling tasks or the use of lifting equipment. Some clients may initially become frightened with the use of lifting equipment. It is important to reassure the person. One of the objectives of care is to assist the individual to maintain his or her independence. But quite often, clients are taken to the toilet in a wheelchair in order to save time. This practice seems to deprive them of the opportunity for promoting and maintaining their independence. An attempt should be made by clients to walk independently to and from the toilet, if possible with an arm support.

At the end of the exercise, always invite the resident to express his or her views and satisfaction about the procedure.

## References

Disabled Living Foundation(1994) *Patient Handling Equipment Advice and Information*. DLF, London
EC Directive (1990) *Manual Handling of Loads*. (90/269 EC) Brussels
Health and Safety Executive (1992) *Manual Handling: Guidance on Regulations*. London
Love C (1995) Managing manual handling in clinical situations. *Nurs Times* **91**(26): 38–39
Royal College of Nursing (1993) *The Code of Practice for the Handling of Patients*. RCN, London
Royal College of Nursing (1996) *Manual Handling Assessments in Hospitals and the Community*. RCN, London
Nursing Times (1992) *The NT Guide to Manual Handling*. NT, London
Confederation of Health Service Employees (1992) *Back-Breaking Work*. COHSE, Banstead
Tarling C (1992) Handling patients. *Nurs Times* **88**(43): 38–40

### Audio visual aids

*Format: VHS video*
Training video: *Handle with Care*: Registered Nursing Home Association
Ref: 350/ CT Parts 1 and 4: *Lifting Patients — Lifting and Carrying in Hospitals*
Oxford Educational Resources Ltd

## Assignment

The purpose of this homework is to assist you in preparing for your Workbased Assessment of Competence. As there is no pressure on you, feel free to work at your own pace, but avoid the temptation to procrastinate. After you have read your notes and suggested references, submit your work for correction. The completed work becomes part of your Personal Portfolio.

## Lifting and handling (Z7: 1–2)

1. Conduct a survey of your care establishment and list the variety of lifting and handling aids available and their uses.
2. Describe correctly a method you have been shown for lifting and handling clients, which is currently in use in your care environment.
3. Discuss three circumstances in which you would use a mechanical aid in moving and handling residents and your choice of aid.
4. Describe how you would transfer a resident suffering from hemiplegia from a bed into a wheelchair.
5. Discuss how you would move a resident up the bed. What precautions would you observe?
6. List copies of legislation and policies on display in your care establishment, relating to safe handling and lifting of people.

## Exercise and passive movement of limbs (Z6: 1–2)

Exercise is movement of muscles and limbs to encourage the physical, mental, social and spiritual well-being of individuals. Exercise according to ability and capability is necessary. Some elderly people find the activities of daily living difficult because of stiffness in joints. Although the rate at which people age varies, some parts of the body wear out quicker than others. If residents in care homes take limited or no exercise, their muscles will become flabby and this will lead to atrophy (wasting) which, in turn, affects their ability to move. Lack of muscle action, may lead to changes in bone structure. This process is known as decalcification, or osteoporosis. This is a lack of calcium in the bones, and bones may take some time to return to normal if they ever do.

If the joints remain in the same position due to lack of movement for a long time, they stiffen, and the muscles around the joints are shortened, leading to contracture. If the process is not checked by gentle exercises, the situation will become irreversible.

It is essential that attention should be paid to the general alignment of the body, especially the natural hollows in the small of the back when a person is spending long periods in bed. Care should also be taken to prevent foot drop by positioning the feet at right angles to the leg. The use of pillows, sandbags, splints, pads and bedcradles can help to maintain a good alignment and prevent deformity when a resident is helpless or paralysed, or has reduced mobility. Maintain constant observation on the areas that are prone to pressure sores.

### Nature and purpose of exercise

Taking part in regular exercise can improve the body systems, eg. circulatory, alimentary, muscular, and keep the bones strong and the joints flexible. Exercise does not mean taking part in sporting activities, but just to get out into the fresh air, walk to the shops, use the stairs instead of the lift, a walk around the garden, take the dog for a walk or go swimming. Walking is excellent exercise, particularly if it is brisk, and it is one of the easiest ways of fitting more activity into daily living. In fact, any activity which helps to keep a person supple and mobile is highly recommended.

During exercise the muscle contraction involved not only increases muscle strength, it improves circulation, appetite and the movement preserves muscle tone and helps to prevent contracture. The number of times exercise is carried out is not important, but two or three useful exercises are better than ten that do not make the muscles stronger.

### People who need exercise

Elderly people are often completely dependent on other people, eg. relatives or carers, for their mobility. Exercise may be carried out by people themselves (active), or by others, eg. a carer helping the person (passive or assisted). People suffering from arthritis, amputation, obesity, multiple sclerosis, stroke, fractures, incontinence and muscle weakness experience problems with mobility. The blind, deaf and dumb and those with other disabilities, eg. anxiety, confusion, depression or infection need help to cope and lead as normal a life as possible. Their need for exercise should be based on assessment of their physical, mental, and social well-being, and recorded in their individual care plans.

### Preparing clients for exercise

*Guidance*
- consult the person-in-charge or appropriate paramedical staff, eg. physiotherapist
- discuss the care plan for the type, frequency and duration of exercise prior to embarking on the activity
- be aware of local policy and procedures for carrying out this type of activity

- develop and maintain a good interpersonal relationship with the client by seeking his or her co-operation, and explain the reasons for the exercise. Respect the client's rights and wishes
- demonstrate knowledge and skills in the type of exercise prescribed for the person
- ensure that the client is well prepared, eg. with a walking aid, and is wearing appropriate footwear; persuade the client not to eat a large meal before exercise but make it something to be enjoyed
- encourage or offer the use of toilet facilities before starting any exercise, followed by good personal hygiene, eg. handwashing
- assist the client in choosing appropriate clothing for the exercise with due attention to the weather
- ensure that the immediate environment has plenty of room and good ventilation
- teach and encourage the client to be self-managing as far as is possible and provide help where necessary and support and encouragement for every effort made by the person. Demonstrate knowledge about seeking help in the case of an emergency
- report any untoward effects which may be experienced through exercise to the person-in-charge and make an appropriate and accurate record.

## Provision of exercise

For some elderly people the actual performance of exercise involves the process of learning. The old saying of not being able to teach an old dog new tricks is not true — it just takes longer. The need for exercise is based on assessment of individual functional ability and capability in relation to physical, mental and social well-being. As members of the health care team, the physiotherapists and occupational therapists will assess, prescribe and provide the type of exercise each individual client requires. In their absence, care staff assume responsibility within the concept of total client care. Exercise may be permitted within certain limits, but it is not the remit of care assistants to decide what those limits will be. It is important to consult the person-in-charge or team leader before embarking upon any form of exercise.

### *Guidance*

There are a variety of simple, age-related exercises which can be carried out when lying down, standing or sitting throughout a span of duty. Encourage people to perform the exercises themselves as far as possible, but the idea is to involve the whole body and to bring about:

**Flexion:** bending parts of the body, eg. limbs (elbows, knees), wrists, back

**Extension:** stretching various parts of the body, eg. the arm, leg, shoulders

**Rotation:** turning the head and neck, foot, knee, hip or shoulder joints inwards and outwards

**Abduction:** moving parts of the body away from the body, eg. arm and leg

**Adduction:** moving parts of the body towards the body, eg. arm and leg

## Discomfort with exercise or mobility

### *Sudden severe pain*

The pain is experienced by a person when a limb is fractured. It may result from muscle spasm and tissue damage, and may produce deformity and shortening of the limb.

**Action**: stop any exercise, reassure the client and report the symptom immediately to the person-in-charge.

### *Chronic pain*

This type of pain is often associated with the musculo-skeletal system as a result of muscular rheumatism (fibrositis), low back pain (lumbago) and joint pain (arthritis).

**Action:** stop the exercise, reassure the client and report the symptom to the person-in-charge.

### Sharp shooting pain

This pain occurs when there is injury to an inter-vertebral disc. The person usually finds that a particular movement causes a sharp shooting pain which is experienced along the pathway of the sciatic nerve, through the buttock and down the back of the leg.

**Action:** stop the exercise, reassure the client and report the symptom to the person-in-charge.

### Deep boring pain

Pain in the bone is usually described as excruciating. Since the bone is a relatively dense structure, it has little space to accommodate the swelling caused by inflammation or extra tissue from a new growth like cancer. Carefully position and support the part relative to the rest of the body.

**Action:** stop the exercise, reassure the client and report the symptom to the person-in-charge.

### Phantom pain

A discomfort which is particularly disturbing to a person who has had an amputation. It is generally known as 'phantom limb pain'. The pain is a subjective experience which is psychological with no physical location. Usually the experience is temporary, but while it lasts the person requires special care and attention to help him/her with this pain, which is very real to the person concerned.

### Social and emotional discomfort

When mobility is impeded, there is emotional discomfort and upset because of the loss of freedom, loss of independence and loss of self-respect and personal dignity. In addition, there is anxiety about the state of immobility and its cause. Reassure clients, report and record accurately any untoward effects or experiences.

## References

Hooker S (1981) *Caring for Elderly People. Understanding and Practical Help.* Routledge and Kegan Paul, London: ch 8

Darby C (1984) *Keeping Fit while Caring. A Step-by-Step Guide for Carers.* The Family Welfare Association, London

### Audio visual aids

#### Format: VHS video

Ref: 172CT: *Exercise for the Over 60s*
Ref: 248/1-2CT: *Keeping Well in Old Age*
Ref: 194/1-4 CT: *Training for Independence*
Oxford Educational Resources Ltd

## Prevention of pressure sores (Z7: 2–3, Z19: 1–2)

Pressure sores are a major nursing care problem which cause great pain and suffering and, in some cases, can be a major factor contributing to death. Pressure sores are an ulceration of the skin and underlying tissues due to extreme and prolonged pressure and compression between a bony prominence and a hard surface such as a bed or chair. The blood supply to the area is restricted, resulting in death of tissues. It can occur in any part of the body where external pressure acts upon a bony prominence. Dealey (1992) defines pressure sores as damage to the skin caused by pressure, shearing forces or friction, or a combination of any of these.

## Predisposing factors

Research has shown that many factors are responsible for the development of pressure sores including:
- heat: friction and pressure combined produce increased temperature
- excessive moisture on the skin from sweat, urine and faeces as a result of poor personal hygiene
- abrasion and blister formation due to irritation of the skin in a restless person
- shearing force in a patient with a tendency to slide down in his/her chair or bed
- poor physical and general nutritional state of the client, dehydration and reduced mobility
- poor lifting and handling techniques which result in dragging of the individual
- creases, crumbs and other foreign bodies in the bed, causing friction
- unsuitable clothing and positioning
- persistent irritation and scratching of the area and lack of spontaneous body movement
- mental health problems such as confusion, depression, restlessness.

## Clients prone to pressure sores

Everybody is at risk of developing pressure sores but patients most commonly affected are those who are unable to move spontaneously, such as:
- the unconscious, semi-conscious
- the very ill
- those who are totally paralysed, partially paralysed
- those suffering from spinal injury
- patients in plaster or splints
- patients under the influence of alcohol, drugs, eg. hypnotics (sleeping pills).

## Areas commonly affected

These are the weight-bearing areas where the skin and tissues are compressed between the bed and underlying bone, eg:
- sacrum (buttocks), greater tronchanters (hip), heels, foot and toes
- occipital region (back of head), scapula (shoulder blades)
- elbows and knees (anterior and posterior), patella (kneecap), spinous process (spinal column)
- wrists and knuckles, under the breast, around the thighs and genital areas.

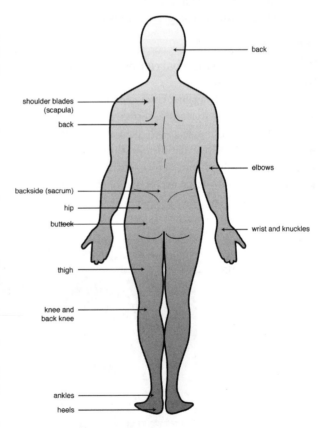

**A diagram showing sites prone to pressure sores**

## The skin

It is necessary to look at the basic anatomy of the skin and the underlying tissues, because it is the skin that is prone to the development of pressure sores. The skin is a sense organ, and one of the largest organs which covers the outside of the body, deep down into its orifices. It is a very complex organ, and is divided into two main parts.

### 1. Epidermis

This is generally known as 'false' skin, and is made up of a number of layers of cells, whose thickness depends upon their location. It is most dense where it is exposed to compression forces, eg. in the palms of the hands and soles of the feet. On the fingertips is a regular pattern of ridges which form the basis of the 'finger print tests' in the investigation of crime. It is continuously discarded and replaced with new cells which form at the base of the epidermis.

### 2. Dermis

This is the 'true' skin comprising connective tissue and elastic fibres. Other structures which can be found here include sensory nerve endings, blood and lymph vessels, sweat glands and ducts, hair, pores, hair follicle, hair roots, sebaceous glands, involuntary muscle. Beneath the dermis is a fatty tissue (adipose) known as a subcutaneous layer which is attached to underlying structures such as muscle and bone. The female has more fatty tissue than men, and for this reason women are always assessed as being at the greatest risk of developing of pressure sores.

### Functions of the skin

When intact, it forms a barrier between the body and the outside environment. Its main duties are to:

- protect the body against cold, infection and act as a waterproof covering
- regulate body temperature, secrete sweat, insulate the body by fat (adipose tissue)
- provide sensations, ie. touch, pain and pressure
- make vitamin D by reaction with the ultraviolet rays of the sun
- absorb a small amount of oily substances and lotions
- communicate — facial expression of pain, changes in colour of skin, eg. blushing.

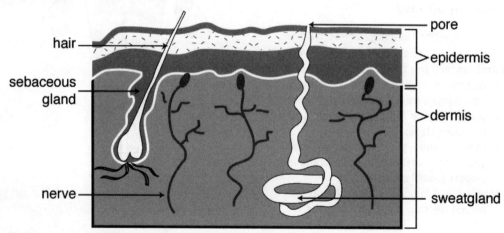

**A simple diagram of the skin**

### Recognition of pressure sores:
- signs of redness to the area which remains red when pressed
- dusky blue or grey areas. There may be partial loss of the true skin (dermis)
- swelling (oedema) and blister formation, deterioration or a complete break in the skin
- pain and loss of function in the area due to pain and swelling (oedema).

### Principle of pressure relief

Pressure sores can form very quickly and treating them takes a lot of time and money, and is very distressing for the client concerned. Emphasis should be directed to eliminate shearing force and friction and help weight distribution to the whole body by supporting the areas where pressure sores can form. But once a person is identified as being at risk of developing pressure sores, a care plan should be designed by members of the health care team. The following points should be taken into consideration:
- changes in position should be made, indicated by:
    - risk assessment and monitoring by using a pressure areas check list
    - the effect of pressure on the skin, eg. skin marking
    - the promotion of rest and comfort
- regular position changes and handling techniques that avoid shearing
- choice of appropriate pressure-reducing aids for beds and chairs
- patient/client and carer education programme
- the promotion of good nutrition
- the management of wounds and incontinence.

### Positioning

The position chosen should be the one which is the safest and most comfortable for the person's medical condition. It should be chosen to reduce the pressure on those areas at greatest risk apart from during rest periods and meal times. Consideration should be given to a client with a sacral sore, and attempts should be made to sit him or her correctly to remove pressure from this area.

### Pressure reducing aids

| Risk | Aid |
|---|---|
| Low | Foam mattress replacement |
| Medium | Alternating-pressure mattress |
| High | Air-fluidised bed or low air-loss mattress |

**Others** include the use of:
- pressure relieving cushions
- heel pads, foam mattress.

### Nutrition

This has an important role in the prevention and treatment of pressure sores, as malnutrition increases the individual's chances of developing pressure sores. A change of diet may be necessary, eg. to one with increased protein such as eggs, meat with plenty of vegetables. Encourage adequate intake of fluid. Vitamin C can help the wound-healing process.

## Incontinence

The management of established pressures may be at risk of delayed healing due to contamination from faeces and urinary incontinence. Assessment of residents for short-term catherisation is an important part of the management of pressure sores to allow the wound to heal. Other forms of care may be considered if the problem of both faecal and urinary incontinence continue to interfere with the healing process.

## Management of wounds

The principle of care is based on reassessment of the wound at frequent intervals by qualified staff who will apply dressings in accordance with local guidelines in relation to classification. The aim is to ensure the highest standards and quality of client's or patient's health to bring about an effective healing process, together with relief of pressure. Priority is given to removal of any slough or dead tissue and prevention of infection.

## Preventative measures

There are many types of mattresses, beds, chairs and cushions, as well as moving and handling devices that may be considered as aids to preventive management. They are aids and cannot replace clinical observation and judgement.

### Guidance
- the most important responsibility of carers is to prevent pressure sores from developing. This can be best achieved by:
  - demonstrating a knowledge of all clients, developing and maintaining a good relationship with them and asking them to report any discomfort to a member of the health care team
  - relieving pressure to avoid body weight resting on one particular area, until normal colour returns
  - turning clients every two hours and reassessing 'risk' areas of the skin for improvement or deterioration
  - telling clients and their family about the risks, giving reasons for nursing interventions
  - documenting findings accurately in the care plan
  - being aware of local policies for preventing pressure damage. Asking the person-in-charge to provide a policy if one does not exist
  - keeping clients dry and avoiding excessive heat and moisture, eg. incontinence
  - maintaining client's good personal hygiene by regular washing and patting dry, with particular attention to the breasts, genital areas, groin, armpits, between the toes
  - ensuring the client maintains adequate and good nutritional status
  - using a good lifting technique to prevent shearing force ie. hoists, Ambulift®, Mecalift®
  - monitoring the areas prone to sores by the use of pressure area check lists.

## Preventive aids

There are many types of aids, such as mattresses, beds, chairs and cushions as well as moving and handling devices which may be considered as preventive aids. These include:
- mattresses eg. ripple mattress, floatation mattress, pressure-relieving mattress eg. Fab Foam
- Mecabed® (net suspension bed)
- ripple bed (electrically controlled and operated)
- supportive, ie. water beds — assessment is suggested before using one for a client or patient
- bed attachments, ie. bedcradles
- low air-loss beds that provide a constant low pressure support.

Generally, beds should be checked regularly to ensure that there are no foreign bodies, eg. coins, false teeth, wrinkles or seams which may cause damage to the person's skin. Also, check that bedding is not tucked in so tightly that it restricts the client's movement.

### Client education

Ideally, the individual should be taught a risk-free way of moving themselves. There should be full liaison with the physiotherapist at all times.

### Clothing

It is important to avoid clients wearing tight clothing; cotton, two-way stretch underwear is recommended.

### Classification of pressure sores

#### Grade 1
There is superficial damage to the skin. It remains red when gently pressed.

#### Grade 2
The dermis is exposed due to a partial loss of the thickness of the skin, causing great pain. The area is swollen and dark red/black with possible blister formation.

#### Grade 3
Full thickness skin loss and damage extends to underlying tissues. Dead tissue is present in the form of slough (yellow) and dead black tissue. Wound edges are clearly defined.

#### Grade 4
Full thickness skin loss with extensive destruction and death of tissue or damage to muscle, bone or supporting structures.

### Pressure sore risk assessment

This involves careful observation of the physical, mental, nutritional and incontinence state of all those clients or patients at risk of developing pressure sores. The factors considered are build, skin condition, mobility, sex, age, continence, nutritional status. The most popular risk indicator is Norton (1975). Others include Waterlow and Braden scales. The outcome of assessment is recorded in the care plan and reviewed at set intervals or whenever necessary. The score is totalled and the lower the total the higher the risk of a patient developing pressure sores. A score of 14 or less indicates patients who are 'at risk' and require preventive measures.

| Norton scale | | | | | | | | | |
|---|---|---|---|---|---|---|---|---|---|
| A | | B | | C | | D | | E | |
| Physical condition | | Mental state | | Activity | | Mobility | | Incontinence | |
| Good | 4 | Alert | 4 | Walks | 4 | Full | 4 | Does not have | 4 |
| Fair | 3 | Apathetic | 3 | Walks with help | 3 | Slightly limited | 3 | Has occasional | 3 |
| Poor | 2 | Confused | 2 | Chairbound | 2 | Very limited | 2 | Usually urinary | 2 |
| Very bad | 1 | Stuporous | 1 | Bedfast | 1 | Immobile | 1 | Double | 1 |

## Pressure areas check list

Name:  Date of birth:

Date of admission:

Care establishment:

| Date | Time | Rt heel | Lt heel | Rt hip | Lt hip | Sacrum | Specify if other | Signature |
|------|------|---------|---------|--------|--------|--------|------------------|-----------|
| **On admission** | | | | | | | | |
| | am. | | | | | | | |
| | pm. | | | | | | | |
| | am. | | | | | | | |
| | pm. | | | | | | | |
| | am. | | | | | | | |
| | pm. | | | | | | | |
| | am. | | | | | | | |
| | pm. | | | | | | | |
| | am. | | | | | | | |
| | pm. | | | | | | | |

**Key**  0 = no pressure damage
1–5 = grade of pressure tissue damage (Torrance, 1983)

### The role of care assistants

Care assistants should use their knowledge of the caring skills and attitudes essential in helping to assess the needs of clients and for supporting them when carrying out these therapeutic activities. They should assist in recording observations on the pressure areas check list. It is advisable to report or consult the person-in-charge at any time, if and whenever you are in doubt.

## References

Andrews C, Smith J (1989) *Nurses Aids Series — Medical Nursing,* 11th edn. Bailliere Tindall, London

Dealey C (1989) The pressure debate. *Nurs Times* **85**(26): 75

Dealey C (1991) The size of the pressure sore problem in a teaching hospital. *J Adv Nurs* **16**: 663–6670

Flack M, Johnson M (1986) *Handbook for Care.* Beaconsfield Publishers Ltd, Bucks

Hibbs P (1988) *Pressure Area Care for the City and Hackney Health Authority. Prevention Plan and Policy for Management.*

Norton D et al (1975) *An Investigation of Geriatric Nursing Problems in Hospital.* Churchill Livingstone, Edinburgh

Torance C (1983) *Pressure Sore: Aetiology Treatment and Prevention.* Croom Helm, London

Waterlow J (1991) A policy that protects. Waterlow pressure sore prevention/treatment. *Prof Nurse* **6**(5): 258–264

## Audio visual aids

**Format: VHS video**
Ref: CNE 4403: *Wound Care Series: Part 3 — Prevention and Management of Pressure Ulcers*
Ref: CNE 9923: *Controlling Transmission of Infection*
Ref: DSI/1-4: *Prevention and Healing of Pressure Sores*
Ref: FHM1: *Pressure Ulcer Prevention*
Oxford Educational Resources Ltd

## Assignment

The purpose of this homework is to assist you in preparing for your Workbased Assessment of Competence. As there is no pressure on you, feel free to work at your own pace, but avoid the temptation to procrastinate. After you have read your notes and suggested references, submit your work for correction. The completed work becomes part of your Personal Portfolio.

## Prevention of pressure sores (Z7: 2–3, Z19: 1–2)

1. What is the skin? Draw and label a simple diagram of the skin.
2. List five functions of the skin.
3. Explain what you understand by a pressure sore?
4. Give an account of the causes of pressure sores.
5. Name six possible areas which are prone to the development of this problem.
6. Describe observations you would make and report on the general condition of the elderly resident in an attempt to prevent the development of pressure sores.
7. How would you assist the healing process of a wound?
8. Discuss your care of an elderly resident who has developed a pressure sore.

## Care of mobility aids (CU6.1: 1–3, Z6: 1–2)

People should move around in order to maintain their mobility. Some may need walking aids if they suffer from disabilities caused by disease or physical infirmity. These aids are usually suggested by the doctor, and the physiotherapist will assess each individual client for height and weight and prescribe appropriate walking aids. The best way to maintain mobility is to encourage clients to help themselves, but reassure them that assistance is at hand if it is needed. There are a variety of walking aids, but those in common use are:

### 1. Walking stick (folding or straight)

This may be a cane which is suitable for balance and support, or made of metal and adjustable. A walking stick is used if the person has no disability in his/her upper limbs.

*Care of walking sticks*
- check the tips for worn rubber ferrules
- check canes for cracks or loose screws
- be sure that the person is using the cane correctly

- be sure that the person using the cane is the owner.

## 2. Sitting aids

Wheelchairs of various designs are usually prescribed to suit the needs of people who may not be able to walk with a walking aid. They are equipped with a number of options and, when using a wheelchair, the carer should ensure that the person is properly positioned for comfort and safety.

Wheelchairs should not be used instead of an ordinary armchair if transfers are possible. A cushion must always be used, and check that the footplates are in position and brakes are secured before helping the client in or out of the chair.

### Care of wheelchairs
- check inflatable tyre pressures regularly
- check the brakes for loose, worn or missing parts
- check regularly, especially if electrically operated, and follow the manufacturer's guidance for use and maintenance
- keep the chair clean and oil moving parts regularly
- ensure that the chair is properly adjusted for the user.

It is important to ensure that permanent wheelchair users who are at risk of developing pressure sores are regularly assessed, and provision is made for replacement of special cushions for wheelchair users.

## 3. Zimmer frames

These are fixed for height and are adjustable to suit the client's need and disability. Frames are ordered by the doctor/physiotherapist.

### Types
There are two main types: the standard Zimmer frame which is rigid, with four legs and is used for balance, and the gliding Zimmer frame which has wheels on the front legs. It can be pushed along without having to lift it off the ground.

### Care of Zimmer frames
- make sure that the Zimmer frame is the correct size for the person using it
- check for loose screws and worn tips
- ensure that the wheels cannot roll out from under the person and cause a fall.

## 4. Crutches

Occasionally people have to use crutches and they should be checked regularly for friction sores under the armpit or on the elbow.

### Care of crutches
- check the tips for worn ferrules
- check the padding for wear
- check for loose screws or cracks.

## 5. Walking up the stairs

Most people can negotiate the stairs using their walking aid, although some may have difficulty. The aim is usually to establish a normal pattern of one leg before the other, but where one leg is injured or lame this method may not be appropriate. Therefore:
- seek guidance on how best to help an individual client

- allow the person to hold onto the handrail for support
- support the person from behind and round the waist to give confidence
- stand in front of the person when going downstairs to prevent him/her falling forward.

## General approach and support

### *Guidance*

In order to enable clients to maintain and improve their mobility, it is important to:
- have an in-depth knowledge of the person's needs for mobility and develop a good interpersonal relationship with him or her
- check with the care plan regarding the client's mobility needs
- encourage the client to be independent as far as possible but to seek help when necessary
- ascertain that the client does not experience any discomfort, reporting any complaints to the person-in-charge
- allow the client adequate space to manoeuvre by ensuring that all potential hazards are removed or minimised, eg. worn carpets, rugs, steps
- pay special attention to the arrangement of furniture to prevent falls
- support the client when negotiating stairs, if there is no lift to use
- reinforce the importance of using mobility aids at all times, and offer practical support as necessary
- maintain accurate records of clients' progress
- label any defective appliance, take it out of use and report to the person-in-charge
- request a replacement if necessary
- store all walking aids in a designated place, for the convenience of clients
- be familiar with individual clients' walking aids which are provided to enable them to move freely in the care environment.

## References

Community Outlook (1979) Getting the right piece in the right place. *Nurs Times* **75**(8): 33–42

HB6 (1990) *Equipment and Services for People with Disabilities.* Health Education Publications Unit, Heywood Stores, Heywood

McMahon C et al (1993) *Knowledge to Care.* Blackwell Scientific Publications, London

**Section V: The delivery of care — option group B**

At the end of this section, candidates should aim to demonstrate an understanding of the basic principles of delivery of care defined by the following units of learning.

|  | Units and elements of learning |  |
|---|---|---|
| **Unit 12: Assist in clinical activities: investigations in care** | *X12, X13, Y4, Z19* | 267 |
| o Measuring temperature, pulse and respiration | *X12.2, X13.3, Z19.2* | 267 |
| o Collecting body wastes | *X13.3, Z11.3, Y4.2* | 272 |
| o Urine testing | *X13.3, Y4.2* | 276 |
| o Take and record blood pressure | *X13.1, 4* | 279 |
| o Measuring weight and height | *X13.1, X19.4, Y4.2* | 281 |
| **Unit 13: Assist in clinical activities: delivery of care** | *CU3, CU4, CU6, X13, Y4* | 284 |
| o Administer clients' own medication | *X13.5, Y4.3* | 284 |
| o Maintenance of materials and equipment | *CU6: 1–3* | 288 |
| o Cleanliness of the care environment | *CU3: 1–3* | 290 |
| o The missing person and his or her belongings |  | 295 |
| o Support and control of visitors | *CU4: 1–3* | 300 |
| **Unit 14: Assist clients to participate in leisure activities** | *X14, Y1, Y3, Z5, Z7, Z13* | 304 |
| o Rehabilitation | *X14* | 304 |
| o Personal, domestic and financial resources | *Y1: 1–5, Y3: 1–3* | 309 |
| o Concepts of mobility | *Z5.1, Z7.1* | 313 |
| o Preparing clients for a journey or visit | *Z5: 2–3* | 316 |
| **Unit 15: Health education and promotion** | *NC7* | 319 |
| **Unit 16: Assist clients to express sexuality** | *W1* | 324 |
| o Nature and purpose of sexuality in later life | *W1: 1–4* | 324 |
| o Helping the elderly to express sexuality |  | 327 |
| **Unit 17: Community care** | *W4, Y2* | 330 |
| o National Health Service and Community Care Act 1993 | *W4: 1–2, Y2: 1–2* | 330 |
| o Primary health care team | *W4.1* | 331 |
| o Services and facilities in the community for the elderly | *W4: 1–2, Y2: 1–2* | 333 |
| **Unit 18: Support clients in the activity of dying** | *NC1, NC3, Z14, Z15* | 336 |
| o Nature and purpose of dying | *NC1.1* | 336 |
| o Bereavement and grieving | *NC1.1* | 337 |
| o Management of problems | *NC1.2, NC3.3* | 339 |

- Last offices — Z15: 1–2 — 344
- Support for relatives — NC1: 2–3, NC3: 1–3 — 346

## Unit 19: Special care needs (mental health) — CL7, NC10, W2, X2, X16, Z8 — 348

- Mental health problems in the elderly — W2.1, Z8.1 — 348
- Assessment of functional abilities — X2: 1–3 — 353
- Management of mental health problems — X1: 2–3, X2: 2–4, X16: 1–2 — 356
- Specific treatment programme — X2: 2–4, X16: 1–3, NC10.3 — 360
- The depressed elderly person — W2.1, Z8: 1–2 — 363
- The confused elderly person — CL7: 1–2, Z8: 1–2 — 366
- The overactive elderly person — NC10: 2–3, NC11: 1–3 — 367
- Mental Health Act 1983 — 370

# Unit 12
# Assist in clinical activities: investigations in care (X12, X13, Y4, Z19)

## Measuring temperature, pulse and respiration (X12.2, X13.3, Z19.2)

Temperature, pulse and respiration are called **vital signs** because they provide important information about the health of an individual. It is recognised that variations may occur which are significant in care, therefore accurate measurements are absolutely essential, especially for clients who are acutely ill. As a result, the measurements of these vital signs are regarded as a delegated function. It is essential that results should be checked in the first instance with a qualified nurse, and at any subsequent time if there is any doubt whatsoever.

### Body temperature

This is the state of warmth or coldness of the body as measured with a thermometer which may be a calibrated glass filled with liquid mercury or a disposable thermometer, eg. Tempo Dot single use thermometer. Care must be taken not to drop or damage the glass calibrated thermometer. The normal oral temperature is 37.1°C with a slight decrease early in the morning and a slight increase at night. The process indicates a balance between heat production and loss.

### Routes for measuring temperature

Temperature may be taken orally, axially, per rectal or at the groin, according to age, condition of the client and nature of the illness.

### 1. Oral route

This is taken when a client has no difficulty holding the glass calibrated thermometer in his/her mouth.

*Requirements*
- a clinical thermometer, a watch with a second hand, a pen
- the client's temperature chart for recording the result
- a spirit swab for wiping the thermometer, and a disposable bag.

*Procedure*
- wash and dry your hands thoroughly before and after the procedure
- inform the client what you are about to do and seek his co-operation
- make the person comfortable either in bed or sitting in a chair
- delay the procedure for about 15 minutes if the client has had a hot or cold drink, has taken exercise, had steam inhalation, a bath or a shower or has been smoking.

*Measurement of oral temperature rate*
- read the clinical thermometer, examine for cracks, shake the mercury down to below 35°C and insert the bulb end in the client's mouth under the tongue

- advise the person not to suck, talk or bite the thermometer, but to close his/her lips
- leave the thermometer in his/her mouth for about 3–5 minutes
- remove the thermometer, read the result, shake the mercury down, wipe with a spirit swab and return it to its container
- record the result on the TPR chart and show it to the appropriate person-in-charge who asked you to carry out the procedure.

## 2. Axial route

- wash and dry your hands thoroughly before and after the procedure
- follow the initial procedure, ie. seeking client's cooperation
- wipe and examine the thermometer for cracks
- ensure that the skin under the axilla is dry and free from perspiration
- place the thermometer in the axilla. Position the arm carefully so that the skin surfaces are directly in contact with the bulb end of the thermometer
- leave for about 10 minutes, remove, read the result, shake the mercury down, wipe with a spirit swab and return the thermometer to its container.

It is important that each client has his or her own thermometer, to be stored either in a dry or wet container. In some areas disposable thermometers may be used either orally or placed on the client's forehead, eg. Tempa Dot. Electronic thermometers may also be used. Clear instructions should be given by the nurse-in-charge if you are required to use these.

## Care plan for clients with a 'temperature'

### *Guidance*

- nurse ensures the client is in bed. Removes excess clothing or extra bedclothes
- limits activities and offers frequent drinks and mouth washes
- tepid sponge may be ordered in the case of rigor and hyperpyrexia to help reduce body temperature. Treat pressure areas in the process
- assist in maintaining a hourly TPR chart and fluid balance chart.

## Pulse

This is the heart rate most conveniently taken at the wrist. Each pulse represents a cardiac cycle and may be felt at any point where an artery passes superficially and lies under a bone. It is most conveniently felt at the radial artery just below the root of the thumb. The pulse may also be felt at the temporal artery below the ears and carotid artery below the chin.

## Normal pulse

The normal adult pulse rate is about 72 beats per minute. In childhood it is more rapid and varies from 130 in infants to about 80 in older children. In old age the pulse rate usually becomes slower and it may quicken again in extreme old age.

## Measuring pulse rate

The pulse is usually counted at the radial artery of the wrist and is counted for a full minute. If you are required to take and record the pulse rate, rhythm (regularity) and volume (fullness), the qualified nurse will instruct you on these measurements. 'Critikon' Dinamap an electronic instrument may also be used.

## Respiration

Respiration is the exchange of gases in the body tissue as a result of breathing in air (oxygen) and breathing out carbon dioxide. The process is known as inspiration and expiration.

### Normal respiration rate

Normal respiration is quiet, regular, comfortable and rhythmic. The rate varies with age and sex. A new-born infant is about 40 and an adult varies from 18 to 20 per minute, but it is slightly faster in a woman.

### Measuring respiration rate

This is counted by observing the rise and fall of the client's chest wall.

### *Procedure*

This needs to be carried out unobtrusively when a client is at rest. The rate may alter if he/she is aware that you are watching him/her. The easiest way is to 'take' the respiration rate while the thermometer is still registering, or by continuing to hold his/her wrist after counting the pulse rate. Any alteration must be reported. Observe and report any changes which the client may show, such as loud snoring, a harsh grating sound (stidor), grunting or wheezing.

### Factors which may influence temperature, pulse and respiration

Adverse factors may include:
- extreme temperatures (hot and cold)
- exercise, drugs, smoking, a variety of diseases, old age
- psychological reactions, eg. anxiety
- reactions associated with body temperature.

The most common adverse reactions associated with body temperature are:

### *1. Pyrexia*

This is fever characterised by a rise of body temperature to any point between 37° and 40°C. The skin is flushed with increased perspiration and client may complain of feeling unwell. The pulse and respiration rates are increased, with loss of appetite, decreased urinary output and mild mental confusion.

### *2. Hyperpyrexia*

The body temperature is about 40°C.

### *3. Rigor*

An attack of intense shivering occurring when the heat regulation of the body is disturbed. The temperature rises rapidly and may either stay elevated or fall rapidly as profuse sweating occurs.

### Hypothermia

This is an abnormally low decline of body temperature dropping below 35°C. It becomes serious if the reduction of temperature is so drawnout that the person falls ill and fails to take adequate nourishment. Hypothermia is normally associated with severe cold weather conditions followed by frostbite. It is prevalent among babies and the elderly, especially elderly people living alone in the community.

## Causes

With ageing, the ability of the body to create and maintain body temperature decreases, and the blood supply to vital organs of the body, eg. brain, is reduced. The condition may be due to:

- prolonged exposure to a cold or damp environment. During this period the body temperature drops, resulting in the slowing of the metabolic rate of both mental energy and activities of the body. If untreated the person goes into coma
- illness reducing the awareness and ability to care for self. This may result in falls
- the effects of ageing on temperature control
- the use of certain drugs, such as hynoptics (sleeping tablets)
- social factors, eg. poverty due to a reluctance to spend money on food and heating and fear of getting into debt

## Clinical features

- parts of the body covered with clothing feel extremely cold to the touch
- skin looks waxy and greyish blue
- slow pulse rate and fall in blood pressure
- voice is hoarse if the client is able to talk and he/she breathes with difficulty
- anorexia — lack of appetite
- restlessness, with difficulty in maintaining desirable posture
- mental confusion and sleepiness, which may lead to coma
- severe shivering attack resulting in loss of memory (amnesia).

### Care plan for clients with hypothermia

The aim is to help the victim to regain normal body temperature by the use of rewarming methods.

## Guidance

- help the victim into bed and ensure that the room temperature is between 18°–24°C
- wrap the client with a heat retaining metalised (space) blanket
- use insulating materials, eg. cotton blanket or thermal clothing
- offer plenty of warm drinks and maintain a fluid balance chart
- give a light nourishing diet containing protein, fruit and vegetables
- assist in maintaining hourly TPR and blood pressure
- turn the client and treat pressure areas four-hourly
- ensure that the client moves about as he or she improves, but maintain observation for several days
- talk to the person, reassure and encourage him or her to express personal wishes.

## Prevention of hypothermia

Hypothermia is not a disease but a condition which can be prevented through education of clients. It is often seen in elderly people who live alone and lack knowledge of the risks of hypothermia. This is because they are afraid to spend their pension on heating or on food. The outcome is that they become malnourished, the body cannot generate heat, and their temperature falls. They are unaware of becoming cold and this leads to the onset of hypothermia. Nowadays this is rarely seen in residential care establishments.

## Guidance

It is important that clients are given information and planned preventive care. Carers have an important role to play in explaining the incidence of hypothermia to the client to prevent a recurrence. It is important to:

- make regular visits to people at risk of suffering from hypothermia, such as those suffering from dementia or other mental health problems
- ensure that the bedroom and living-rooms are warm and at a constant room temperature of 20°–24°C
- ensure that the individual maintains an adequate diet with vegetable, fruits and copious fluid intake. Meals on Wheels could be arranged, if required, to ensure that the individual has one good meal a day
- encourage the person to wear layers of light warm wool material, particularly woollen bobble hats to prevent heat loss through the head
- revitalise the person with age-related exercises, eg. gentle walks in the park
- advise and check whether the person is aware of the Government Income Support scheme which is intended for elderly people who do not have enough money on which to live
- promote contact with local branches of Help the Aged and Age Concern
- provide information on prevention of hypothermia.

## Measuring temperature, pulse and respiration

### General guidance

There are a number of clinical thermometers in use today. If the calibrated glass filled one is in use in your area of work, then follow these suggestions. Otherwise, observe manufacturer's instructions for use.

1. Always inspect the clinical thermometer and never use one that is chipped or cracked. **Never touch the bulb end**, if a calibrated glass thermometer is used.
2. Mercury is poisonous and can be absorbed through the skin. Use special care in cleaning up a broken thermometer.
3. Never leave a client unattended with a clinical thermometer in place.
4. Always wash your hands before and after the procedure.

## References

Irvine RE et al (1986) *The Older Patient, 4th edn: An Introduction to Geriatric Nursing*. Hodder and Stoughton, London.

Robertson B (1992) *Study Guide for Health and Social Care Support Workers NVQ in Care Level 2*. First Class Books Inc, USA

Roberts A (1989) Hypothermia. Systems of life No 168 Senior Systems — 33. Hypothermia. *Nurs Times* **85**(6): 59–62

Vyvyan MY (1992) Making sense of hypothermia. *Nurs Times* **88**(49): 38–40

Vjdelingum V (1990) The elderly and hypothermia. *J Dist Nurs* **8**(7): 5–7

## Audio visual aids

### Format: VHS video

Ref: *Basic Observations A: Temperature, Pulse and Respiration*
Ref: 425CT: *Healthy Eating for Elderly People* (tape slide)
Ref: 315CT: *Accidental Hypothermia in the Elderly*
Oxford Educational Resources Ltd

# Collecting body wastes (X13.3, Z11.3, Y4.2)

A variety of body wastes are dealt with in this section. Collection of specimens is a delegated function which care assistants may be asked to help with from time to time The most common specimens are urine, stools, sputum and vomit. It is important that during this procedure, the need to maintain a client's self-respect, privacy and dignity are observed at all the times. Clients need information on reasons for the procedure, instruction on what to do and time in which to do it. Carers must recognise the need for a high standard of personal hygiene, in order to prevent the spread of infection to themselves and others.

## Purpose of collection of specimens

**Examination** of specimens will be necessary for a number of reasons, such as:
- diagnosis and progress of disease such as diabetes mellitus
- observation of the effect of a specific treatment or drug
- bacteriological examination in the case of infection
- routine examination on admission of a patient, and admission pre and post operations.

## Collection of specimens

Samples of body waste may be collected at any time. On admission these should be obtained as soon as the client is reasonably settled. Where appropriate, protective clothing, such as disposable aprons and gloves should be worn. Specimen containers must be clearly labelled with the client's name, the date and time of collection, the ward/home and sent to the pathological laboratory with the request form written and signed by the doctor. It is important to be aware that the best result is obtained when specimens are fresh.

## Urine

Urine is fluid secreted by the kidneys and excreted through the bladder and urethra. It consists of about 96% water and 4% solid. The average amount passed daily is about 1,500 mls (52 ozs) and varies according to the fluid intake and needs of the body. Normal urine is clear, pale amber in colour and has a slightly acid reaction.

### *Abnormalities in urine*
These relate to:
- **volume** (quantity) which may increase in certain conditions such as diabetes, anxiety, diuretic drugs, intake of fluids or decreased in febrile conditions, heart and kidney diseases, the use of certain drugs
- **colour** — varies with quantity. If there is injury, blood renders it smoky or red and some drugs may make it bright orange or yellow. At times it may turn beetroot coloured after a meal of salad
- **clarity** — a cloudy appearance may indicate the presence of infection
- **odour** — this may be slightly 'fishy' when it has decomposed. The presence of acetone may suggest a smell of newmown hay
- **concentration** — normally it will be clear if the client passes a large volume, but during the hot summer months, it may be concentrated. Also a client who is dehydrated will pass urine with a darker appearance, especially if he or she is not drinking sufficient fluid.

### *Procedure for collection of urine specimens*
Explain to the client the need to provide a specimen of urine for routine examination and seek his/her co-operation:
- wear a disposable apron and gloves

- give him/her a clean and dry specimen bottle labelled with his/her name, the date and time of collection.

### Female client:
- provide her with a clean receptacle, eg. bowl, bedpan and cover or commode
- ask her discretely if she is menstruating. If so, provide her with small, clean cotton wool balls and ask her to:
  - wash and dry her hands thoroughly
  - place a cotton wool ball firmly in the entrance to the vagina to prevent blood passing into the urine specimen, and then to pass urine into the clean receptacle
- wash and dry her hands thoroughly
- transfer the urine specimen from the receptacle into the clean, dry specimen bottle labelled with her name.

### Male client:
- give him clean urinal if he is not able to use the toilet, and request him to pass urine into it
- provide the client with handwashing facilities
- transfer the urine specimen from the urinal into the clean specimen bottle
- observe the colour and appearance of the urine specimen
- wash and dry your hands thoroughly.

### Mid-stream specimen of urine
The procedure requires a specific technique, to avoid contamination of the specimen. The aim is to identify the cause of infection. Provide client with the following articles and ensure that he/she understands the procedure.

#### Equipment:
- handwashing facilities, eg. soap, wash bowl, disposable towel
- clean the specimen bottle labelled with the client's name, date and time of collection
- a bedpan and cover or commode if the client is unable to go to the toilet

#### Procedure:
- ask the person to wash and dry his or her genital area with warm soapy water before using the toilet, bedpan or commode
- ask the client to start passing urine into the toilet/bedpan/commode, then switch to passing urine into the specimen bottle during the flow and, finally, to remove the bottle and continue to empty the bladder in the toilet or bedpan or commode
- ask the client to secure the lid of the specimen bottle and hand it to the carer
- provide the person with handwashing and drying facilities.

### 24-hour collection of urine specimen
A 24-hour urine specimen may be required to:
- determine the function of the kidney and the content of the urine
- record body fluid balance.

#### Equipment:
- measuring jug
- a large urine container obtained from the pathological laboratory. If it has solution in it, do not discard before adding the urine specimen, as it is a necessary part of the laboratory test.

**Procedure** Everyone involved in the care, must be aware that 'a 24-hour collection of specimen is in progress'. A large specimen container with preservatives which has been labelled with the client's name, the date, time, ward or home is required. Also a laboratory request form bearing details of the

client and investigations required. A starting time is agreed, eg. 7.00 am and then the following procedures are taken:
- discard the first specimen of urine the client passed at 7.00 am. This is because it is not known how long it has been in the bladder and is likely to be stale
- measure and record every subsequent urine specimen passed during the following 24-hours and pour it into the specimen container. The container is collected or sent to the pathological laboratory accompanied by the laboratory request form according to local arrangement.

## Sputum specimen

Sputum is material which is expelled from the respiratory passages through the mouth as a result of irritation of the tract. It is usually the outcome of coughing and is not produced in a healthy person unless he is a smoker or has some form of throat infection.

### *Abnormalities*
Sputum consists chiefly of mucus and saliva, but in diseased conditions of the air passage it may be:
- purulent, ie. consist of pus which occurs in a lung abscess
- blood stained. This usually appears as rusty-coloured sputum, eg. in people suffering from pneumonia
- frothy sputum is a characteristic of acute oedema of the lungs and may occur in cases of heart or kidney failure
- haemoptysis. This is a term used to describe the coughing up of blood in any quantity, eg. in pulmonary tuberculosis.

### *Procedure for collection of sputum specimen*
The specimen is best collected first thing in the morning before the person has had breakfast. Explain the procedure to the person and seek his or her co-operation:
- give a clean specimen jar already labelled with the name, date and time of collection
- ask the client to expectorate into the bottle without moving the sputum about in the mouth to collect saliva
- send the specimen to the laboratory accompanied by the laboratory request form
- offer client handwashing and drying facilities, and a mouthwash if it is considered necessary.

### *Guidance*
Care must be taken to avoid soiling the sides of the specimen jar. Report any sign of discomfort the client may complain of to the person-in-charge immediately.

## Faeces or stools

A specimen of faeces may be requested for laboratory investigation over a number of days.

### *Abnormalities*
These could be:
- green, loose or watery and foul smelling, black or clay coloured
- hard and dry
- accompanied by mucus, blood or containing foreign bodies, eg. worms.

### *Collection of specimen of faeces*
#### *Equipment:*
- bedpan with cover
- a labelled specimen jar with a small spoon attached to a screw cap
- handwashing facilities, eg. towel, soap, wash bowl, disposable towel.

#### *Procedure*
- explain the procedure to the person and seek his or her cooperation

- offer him or her the use of a bedpan
- remove the bedpan after defecation and give him or her handwashing facilities
- take the bedpan to the sluice and spoon a specimen of faeces into the specimen jar. Faeces may be of different colours and a small sample of each colour should be collected
- make sure that the specimen jar has been labelled with the patient's name, the date and time of collection, the ward, nursing home/hospital, and send to the pathological laboratory with the request form signed by the doctor
- wash and dry your hands after collecting the specimen and report the result of your work and observations to the nurse-in-charge.

## Vomit

This is matter ejected from the stomach through the mouth, and may be coffee coloured with small quantities of altered blood. It may also be dark brown with an unpleasant odour. Quite often it is preceded by nausea and excess secretion of saliva due to irritation of the stomach. Vomiting may occur as a result of pregnancy, psychological reaction and other causes.

### Abnormalities
- bile, which gives it a yellowish or greenish colour
- faecal matter, which may be due to intestinal obstruction
- blood as a result of damage to the stomach.

### Collection of vomit specimen
As a general rule, vomit is kept in the bowl in which it is received. It should be covered as it is moved about the ward or conveyed to the laboratory for examination.

## General guidance for collecting specimens

1. The process of collection of all specimens should be undertaken in private, maintaining the dignity and views of the clients throughout.
2. All specimens must be:
   - labelled correctly with the name of the person, date and time of collection, hospital ward and/or nursing or residential care homes
   - sent immediately collected to the pathological laboratory accompanied by a pathological request form(s) duly completed and signed, eg. by doctor. They should never be left lying about for other people to see.
3. Disposable apron and gloves should always be worn; wash and dry your hands thoroughly during and after carrying out the procedures.

## References

Flack M, Johnson M (1986) *Handbook for Care*. Beaconsfield Publishers Ltd, Bucks

McMahon CA (Ed) et al (1994) *Knowledge to Care. A Handbook for Care Assistants*. Blackwell Scientific Publications, London

Robertson B (1992) *Study Guide for Health and Social Care Support Workers. NVQ in Care Level 2*. First Class Books Inc, USA

**Audio visual aid**

*Format: VHS video*
Ref: NT 14: *Basic Observations: D Specimen Collection*
Oxford Educational Resources Ltd

## Assignment

The purpose of this homework is to assist you in preparing for your Workbased Assessment of Competence. As there is no pressure on you, feel free to work at your own time and pace, but avoid the temptation to procrastinate. After you have read your notes and suggested references, submit your work for correction. The completed work becomes part of your Personal Portfolio.

## Collection of body wastes (X13: 1–3, Z11.3, Y4.2)

1. Describe how you would go about collecting a clean specimen of urine from the following clients, and what containers would you use.
    a) a female client
    b) a confused elderly gentleman.
2. State what abnormalities you expect to find in the following specimens.
    a) faeces
    b) sputum
    c) urine.
3. Make a list of things you would get ready for a 24-hour collection of urine. How would you prepare a client for this procedure?
4. What precautions would you take to prevent contamination of your uniform, and spread of infection when collecting specimens?

## Urine testing (X13.3, Y4.2)

Analysis of urine is one of the most important procedures care assistants may be asked to undertake. The findings should be discussed with the responsible qualified staff who delegated the task, as there may be a need to verify the result.

### Reasons for urine testing

1. Admission: provides an overview of the patient's general well-being and may help to reveal certain conditions for the first time.
2. Diagnosis.
3. Pre-operative preparation.
4. Monitoring of treatment.

### Characteristics of a urine specimen

After collecting a specimen of urine it is important to let it stand for a while and make the following observations. The normal characteristics of urine are:

**Colour:** pale amber or pale straw, but changes can occur if there is bleeding. Drugs, protein, beetroot, can make urine coloured

**Odour:** very little smell but on standing may develop ammonia smell

**Quantity:** about 40–60 ounces

**Reaction:** slightly acid

**Specific gravity:** 1010–1025

**Appearance:** This should be clear, but may be cloudy in certain diseases.

## Testing urine using reagent strips

Urine testing has now been made easier by the development of multiple strips by Ames. They give clear indications of urinary abnormalities which may require more definite tests in the pathological laboratory. It is therefore important that care assistants should be aware of and report these abnormalities so that care may be planned to tackle them.

### *Guidance*

1. Ascertain that there is a sufficient quantity of a fresh specimen of urine.
2. Note the colour and clearness and the presence or absence of deposit.
3. Take reaction using a litmus paper. Acid urine turns blue litmus paper red, and alkaline urine turns red litmus paper blue.
4. Take pH Factor — this denotes how acid or alkaline the urine is. It is expressed numerically 1 to 14: 7 is neutral, above is alkaline, below is acid. A normal reading is usually 5 to 8. Vegetarians usually have a more alkaline urine at approximately pH 8.
5. Take specific gravity or density.

The specific gravity of urine is a measure of the ability of the kidneys to concentrate urine. It may be low if the fluid intake is high. A high specific gravity may indicate dehydration. This is normally measured by the use of a urinometer — a small glass measure with a graduated stem. Specific gravity of water as 1000 and the specify gravity of urine is normally 1010–1025.

### *Equipment:*
Reagent strips or a urinometer, a clean specimen jar, clean specimen of urine.

### Procedure

#### *Using a urinometer:*
- stand the specimen jar on a flat surface and pour the urine specimen into the jar
- place the urinometer gently into the urine specimen in the jar
- ensure that the urinometer floats freely in the urine and its base does not touch the bottom of the container.

**Read the result:** The density of the urine is determined by reading the digits on the urinometer at the highest level of the urine that forms the stem (Meniscus).

### Testing the urine specimen

#### *Guidance*
Marked changes may occur in the composition of urine if it is allowed to stand for a long time. So if you are asked to test a routine urine specimen, the guideline is to:

- follow the manufacturer's instructions correctly, especially in using and storing the strips which should not be used after the expiry date
- wash and dry your hands thoroughly and put on a disposable apron and gloves
- chose the reagent required for the test to be undertaken, eg. glucose
- read the manufacturer's instructions on the reagent containers
- check expiry date and use reagents from containers that have been closed
- remove a dip stick carefully and replace the lid immediately. Do not touch the coloured squares of the stick with your hand or put it down on a wet surface
- dip the stick in urine, remove and tap it lightly to remove excess urine
- check the result without allowing the wet stick to touch the chart or coloured squares
- note the findings
- wash and dry your hands thoroughly and put the equipment away
- record or report findings to the person who delegated the task.

## The results

Examination of specimens of urine may be able to provide useful information which may assist diagnosis and monitoring of diseases. Quite often results of urine testing in the clinical area indicate the need for a more detailed investigation to establish a diagnosis of the client's condition. A routine urinalysis may detect any of the followings substances:

**Protein:** A morning specimen is required when testing for protein. Evidence may indicate congestive cardiac failure, pregnancy, febrile conditions, infections, damage to the kidneys.

**Glucose:** This is not normally present in urine. Presence may be due to diabetes mellitus.

**Bilirubin:** This may be present in damage to the liver (hepatic), jaundice, gall stones.

**Blood:** This may be due to stones (calculi) in the kidney, injury, menstruation in women, or some drugs.

**Pus:** This may be due to infection of the genito-urinary system.

**Acetone and diacetic acid:** The presence of acetone and diacetic acid in the urine may indicate the onset of a diabetic coma.

## Special precaution

Never throw away a specimen of urine until asked to do so as a qualified member of staff may wish to examine or confirm your findings. It is also important to maintain a high standard of personal hygiene at all times by wearing appropriate protective clothing and thoroughly washing and drying your hands before and after each procedure.

## References

Cook R (1996) Urinalysis: ensuring accurate urine testing. *Nurs Stand* **10**(46): 49–52

Flack M, Johnson M (1986) *Handbook for Care*. Beaconsfield Publishers Ltd, Bucks

Laker C (ed) (1994) *Urological Nursing*. Scutari Press, London

McMahon CA (Ed) *et al* (1994) *Knowledge to Care for Health and Social Care Support Workers*. Blackwell Scientific Publications. London.

## Audio visual aid

*Format: VHS video*
Ref: NT 13: *Basic Observation: D Urine Testing*
Oxford Educational Resources Ltd

# Take and record blood pressure (X13.1, 4)

Traditionally, taking and recording a client's blood pressure was the routine responsibility of qualified nurses, using a sphygmobolometer or 'Critikon' Dinamap® — an electronic instrument. However, it is gradually being delegated to care assistants under guidance. It is, therefore, important to discuss the findings with the staff who delegated the task, as these usually fluctuate.

## Blood pressure

Blood pressure is the degree of force which the circulating blood exerts upon the walls of the arteries. This force is maintained by the:
- strength of the heart beat
- tone of the vessel walls
- amount of fluid in circulation
- viscosity (density) of the fluid.

Normal blood pressure is estimated to be 120/80. The average force of pressure in large arteries is said to be when the heart is actively pumping sufficient blood to support a column of mercury 120mmHg high. This is the working period of the heart and is known as the systolic pressure. The pressure when the heart is resting is known as diastolic pressure and is about two-thirds of the systolic pressure, which is about 80mmHg.

### Factors which may affect blood pressure
- exercise: the pressure is raised
- psychological, eg. excitement, which also raises the pressure
- change of position: the pressure is lower in a recumbent than in an erect position
- other factors such as heart disease, nutritional status, drugs, alcohol.

## Sounds of the heart

The heart beats continuously for the whole of a person's life and its only period of rest is after each contraction, which is during diastole. The contraction of the heart and closure of its valves gives rise to:

### Systole
This is the working time of the heart and gives rise to the first heart sound 'lob'. The average systolic pressure is 120 and lasts for about $0 \cdot 3$ seconds.

### Diastole
This is the resting time of the heart, shorter than and giving rise to the second heart sound 'dup'. The average diastolic pressure is about 80mmHg, and it is believed that it lasts for about $0 \cdot 8$ seconds. Therefore, the cycle of the heart lasts for about 0.11 seconds.

## Taking blood pressure

Equipment required:
- sphygmobolometer or 'Critikon' Dinamap® — an electronic instrument
- stethoscope
- blood pressure and temperature, pulse and respiration (TPR) chart and a pen.

### *Guidance*

1. Explain to the patient what you are about to do and seek his/her co-operation.
2. Encourage the patient to relax in a sitting or lying position with the arm supported by a pillow placed on the bed or table.
3. Place the sphygmobolometer on a firm surface approximately at the same level as the arm.
4. Put the cuff evenly around the upper arm, taking care that the tubes of the cuff are put over the brachial artery (inner aspect of the upper arm).
5. Feel the patient's pulse at the radial artery and at the same time inflate the bag until the radial pulse disappears. Then raise the pressure another 5mmHg above the figure noted at the first reading.
6. Place the stethoscope over the brachial artery in front of the elbow and reduce very gradually by letting air escape until the pulse becomes just perceptible.
7. Listen very carefully and when a first thumping 'lob' is heard, take the reading for the height of the mercury column, this is known as the systolic pressure. When the second soft sound becomes a muffled 'dup', this is the diastolic pressure and is recorded. The level of the mercury gives the diastolic pressure.

### Recording of blood pressure

Blood pressure should be charted in a graphic manner in the TPR chart and should clearly indicate any change at a glance.

If the pressure was recorded with the client standing (as is sometimes requested), then this fact should be indicated on the chart. Secondly, if a series of readings is to be taken, eg. after injury or surgery, then the sphygmomanometer cuff could be left in position to lessen the disturbance to the person, but not inflated. The measurement of blood pressure requires much practice, guidance and supervision for one to become proficient. It is important to observe the client all the time for any sign of discomfort; to be able to stop the procedure immediately the person complains of any discomfort and to reassure him or her and report to the person-in-charge.

## Reference

Nursing Times (1990) Nursing observations. *Nurs Times* **86**(50): 56

### Audio visual aids

#### *Format: VHS video*
Ref: NT 12: *Basic Observations: B Blood Pressure*
Ref: 209CT: *Blood Pressure*
Oxford Educational Resources Ltd

# Measuring weight and height (X13.1, X19.4, Y4.2)

Weight is the expression of the body or any substance in a quantitative way using a well- defined and suitable scale. In humans the body weight may be stationery, decrease or increase but, whatever form it takes, if change occurs suddenly, it should be regarded as unsatisfactory. Children and infants require a regular and gradual increase as they grow older, and any weight loss may need investigating. In adults, changes in weight may indicate health problems associated with diseases such as tuberculosis. Weight loss or gain provides a good indication, and forms an important aspect of client care. If change occurs rapidly, especially in children, it may be the result of large fluid losses. Weight gained during illness can be a sign of fluid retention, ie. in the case of pulmonary or generalised oedema.

## Weight loss

Loss of weight may occur to anyone and at any time. In some cases, weight loss may be the result of lack of appetite. There is a reduced intake of nourishment and as the body requires more energy than is available in the food eaten, there is a decrease in weight. In the elderly, due to ageing processes, the body slows down, reducing the amount of energy required for the body to function properly. This may result in a reduced intake of nourishment leading to loss of weight with signs of malnutrition. It should be remembered that a reduction in body weight is only a pointer to a poor diet and only relates to energy intake. Lack of sufficient nutrients can occur even when the body weight remains constant. Changes in the skin caused by a loss of weight may result in delayed or poor wound healing and anaemia, and self-neglect may indicate lack of or inadequate dietary intake.

## Management of weight loss

Appetite can be increased by encouraging small and frequent meals to be taken regularly throughout the day. These should include foods which are enjoyable and attractively served. If a client is poorly nourished, he/she should be assessed by a dietician who may encourage him/her to take a high energy and high protein diet in order to meet his/her nutritional needs. In the elderly, weight loss gives a clear indication of poor intake of nourishment and must be monitored regularly.

In children, weight is an important indicator of growth and should be measured every time the child is seen at the clinic and whenever the child is sick.

## Measuring weight and height

### Infants

They are weighed without any clothing, on a balance infant scale. Older children may remain dressed but without shoes and be weighed on an adult balance scale. Depending upon the child's age and the amount of privacy available, the child can undress down to his/her underwear.

### Adults

Record of residents' weight is important as a guide to progress. Long-stay elderly patients should be weighed monthly, others every week or fortnightly as may be ordered. The weight should be recorded in the nursing or medical notes. Some skill is required to weigh an elderly person accurately and in private.

## Procedures for weight

The most commonly used is the standing scale with a measuring rod. For people who cannot stand, there is a wheelchair type and mechanical lift scales.

## *Guidance*

### *1. Wheelchair type scales*
- explain what you are about to do
- ensure privacy
- assist the patient to sit upright in the middle of the chair
- make sure that he or she does not lean or slump too far forward
- slide the bottom weight until the balance drops and centres
- the correct weight is shown when the bar floats horizontally between the stops
- chart the weight and report any major changes to the person-in-charge.

### *2. Standing balance scales*
- explain what you are going to do
- ensure privacy
- assist the person onto the scale
- be sure that he/she is not holding onto you or the scale
- slide the bottom weight until the balance drops and centres
- the correct weight is shown when the bar floats horizontally between the stops
- chart the weight and report any major changes to the person-in-charge.

### *Guidelines for weighing*
- weigh at the same time of day each time
- encourage the person to wear the same or a similar weight of clothing
- weigh with an empty bladder if possible
- remove client's shoes.

### Measuring height
- explain what you are going to do
- assist him/her onto the scale and ask him to stand straight, turning away from the scale
- place the measuring rod against the top of his/her head
- read and record the person's height

- assist the person in getting off the scale, if necessary
- record the height.

### General guidance

Once a measurement has been taken, it is either plotted on the chart or recorded in accordance with local practise in the client's case notes. Weight usually follows the same pattern each time the client is weighed, but any sudden decrease or increase should be evaluated. Any decrease may suggest malnutrition, acute illness, dehydration, emotional problems or chronic illness. An increase in weight may be related to overeating, oedema or endocrine disorders. It is important that any weight measurement is brought to the attention of the person-in-charge as a drastic decrease may indicate nutritional deficiencies, especially in the elderly.

# References

Department of Health and Social Security (1992) *The Nutrition of Elderly People. Report on Health and Social Subjects, 43*. HMSO London,

McMahon CA, J Harding (1994) *Knowledge to Care*. Blackwell Scientific Publications, London

Robertson B (1992) *Study Guide for Health Care Workers*. First Class Books Inc, USA

# Unit 13
# Assist in clinical activities: delivery of care (CU3, CU4, CU6, X13, Y4)

## Administer clients' own medication (X13:1, 2, 5, Y4.3)

Medicine is the science of introducing substances into the body for the purpose of healing, treating or preventing diseases. They are handled within set procedures with particular attention to the health and safety of everyone concerned. Failure to observe these procedures may lead to accidents, fire, explosions, radiation leakage, allergy or poisoning, ill-health and exposuring others to danger.

### Administration

The process is a significant aspect of care in which mistakes are often made. It requires an in-depth knowledge of the procedures, individual clients and relevant policies. It also demands competency, in skills and experience to prevent failure of treatment and an ability to instruct clients about their care in order to improve their health. Experience has shown that with the advent of NVQs, care assistants with these qualifications, are increasingly required to assist with this procedure, especially in residential care homes. The UKCC (1992) is opposed to the involvement of unqualified staff in the administration of medicines, because 'it gives a false sense of security'. But, local policies exist in some settings, and the overall responsibility for this procedure rests with qualified staff who are expected to use their professional judgement in accordance with the UKCC policy guidelines. Therefore, the aim of this section is to offer guidance for those who may be directly or indirectly involved in the administration of medicines. The process involves:

#### 1. Prescribing:
All medicines are prescribed by the doctor.

#### 2. Dispensing:
The pharmacist dispenses medicines in response to a doctor's or a nurse's prescription. These may be in liquid form such as solutions, mixtures, linctus, suspension, syrup, emulsions or oils. They may also be dispensed in solid form such as pills, lozenges, tablets, suppositories, capsules, powders.

### Supplies

Arrangement should be made with a local pharmacist to supply medicines. On delivery, the supplies should be checked and an accurate record maintained. Medicines should never be transferred from one container to another. When a container is to be replenished, the remaining unused medicines should be returned in the container to the dispensing pharmacist. When a particular course of treatment is completed or discontinued, any remaining drugs must be returned to the pharmacist. **Never take the drugs into stock.** Where controlled drugs are concerned, these should be returned to the pharmacist and an accurate record kept.

## Monitored dosage system

Many pharmacists use this system to dispense full prescriptions for specific clients. Within these systems, medicines are provided in a special container with sections for days of the week and times within those days. This approach is best suited for clients in residential care homes where the containers are delivered. Quite often all solid dose and oral medicines are dispensed either in child-resistant containers which comply with the British Standard or in unit packaging of strips.

### 3. Storage:
All medicines must be stored as recommended by the manufacturers. They should be stored in an appropriate medicine cabinet large enough for the medicines of each client to be kept separately. In care homes, medicines should be stored in an immovable locked container out of the reach of clients. Cleansing agents and disinfectants are kept separately in another cupboard. Controlled drugs should be stored in a lockable compartment to comply with the Controlled Drugs Regulations. Keys are always in the safekeeping of the person-in-charge. In clients' homes, arrangements should be made for the safety and security of medicines with access limited to a named client only.

### 4. Administration:
Medicines prescribed and dispensed should be administered in accordance with the instructions of the prescribing doctor. Medicines may be given by any of these routes:
- mouth, injection, rectum, inhalation
- topical application, eg. substances used in wound dressing, eye and ear drops
- inunction, which is the application of a local preparation or spray to the skin, eg. Algipan®.

### 5. Receiving:
This relates to clients receiving the prescribed medicine. It is important to ensure that the person understands and gives consent to receiving the medicine. It may also involve instructing the client and his/her relatives and others involved in care about the drug.

## Procedures for administration by mouth

The procedure should be carried out by the person-in-charge, who is also accountable for the total client care, or by a competent member of staff who has been trained and assessed in accordance with agreed local policy. It is, however, safer and more efficient for two people to carry out the procedures, and a care assistant may help the person-in-charge who should be able to carry out the following:

### *Guidance*
- promote and maintain good interpersonal relationship with clients
- identify the client for whom the medicines is intended and check the prescription card
- read container information in terms of correctness of instruction regarding:
  - to whom it has been prescribed, ie. name of the client
  - what has been prescribed, ie. the type, form and route, eg. tablet to be given by mouth, dosage, frequency or timing (one tablet, three times a day after meals)
- check the expiry date on the container or medicine bottle
- give only drugs that have been prescribed by doctor or nurse on a prescription card; withhold administration if you are in doubt and seek further clarification
- refuse to give medicines which are not in a container with the client's name on the label
- give medicine to the correct client and ensure that it is taken immediately it is given
- ensure that the medicine trolley or tray, if used, is not left unattended at any time

- maintain accurate records in relation to date, time of administration and signatures of those involved in the process in accordance with local policy or statutory requirements
- make written note of any client who refuses or deliberately withholds his or her medicine and give reasons for which medicine was not given. Report any mistake on your part
- report and hand over any tablet found on the floor to the person-in-charge
- observe and report any side effects such as dribbling, shaking, restlessness, rashes.

***Generally, the rule is that the right drug and the right dose should be given to the right client, by the right route and at the right time.***

### Self-administration

This practice of administration of medicines relates to self-administration of medicines by clients in their own homes. The monitored dosage system is useful and highly recommended for self-administration, especially in residential care homes. It provides a safer and easier system of drug control, particularly in keeping medicines out of the reach of children. The process encourages empowerment of clients in their care, and also involves educating relatives and informal carers in their role. It involves assessment and preparation of client to ensure that he or she is able to:

- consent to receive the prescribed medicine
- read and understand the directions on the label and open the container
- recognise the composition of medicine as the size of the tablet or capsule and taste of the liquid may contribute to refusal of the medicine. If there is any problem, an agreeable dosage or other form of preparation may be provided.

In health care homes, arrangement for storage is always the responsibility of the person-in-charge with access to specific clients.

### *Monitoring*

Where a client is receiving medicines from a personalised container, the carer should ensure that he/she understands the principles of safe administration. Accidental poisoning may occur as a result of carelessness, confusion or not being able to read labels due to poor eyesight. It is also essential for staff to be aware of ways of disposing of used syringes and needles, and dealing with spillage, eg. blood. They should guard against misuse of the drugs by others.

### Application of creams and ointments (inunction)

These are applications containing medical ingredients that are always prescribed by a doctor. The procedure is a delegated function, which must be treated with great care. Most of these preparations are in individual containers or jars and must be labelled with the person's name. If you are asked to carry out this task, it is important to refer to the person's prescription card and care plan for direction. Check with the person-in-charge if there are additional instructions to follow.

#### *Guidance*
- wash and dry your hands thoroughly before and after application
- explain to the resident what you are going to do and seek his or her co-operation
- protect your hands with disposable gloves to prevent cross-infection and unnecessary contact with the drug component of the cream or ointment
- read and follow instructions on the container, and apply ointment or cream to the affected part as prescribed
- never use the cream or ointment on anyone else as it could be harmful

- make client comfortable. Observe and report any side-effect, eg. redness, itchiness
- remove disposable gloves, wash and dry your hands thoroughly
- return the container to the appropriate compartment in the medicine cupboard.

## Legal aspects of administration of medicines

### *Inspection*

From time to time, and in accordance with the Medicines Act 1968 and the Misuse of Drugs Act 1971, stock will be inspected by a quality assurance team comprising a dispensing pharmacist, in conjunction with a pharmacist from the Health Authority.

### *Stock of poisons*

A register must be kept on the premises for receiving new stock, the date it was obtained and dispensing of any of the stock to residents. Out of date or unwanted controlled drugs may only be destroyed by persons authorised under the Act. It is important to check the stock before ordering and delivery to ensure that there is no wastage. Maintain accurate records. Orders should not be excessive. All surplus drugs or those belonging to deceased clients should be returned to the pharmacist in accordance with established policy.

## Role of care assistants

### *Guidance*

In some cases, where there is a frequent use of agency staff as senior staff on duty, there is a lack of knowledge of the residents. In order to provide a continuity of care, experienced care assistants with in-depth knowledge of the residents and the care establishment, could be asked to assist by identifying the right clients during the process. If this is the case, then it is important that they should:

- maintain good interpersonal relationships with all of the clients
- use their knowledge, skills and attitude to help the nurse-in-charge
- report and hand over to the person-in-charge any tablet found on the floor
- reassure clients about any negative feelings which may adversely affect the rights of others
- encourage clients to express their feelings, beliefs, wishes, talk and ask questions about their care and treatment, by doing so, they are more likely to report any side-effects earlier
- observe, record and report any unusual behaviour, mannerisms, rashes.

In any care setting, it is important to ensure that relatives and friends do not give any medicines without the prior knowledge of the person-in-charge, and the agreement of the prescribing doctor. Those who are not satisfied should be advised to raise the issue within the complaints procedure

## References

Booth B (1994) Management of drugs errors. *Nurs Times* **90**(15): 30–31

British Medical Association and the Royal Pharmaceutical Society of Great Britain (1992) *British National Formulary*. BMA, London

Cotterell N (1990) The view from pharmacy. *Nurs Times* **86**(43): 55–57

Department of Health (1989) *Guide to the Misuse of Drugs Act 1971 and the Misuse of Drugs Regulations*. HMSO, London

Dowine G *et al* (1987) *Drug Management for Nurses*. Churchill Livingstone, Edinburgh

Hatch AM, Tapley A (1982) A self-administration system for elderly patients at Highbury Hospital. *Nurs Times* **78**(42):1773–1774

Help the Aged (1992) *Managing your Medicines*. Community Services Pharmacists, Glaxo Holding, UK Ltd

Pembrey S (1984) Drug administration policy. *Nurs Times*, April 1994:14

Sutherland K, Morgan J, Semple S (1995) Self-administration of drugs: an introduction. *Nurs Times* **91**(23): 29–31

Trevelyan J (1988) Taking their own medicine. *Nurs Times* **84**(45): 28–32

United Kingdom Central Council of Nursing, Midwifery and Health Visiting (1992) *Standards for the Administration of Medicines*. UKCC, London

United Kingdom Central Council of Nursing, Midwifery and Health Visiting (1992) *The Code of Professional Conduct for the Nurse, Midwife and Health Visitor*. UKCC, London

## Audio visual aids

### Format: VHS video

Ref: CMEUA 811: *Drugs and the Elderly: Problem Drugs in the Elderly, Part 1*
Ref: NT 16: *Storage, Custody and Administration of Drugs*
Ref: CNE 7508: *Medicating the Elderly*
Oxford Educational Resources Ltd

## Maintenance of materials and equipment (CU6: 1–3)

Equipment is simply the tools that may be used for diagnostic purposes, treatment and prevention of illness or injury. It can be a clinical thermometer, wheelchair, catheter, dressing pack, incontinence products, toilet facilities or a weighing machine. The individual uses of equipment forms an essential part of maintaining standards and quality of care, irrespective of the setting. However, the way it is used should do both the client and carers no harm.

### Inventory

Each care establishment has its own scheme for maintaining an inventory, which is a detailed list or stock of the equipment and materials necessary for the smooth running of the service. It is, therefore, essential that the carer should know where the stock is at any time, and whether the oldest stock was used first. Supplies can become less effective as time passes. This may seem like common sense, but it is all too easy to overlook what is familiar.

Certain materials such as dressings, incontinence products, cereals, which are used daily, must be routinely checked by someone responsible to ensure that stock does not run out. Furthermore, inadequate stocks can cause frustration to everyone concerned, especially the clients, as it may result in poor standards of care. Therefore, it is advisable to have at least a package or two of the essential items in stock at all times, and report any deficit to the person-in-charge. The majority of equipment, household goods and materials carry manufacturers' guidelines on storage, how the equipment works, service requirement or use by date. It is important that these specifications should be observed. Check supplies of materials used regularly and report any shortfalls to the person-in-charge, eg. stationery, cereals, incontinence aids.

### Receipt of equipment

Every care institution should have someone to monitor the receipt of goods, and, on receiving the items it is important to check these against the delivery note or a copy of the original order form, eg.

medicines from the pharmacist. A record of goods received should be made and any shortfall reported to the person-in-charge. It is important to take note of guidelines for storage in case of explosive goods, eg. aerosol cans. Take note of manufacturers' recommendations on storage with respect to the Health and Safety at Work Act 1974 and local policy.

## Safety of equipment

Apparatus which is used daily must be checked before use. Before doing so, it is important to answer the following questions:
- is the equipment still safe to use, eg. wheelchair?
- who checked it last and when?
- were the staff properly trained to operate all the devices used in the home?
- did they first learn how to use it up by watching or by others answering their questions?

The key rule is to ensure that all equipment and materials used are safe. Each time a device is used, the carer takes ultimate responsibility for its effects on clients or colleagues. It is wise to adopt a much wider questioning approach to know the capability and limitation of the device you use, as it is not correct to assume that it will always be safe. Carers should aim to:
- check the new supply received against the delivery note, ensure that all items signed for are received and entry made in appropriate records in accordance with local policy
- handle the devices you have been trained to use correctly and do not use anything unless you are sure it is safe to use. If you have any doubt, get it checked and serviced. Read all instructions and check warning labels thoroughly and check them again as they may have changed. It is your duty to safeguard the interests of your clients, so next time you reach for any device think before you use it
- enquire about the way devices are acquired and stored and finally disposed of as inappropriate conditions, such as heat or light could cause damage
- take a close look at the health care equipment in the home and use it only for the purpose for which it was intended, never improvise. The person-in-charge will ensure that serviceable equipment is maintained in accordance with any contractual agreement, eg. lifts, washing machines and that accurate service records are maintained
- do not use devices more than once if manufacturers intended these to be used once only. There should be someone to ensure that it is working in accordance with manufacturers' specifications. Use it without proper training and you can be held personally responsible for the consequences, as can any staff who report to you
- check that the device is in good working condition, know the correct way to use it before helping someone else use it, and make sure that the person knows how to use the device. Do not let anyone use a defective device
- check and report any loss or faults and keep the device properly cleaned
- store and maintain potential dangerous medical devices, including medicines, in accordance with statutory regulations and local policy, eg. the Medicines Act 1968.

## Equipment for personal use

This is material specifically prescribed for a particular individual for his or her treatment, and should not be used for anyone else. It is correct to:
- mark the device with the person's name in an inconspicuous place for identification, such as walking aids, wheelchair, hearing aids, spectacles
- mark the removable parts, eg. foot rest/paddles on the wheelchairs
- keep the equipment within easy reach of the person using it
- observe clients for signs and symptoms of any physical problems that might develop with the use of equipment, eg. redness, pinching, rubbing, swelling, sore spots.

Any device which places someone at risk must be reported. It may be that nothing is wrong with the device itself, but storing or operating instructions may be confusing or misleading. No matter how serious the emergency, you can always make it worse. So report all problems, not just safety related incidents, as minor accidents or abnormalities might indicate quality assurance problems that could have widespread implications.

**Faulty equipment**

Everyone has a duty to report all devices that do not work as they should, especially if clients and staff are put at risk. Also, any equipment which is used inappropriately, maintained inadequately, adjusted incorrectly or modified without permission, poses a potential health hazard. If the fault is not reported, it is likely to happen again. So inform the right person, and ensure that you have knowledge of your local procedures for reporting incidents.

*Action to be taken*

If an adverse incident should occur regarding the use of any equipment, the priority is to:
- make sure your client is safe
- keep device and packaging instructions
- leave things just as they were
- make a record of the device settings if they had to be changed to make the device safe
- check the remaining stock, if the device was part of a batch
- contact and report to the person-in-charge
- provide all information about the incident in accordance with local and statutory policies.

The business of health care has become a more complicated service with the advances in the technological equipment at our disposal. So, think before you use any device. Any faulty equipment must be withdrawn from use, labelled and reported to the person-in-charge. Report anything that goes wrong no matter how trivial it seems. Put safety first. This is the only way to ensure that no harm comes to the client, your colleagues and yourself.

# References

Department of Health and Social Security (1994) *Doing The Patient No Harm* (DNH 2). Health Publication Unit and Distribution Centre, Heywood, Lancs OL10 2ZP

Robertson B (1992) *Study Guide for Health and Social Care Support Workers*. First Class Books Inc, USA

# Cleanliness of care environment (CU3: 1-3)

Hygiene is the science of health, and the action necessary to achieve it can only be taken by the individual and a group of people with the power in the society to enforce it. The government delegated responsibility for the protection of the health of the nation to local authorities, giving them the power to make any necessary additions under the title of 'regulations' as well as to implement the Act in their respective localities. However, it is said that, despite the work which is being done under the Environmental Protection Act regarding disposal of spillage, wastes and dressing, adequate observation of hygiene continues to fail, especially in the health care setting. Personal hygiene is the duty of the individual and has been dealt with under 'Personal hygiene' (*Unit 10* ). Here, we focus on the care environment.

The Health and Safety at Work Act 1974 applies to all persons at work and sets out their duties, which includes a requirement to report accidents and serious injuries to the registration authority. The idea is to promote a safe environment, improve accommodation and services for staff and residents, taking into consideration other safety aspects, such as fire prevention. The understanding is that the duty of keeping the living accommodation clean, tidy and in a good hygienic state will be carried out by ancillary and domestic staff and not by the nursing or caring staff. However, due to unforeseen circumstances they may be obliged to undertake some of these duties in an attempt to maintain high standards and quality of care. It is, therefore, necessary that everyone concerned should contribute to the maintenance of a good hygienic state of the care environment.

Entering a health care home, nursing or residential home should be a positive step forward towards better health and a new lifestyle for the residents. It follows that care establishments should provide better standards and more comfortable accommodation with space and amenities, as required by the Nursing Homes Act 1984, in order to maintain self-respect, dignity and a quality of life according to the differing degrees of individual residents' needs.

## Individual bedrooms

It is normal practice for residents to enjoy the maximum possible use of the accommodation provided for them. They should have the sole use of their own bedrooms with good furniture appropriate to the size and layout of the room, and suitable to the needs of the individual resident. Each resident should be provided with sufficient furniture to use, and each bedroom should have a hand basin with hot and cold running water. They should be consulted on choice, use and positioning of furniture and fittings wherever possible. The wear and tear to fittings and furnishings should be reported, including furniture and fittings which are likely to cause injury to staff and clients. The alarm call system should be inspected regularly. Residents should be encouraged to bring their own items of furniture, cherished mementoes and possessions, and support should be given to those who may wish to decorate their rooms. Where bedrooms are shared, this must be with the agreement of the residents concerned.

The floors should be carpeted or covered with suitable non-slip material, with the surface free from dirt, dust and debris. The frequency of cleaning should be consistent with local policy and carried out by designated staff. Clients may be encouraged to recognise the need for cleaning and to participate in this activity according to their ability. They should be encouraged to use materials and equipment in a manner which minimises risk to themselves and others in order to maintain an adequate standard of hygiene.

## Kitchen areas

Kitchens should be placed in accordance with the Provision of Food Hygiene (General) Regulations 1990, which applies to all areas. The regulations include procedures for the handling, preparation and storage of food. The kitchen should be equipped with:
- food preparation surface: smooth, impermeable and capable of being easily cleaned
- stainless steel double sink unit
- wash basins with hot and cold water, supplied with soap, towel and nail brush
- adequate sanitary conveniences, efficient lighting and ventilation
- pantry or storage space for dry food, fruit and vegetables
- all equipment should be available for constant use, such as fridge-freezer for protection of food from contamination, utensils, eg. knives, spoons, chopping and boning tools
- dishwasher, refrigeration adequate for the size of the home, which should be serviced regularly. Cookers should be simple to use with large surfaces. The inside of ovens should be readily accessible for cleaning
- first aid equipment

- the floor surface should be of smooth, impermeable material, capable of being easily cleaned and the walls should likewise be smooth and impervious and capable of being easily cleaned.

Special attention should be given to floors because of the obvious dangers which wet, slippery or greasy surfaces present to staff and residents. Spillages must be cleaned up immediately. Daily cleaning of floors and working surfaces is essential.

Waste storage should be situated outside the building, preferably covered, although not necessarily in a totally enclosed area. *It is a legal requirement to notify the local authority of any case of food poisoning*. There should be no smoking or unhygienic practices in the kitchen area.

## Bathrooms

Bathrooms should have locks on their doors which can be opened from the outside in case of emergency. They should be equipped with special bathing equipment, eg. special bath or hoist, grab rails, bath mat, bath seat, back brush, with an alarm call system. Floors should be covered with suitable non-slip material which can easily be cleaned.

Baths can be a source of cross-infection, and the most important single preventative measure is disinfection by thorough cleaning with a fine scouring powder or liquid detergent. They should be cleaned in this way as many times a day as they are used. Bath cleaning is a task shared between the cleaning staff and care or nursing staff. The daily washing and heat disinfection of the brush and cloth used for bath cleaning should be the responsibility of the cleaning staff.

## Showers

Some patients, for safety reasons and to lessen the risk of cross-infection, prefer to have a shower. Showers need less frequent cleaning than baths. A cloth may be used for cleaning the walls but a scrubbing brush must be used to clean the floor and to make sure that it does not become slippery.

Shower curtains, if provided, should be laundered weekly and the cleaning equipment washed and disinfected by heat daily.

## Sluice and toilets

Toilets should be readily accessible to all staff and residents. They should have locks on the doors which can be opened from the outside in case of emergency. They should be equipped with toilet paper, grab rails, facilities for adjusting the height of the toilet seat and a nurse call system. Sanitary equipment must be kept clean and in efficient working order. Walls, floors and ceilings should be smooth and impervious and easily cleaned.

Wash basins should be suitably placed for all patients to use. A notice should be displayed in a prominent place requesting users to wash their hands after using the toilet. The floor should be kept dry at all times and soap and toilet paper frequently replenished.

## Laundry

In most nursing and residential care homes on-site laundry facilities are available. These comprise a laundry room with commercial washing machines and extractors, tumble dryers and sinks for hand washing. Never attempt to open a machine while it is in operation.

It is essential that all machines should be operated in accordance with the manufacturer's instructions and serviced accordingly. The walls and floor of the laundry should be smooth, impervious and easily cleaned.

## Linen

Linen is a word used to cover all items which can be laundered. These are divided into:

**Soiled linen**: that which has been used and is no longer fresh.

**Fouled or infected linen**: that which is obviously fouled or is known to have been in contact with an infection.

Used linen is loaded with bacteria and should be handled as little as possible. It should be put into appropriate laundry bags immediately after it is discarded to await transportation to the laundry. The bags should be taken to the bedside to receive the linen. Once at the laundry, the bags should be emptied directly into the washing machines without handling. Laundry bags should be of two kinds or colours for easy recognition. Some homes may have colour coding and it is therefore important that nurses should understand local policy relating to handling of linen to minimise the risk of cross-infection.

## Disinfectants

These are chemical agents which are capable of destroying germs, proven by standard (BS 2462: 1961. A disinfectant is an agent used in disinfection, which makes things safe for handling. Disinfection can be relied upon to remove some germs, but cannot be depended upon 'to kill all known germs dead', especially the spores forming bacteria.

## Types of disinfectants

These may be called by other names, such as sanitisers, germicides, bactericides or 'sterilants'. Care should be taken to avoid mixing disinfectants with detergents. Bleach derivatives such as domestics are examples of disinfectants which are currently available for use as sanitisers, but they require special precautions to prevent misuse. Other preparations may be dispensed by pharmacists, such as Dettol, Hibitane, Hibiscrub, Savlon, Cetavlon for use in the home. It is important that care assistants should familiarise themselves with local policy for use of disinfectants in their home.

## Methods of disinfection

### 1. Disinfection by heat
Heat is a simple, clean and reliable form of disinfectant. Pressing fabrics with a hot iron will achieve some measure of disinfection. Garments that are washed and dried and pressed will be disinfected to some extent. Other forms of heat include steam and pasteurisation.

### 2. Disinfection by cleaning
The process of normal cleaning removes a high proportion of microbes (germs), including spores forming bacteria.

### 3. Disinfection by chemical solutions
Care and skill are needed in the use of chemical disinfectants if they are to be effective.

## Precautions

Disinfectant containers should never be left unattended, or allowed to be handled by residents. It is important to read the label on the container and to follow the maker's recommendations or the pharmacist's instructions for use. A further check can be made to see whether the relevant British Standard Specification number is quoted on the label. Disinfectants should be stored in the poisons section of a medicine cupboard. It is important that care assistants familiarise themselves with local policy for the use of disinfectants.

### *Guidance*
- treat all household cleaning agents with care; remember they contain powerful chemicals
- always wear protective clothing, gloves are required
- read instructions carefully and use the recommended quantity
- never mix chemicals, especially Harpic and bleach or smoke while using them
- keep aerosols away from heat. Never puncture and avoid breathing the vapour
- report any feeling of illness or drowsiness after using cleaning agents to the person-in-charge.

### Wet mops

Wet mops are used in cleaning. They hold water and provide a breeding ground for bacteria which not only survive but multiply rapidly in wet conditions. Wet mops harbour bacteria and they should be disinfected every day.

### Care of wet mops

There are many ways of treating wet mops, but the most common ones are to stand them overnight in disinfectant, to wash and dry at various temperatures, or to wash, squeezed and soak in strong disinfectant. It is important that nurses familiarise themselves with the method currently used in their care environment.

### Dust

Some germs (microbes) flourish in moisture but die soon after drying. Others are able to survive in a dry state for long periods and are commonly found in the dust in health care homes and hospitals. Germs are present in large quantities in bedding and disturbed during bed making, many falling onto furniture and the floor. Even caring routines and cleaning processes may distribute them through the air or by contact so that they can reach a critical site, eg. an open wound.

### *Control of dust*
There are many methods of dust control, but those commonly used are:
- avoid unnecessary shaking of bedding during bed making, including violent pulling of bed curtains or portable screens
- use vacuum cleaners for cleaning floors and furnishings once a day and when necessary
- avoid the use of brooms, especially in areas frequently used by patients. If possible, keep brooms out of the care environment as they spread germs (microbes)
- use oil-impregnated cotton mops or nylon mops with detachable heads, but their effectiveness depends on the care with which they are used
- damp dusting. This is best done with an attachment to a suitably designed sweeper or with a damp duster The duster may be of paper or other type of disposable cloth, or a sponge. The duster should be dipped in clean water and squeezed until no more water will come out of it, remaining damp all the way through. The dust should cling to the damp duster and the surface should be left slightly damp but not wet. Detergent water will be more effective than plain water on a shiny surface. The addition of a chemical disinfectant to the water used for damp dusting is not recommended because chemical disinfectants are active when they are wet and may harm surfaces.

Finally, maintaining the care environment in a good hygienic state is the work of a team. It includes a flexible working system and the maintenance of good personal hygiene by all concerned.

# References

Maurer M (1985) *Hospital Hygiene,* 3rd edn. Edward Arnold Ltd, London

Walters EM (1980) *The Infection Control Nurse in United Kingdom: Aspects of Infection Control Series.* Pharmaceutical Division, Cheshire

## Audio visual aids

### Format: VHS video

Ref: 188/CT: *Hospital Cleaning*

Ref: 188/CT Part 1: *Daily Ward Cleaning* (VHS Still frame Video)

Ref: 188/CT Part 4 : *Baths*

Part 188/CT Part 5 : *The Lavatory*

Ref: 188/CT Part 6 : *The Ward Kitchen*

Ref: 188/CT Part 7: *Washing Up*

Oxford Educational Resources Ltd

# Assignment

The purpose of this homework is to assist you in preparing for your Workbased Assessment of Competence. As there is no pressure on you, feel free to work at your own pace, but avoid the temptation to procrastinate. After you have read your notes and suggested references, submit your work for correction. The completed work becomes part of your Personal Portfolio.

## Cleanliness of care environment (CU3: 1–3)

1. Discuss what you mean by the word 'hygiene'.
2. Explain how you would contribute to maintaining the cleanliness of:
   a) clients' rooms
   b) laundry
   c) bathroom.
3. What do you understand by the word 'disinfectant'? State precautions to be taken for its use.
4. Discuss how you would handle dirty and soiled linen. What precautions would you take?
5. A confused elderly resident is sick in the lounge. How would you deal with the situation in relation to care of the client, furniture, carpet and yourself?

## The missing person and his or her belongings

From time to time, for a variety of reasons, clients may wander, stray or go missing from the health care home. Some of those who do so, may be at risk of abuse. Newly admitted clients who are mobile may find the care environment and its surroundings rather strange, and set out to explore it in order to satisfy their curiosity. They may wander and go beyond the area they seem to know, and so become anxious, increasing the risk of accidents to themselves.

     Wandering is the term used to describe aimless walking round without a purpose or walking to non-existent destinations. It is believed that although common, wandering is not a feature of every person suffering from dementia but, if it occurs, may lead to serious consequences. In some cases, clients may become agitated and pace up and down the corridor, clearly looking for something in the home. The person may even wander outside to non-existent destinations. They may believe that they are meeting somebody, such as a lost relative who is known to be dead. It is important to understand the driving force behind such wandering and respond with empathy.

## The missing person

Any resident may go missing, but those likely to do so are frail, elderly, children, mentally infirm and handicapped people, who may be confused, disoriented or over-active. Also some clients who are admitted under the Mental Health Act 1983, may make a conscious attempt to go absent without official leave because of restrictions on their access and movement; this includes those who are in secured units for health reasons. More importantly, clients with a previous history of wandering are likely to repeat their past behavioural pattern.

## Reasons for wandering

A variety of factors may account for the person's wandering behaviour, such as:

- separation from familiar surroundings due to recent admission, with an attempt to return to previous place in search of a deceased loved one or something unobtainable
- fear or anxiety of upsetting caring procedures such as bathing. Also attention seeking, believing that he or she is receiving less attention than others
- overcrowding, too much stimulation in the environment due to noise
- an attempt to get away from a restricting order of detention under the Mental Health Act 1983. Therefore absent without leave
- the need to use the toilet or in search of something to eat (hunger)
- the result of side-effects of medication, response to pain, an acute illness or dehydration, recent changes in the person's location leading to a search for the previous home
- boredom and loneliness may result in wandering and the person may lose his/her bearings, due to unfamiliarity with new surroundings which they have been attempting to explore
- a belief that others are trying to control their behaviour or trying to do them harm as a result of delusions and hallucinations.

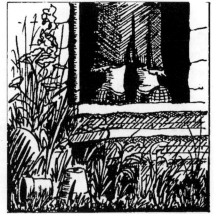

## A framework of care

The principle of care is to create and maintain a safe and secure environment in which clients are assisted and allowed to relax, take risks and use their remaining skills to maintain their individual self-respect, dignity and independence. Locking a door to keep a client in may constitute false detention. This applies to the use of any form of mechanical restraint, eg. double-handled doors, handles set in inaccessible positions. Similarly, physically restraining a client is not permissible. The design of the building and their grounds should allow residents space to wander or move about in safety in an attractive and stimulating surrounding.

The holistic approach to care involves assessment of individual clients' total care needs and risk-taking, and designing care plans to meet these needs. They should constantly monitor and update the caring procedures and practices. Every home should have a written policy for the procedure to be followed if a resident is missing. This policy should be known and discussed with everyone, including relatives and clients' advocates.

One of the most important aspects relates to the safety and security of the care environment in ensuring that the missing person does not suffer harm or injury during this period of absence. It is essential that all members of the care team should have an in-depth knowledge of all their clients, their whereabouts at a given time, and priority should be given to protecting those at risk of wandering, abuse, injury or harm. It is well-known that a missing person could be in danger within the inaccessible area of a care environment, eg. in a basement among the central heating appliances. Staff are, therefore, obliged to constantly watch for hazards within the care environment, reporting and taking appropriate steps to minimise or avoid them. Everyone on duty should accept responsibility for the safety of their particular areas of work, and ensure that the equipment, methods and procedures they use are safe for themselves and others, in accordance with the Health and Safety at Work Act 1974.

## Management of the problem

It may be necessary to develop and foster a good neighbourly relationship in the area in which the home is situated. This will help to ensure that a missing person is quickly found and returned to the home. A resident who is inclined to wander outside the home may become lost or get into danger. The handling of such behaviour should be discussed, agreed by all concerned, recorded in the person's care plan, and reviewed frequently. If a resident is found to be missing, appropriate action should be taken *immediately* within local policy and practices. It is important that all staff should have:

- detailed knowledge of the missing person
- knowledge of the whereabouts of clients who are likely to wander off, at a given time
- knowledge of places regularly visited by the resident and places they have known well in the past.

Generally, everyone on duty should be informed that a client is missing to ascertain when, where and who last saw the person. Using this information as a basis, the person-in-charge should be able to organise a search depending on the time of day, number of staff on duty, and the prevailing conditions. There is a special procedure to be followed regarding clients detained under the Mental Health Act 1983.

## The search

This should be a thorough and systematic inspection of the care environment and its surroundings. Start looking inside the care environment, all bedrooms, cupboards, basements, cellars, ventilation shafts. If the indoor search is unsuccessful, the surroundings should then be searched, eg. the gardens, bushes, hedges, roads. As a result of past history, client's known haunts may be contacted or visited and neighbours requested to look out for him/her. When searching the outside, it is helpful to call out the missing person's name, but remember to give him or her time to answer. The use of a mobile phone or radio is desirable, depending on the area to be covered in order to maintain contact with members of the search party and the base. If none of the searches are successful, then the person-in-charge should inform the police and client's next of kin, advocate, doctor, matron or the proprietor in accordance with the policy.

It is important that everyone involved in the search should carry personal identification cards to avoid embarrassment in trying to explain yourself and your actions to a police officer, as the missing person may complain that he or she is being apprehended by a complete stranger. It can be useful too if likely wanderers carry their name and address in a wallet or handbag.

## Documentation

1. A missing person's form should be completed giving information on the person, eg. description, clothes worn, distinguishing features, known haunts.
2. A photograph, if available, is always useful. All information should be in the client's care plan.

### Return of the missing person

On the return of the missing person, the person-in-charge should be able to inform all those previously informed about the problem, ie. the police, next of kin and advocate, doctor, matron proprietor.

### Guidance

- maintain a good interpersonal relationship with the person
- note time and mode of return
- offer a hot bath and clean clothes and examine feet for blisters, signs of injury
- enquire if the person is hungry and offer a choice of food and drink
- allow the client to rest quietly in his or her room
- encourage the person to express him or herself, including where he or she went, what the person did and reasons for the behaviour. Use a friendly tone of voice; it is important that you do not confront the person. Return at a later time if information is not forthcoming as it is necessary to look for patterns and what triggered off the behaviour. This information should be recorded in the individual's care plan.

### Preventive measures

There is always a temptation to hide clients' personal belongings such as shoes, coats. This is a retrograde step which is always counterproductive and should be avoided at all costs. It is better for those clients with a tendency to wander off to be adequately dressed, rather than for them to be exposed to adverse weather conditions.

### Guidance

- develop and maintain a good interpersonal relationship with every client. If the relationship is good, they will be able to help by observing and reporting any unusual incidents to the caring staff, including the movements of those at risk of abuse or wandering
- be able to assist in identifying the reason(s) for the person's wandering behaviour by using a low key tone of voice when speaking and encouraging the person to express him or herself without embarking on a questioning approach
- occupy residents with simple diversional activities in small groups, and check their presence at regular intervals. Use the principles of reality orientation by showing pictures depicting bedrooms, bathrooms to confused clients in the group
- ensure that special door locks and alarm systems are working properly to alert staff if anyone attempts to leave. Show knowledge of routine procedures for checking clients at the end of each shift of duty
- ensure that there is no gap within any enclosed outside courtyard and that garden furniture, if any, is in good working order
- check and report any faulty doors and windows in accordance with local policy
- provide group care for sensitive individuals who wander and observe them constantly
- organise regular walks to meet the clients' individual needs, as a change of environment may help to calm down some overactive residents. Good luck!
- re-arrange furniture to allow a client to pace up and down a bit, rather than restraining the person. But remember the needs of clients who may have visual impairment
- be aware of the whereabouts of all clients at all times, be aware of any restrictions on client's freedom, eg. under the Mental Health Act 1984
- be aware of clients at risk of abuse and procedures for reporting. Ensure that those who may take them out for a walk or car drive have permission to do so
- demonstrate knowledge of visitors to the care environment, including residents' relatives, look out for, and report, any unauthorised visitors and prowlers to the home.

## Electronic tagging

There is a debate regarding the use of electronic tagging, which is a relatively recent innovation, on ethical and legal grounds. This involves the placing of a tag on an individual. Staff will respond when the alarm is activated. It is similar to those used in shops to prevent theft. The argument is that the tag has the potential to degrade and depersonalise people. However, arrangements for introduction should be the subject of discussion with the residents, their relatives, advocates and the registering authorities as to its positive benefit in care.

## Residents' valuables and other belongings

The policy for care and security of clients' possessions varies from one care establishment to another, but generally, it remains the responsibility of managers, in accordance with the contract of care. Belongings of the missing person are no exception, but it is important that carers are familiar with their local policy and practice. Following admission, it is difficult to know what each individual long-term clients keeps in their possession, because of the need to maintain their privacy, self-respect, independence and freedom of movement. It would be reasonable to seek their permission to carry out an inventory of their possessions periodically, in order to update them, probably for insurance purposes in case of any unforeseen circumstances.

    The current practice is that, on admission, personal possessions brought in by residents are checked, preferably by two members of the staff in the presence of the client or his/her relatives and entry made in the appropriate record. Signatures of those making the entry, including client's and/or relatives may be essential. Valuables are also accurately described and listed in the 'valuable book' in the same way and receipts issued. These may be jewellery, certain sums of money, which should be locked away for safekeeping within local policy. Alternatively, with consent, their relatives may take them home, and receipts should be obtained or a record made in client's case note to that effect.

    In this respect, and for security reasons, the missing person's belongings should be checked immediately he or she is found to be missing. His or her room is securely locked and keys kept in accordance with local policy. On the person's return, the situation should be explained, and an opportunity given for confirmation of the current or emergency inventory.

## Action to be taken

Any loss must be reported immediately to the person-in-charge for investigation in accordance with local policy. In some cases, the police could be informed, depending upon the nature of the loss, and what is involved.

# References

Stokes G (1987) *Managing a Wanderer. First Find Out Why? Psychogeriatrics*. Geriatric Medicine, London

Chapman A *et al* (1994) *Dementia Care. A Handbook for Residential and Day Care*. Age Concern, London

## Audio visual aid

*Format: VHS video*
Ref: *Hazards of Disposal*
Oxford Educational Resources Ltd

# Support and control of visitors (CU4: 1–3)

We have previously discussed the role of the family and benefits to clients and staff in this unit of learning. In this section we hope to focus on support and control of visitors to services and facilities. One of the aims of visiting is to help clients maintain contact with members of their family and others important to them. Most clients have a family and being taken away from it because of ill health can be a distressing experience. It is, therefore, important for clients to maintain contact with the members of their family group and the community in which they live.

## Visiting

Meal times and visiting time are highlights of the day for residents. Visiting is a necessity to all residents and forms a very important aspect of their care and recovery. It makes the day more interesting and is of mutual benefit and pleasure for residents and staff. Information on visiting times is usually given on admission and the way visitors are received can affect the way in which their relatives settle later. There are, of course, some residents whose family may not be able to visit, and for them contact by telephone and letter may help to make up for this lack of visiting. Others, for instance the elderly, may no longer have anyone to visit them, and carers can help by discussing with them whether they would like someone from the voluntary visitors' scheme to come, if this service is available in the area.

## Visiting times

It is a requirement that a notice of visiting times should be displayed in a prominent place. Most care establishments have a policy on specific visiting days and the number of visitors a resident may have at any one time. A flexible arrangement enables visitors to visit at times convenient to themselves. One of the advantages is that it encourages regular visiting, especially in long-stay situations. It also offers both visitors and staff an opportunity to communicate with each other, and build up good relationships. In some instances, during visiting, relatives can be made aware of the beliefs of informal *reality orientation* which they can practice with their elderly relatives to ensure continuity of this approach to care.

## Visiting rooms

One of the most noticeable concerns for visitors and their relatives is lack of suitable visiting rooms and privacy. This is partly a matter of design and partly of practice. Privacy means the right to a room to yourself where you can live as you please. In some care homes there is no place for residents to receive their visitors in private. This problem is more obvious in smaller care homes, when two or more people share a bedroom. In some places, living rooms are used for this purpose, but they tend to become too overcrowded and conversation is inhibited by the distraction of television and other people talking. Dining rooms, in most cases, are available for use by residents and their visitors. A proprietor of one nursing home found it necessary to convert a sleeping room into a visiting area which improved visiting for the residents and their visitors. This room was also used as a quiet room by residents. Making such a provision meant a loss of revenue to the home, but it brought with it an improvement in lifestyle for some of the residents and was of particular emotional benefit to those residents who valued their privacy. In summer months, residents may receive their visitors in the garden.

## Preparation for visits

A spacious, clean and comfortable home will make visitors feel welcome, at ease, and is necessary for the residents' recovery. The homes, generally, are clean and should not require tidying up for visiting, except the rooms in which residents and their visitors meet. It is important that routine cleansing of some residents should be completed before visiting. The appearance of clients is an indication of the standard and quality of care that they are currently receiving. Consideration must be given to the needs of residents from minority ethnic groups, which takes into account their ethnic and cultural traditions. Some clients are generally self-sufficient but will ask for help if they need it.

## Types of visitors

Visitors to hospitals, nursing and residential care homes, may be associated with the general management of the care establishment. These are special visitors who come for professional purposes, but have no direct contact with the residents. They may include inspectors of care homes, doctors, members of the community health council, solicitors, fire prevention officers, pharmacists, service engineers and delivery people. Others may include the parish priests, social workers, voluntary workers and tutors. Anyone who is not a regular member of staff or a resident in the care environment, is a visitor and must be treated as such. It is important how they are received and the assistance given to them. They should be received courteously and made to feel welcome and at ease in the home environment.

However, this section focuses on those visitors who are residents' relatives or friends: to whom the residents turn in time of need. Illness is one of the times when help is needed. These kind of visitors are trusted friends, colleagues or relatives, generally known as 'on hand' visitors, upon whom clients depend, but not necessarily in the financial sense. They are usually calm, unobtrusive and alert to the residents' needs. For these reasons, it is important that carers should recognise who are the 'on hand' visitors for each individual resident.

Carers need to be aware that admission to an institution may not only affect the clients, but also relatives at home. These visitors may at times experience difficulties themselves while the client is receiving care and attention. During visiting times, a visitor may arrive, apparently in need of help and support. He or she may be an elderly person in poor physical health with impaired mobility who previously relied on the spouse for help, but because of admission he or she is now deprived of that support. Carers can help such visitors to cope with this situation by suggesting that they contact their local social services department about home care services (see *Unit 17, Community care*).

## Control of visitors

Some care establishments have liberal visiting facilities for friends and relatives to visit the home at any time. In a larger home, overnight accommodation and catering facilities may be available to visitors at a reasonable cost by prior arrangement. It is important to know who comes into the home and a record of visitors should be maintained in accordance with the local policy of care. As a means of control, some homes maintain visitors' books which are available for inspection during a re-approval visit. This book is used by everyone including special visitors and owners of the care establishments.

## Problems with visitors

Visitors are necessary to the residents although some present problems to the carers when they attempt to justify their value, relationship and loyalty to the residents. Sometimes a visitor may be self-appointed as a resident's spokesman and may ask questions which the carer cannot answer. The visitor may appear to be really annoying the resident and refuse to leave. Such visitors do not like to be seen as a problem, although their actions may suggest the opposite. Handling some of these problems has been discussed in topics of admission, contact with family and significant others, and abuse of residents (*units 5 and 6*).

### *Guidance*
- treat all visitors courteously as guests and offer practical help as necessary
- be aware of the cultural needs of minority ethnic groups in your care and refer any problems to the person-in-charge
- demonstrate a knowledge of local policies relating to visiting and complaints procedures. If necessary, offer visitors an opportunity to make complaints
- do not discuss a particular client with his or her visitors
- refer difficult questions to the person-in-charge
- follow guidance previously given on handling problems relating to admission, contact with family and significant others and abuse of residents
- make a request, but do not order the visitor to leave the room, even if it becomes necessary for them to leave. They are, generally, very co-operative when asked to do something. Give a reason for your request, eg. 'I'm so sorry. I must do the treatment. Would you mind going out for a few minutes?' is so much better than 'please step outside', said in a tone that suggests you will meet them there to settle an argument
- make an accurate record of visits and any potential problems in the resident's care notes.

## Special situations

Visiting in specific situations, such as if the person is dying and infection control, have been covered in the respective units of learning. Each dying client has special visiting needs; if he or she is conscious such wishes should be granted. If unconscious, it is the relatives who need information and consideration about whether or not to stay with the client. Visiting relating to infection control is governed by local policy.

As residential care establishments form part of the local community, residents, as members of that community, should have freedom to invite and receive visitors as and when they wish, depending on their condition. For most of them, continuity of personal relationships is important and carers should ensure that residents are helped to keep whatever patterns of contact they choose to have with their family and friends.

## References

Faulkner A (1996) *Nursing: The Reflective Approach to Adult Nursing Practice*. Chapman and Hall, London
Roper N, Logan W, Tierney AJ (1985) *The Elements of Nursing*. Churchill Livingstone, Edinburgh
Sadler C (1981) Some thoughts on ward visiting. *Nurs Mirror* **153**(11): 4

# Unit 14
# Assist clients to participate in leisure activities (X14, Y1, Y3, Z5, Z7, Z13)

## Rehabilitation

Caring for the growing number of elderly people is a complex and challenging process, and calls for a new direction from custodial care to rehabilitative care. Custodial care is 'doing things' for them thereby fostering dependency on care staff for their every day needs. Research predicts that about 1,047,000 people, aged over 85 years, will be alive in the year 2001, with an increase of about 43% in the ageing population 85 years + group. This means that most of the elderly people will invariably become dependent and require outpatient, day hospital, long-term or respite care in conjunction with community and social services. So there must be movement towards promoting and supporting a client's independence.

The NHS and Community Act 1993 recognises this situation and suggests that appropriate training should be provided, and that designated disciplines should co-operate and work together to tackle this problem. Rehabilitation has become a major factor in preventing the situation from deteriorating both in the care settings and in the community.

Rehabilitation has many meanings and interpretations. Basically, it is a flexible and challenging process in which individuals are helped to regain their independence as quickly as possible, while at the same time maintaining their self-respect, privacy and dignity. The process starts immediately the individual is diagnosed as in need of care, admitted into a health care environment or hospital, and continues throughout his or her stay until discharged back into the community. The principal aim is to restore function by the use of therapeutic schemes, eg. activities based on the assessment of physical, social and psychological functional abilities of the person by a multidisciplinary team. The needs and functional ability of the person are identified and a care plan is designed to enable the individual to learn and adjust to new situations. If this fails, then the aim is to improve the person's ability to use his or her remaining skills in a limited way to carry out activities of daily living unaided — either in the health care home or in the community with support from relatives, statutory or voluntary services as may be necessary.

### Multidisciplinary team work

The care and rehabilitation of the elderly is a multidisciplinary team approach involving experts from various disciplines, such as nurses, occupational therapists, physiotherapists, speech therapists, dieticians, etc. Each provide their own form of treatment, and roles overlap so a carer should not feel threatened, as the success of the treatment depends on an ability to appreciate and understand each other's role. The support and participation of members of the client's family and others significant to them in some activities are always appreciated, especially in social and recreational activities, eg. a coach outing.

## Leisure activities (Z13: 1-2)

These are age-related activities organised with the help of residents to encourage them to maintain their independence and lifestyle as far as possible. The method is based on assessing the normal pattern of clients' individual lifestyles in relation to what they like and what they dislike doing, and planning activities to meet these needs. These activities are dealt with under occupational therapy.

## Management of activities

The organisation of leisure activities involves an in-depth knowledge of the person, his or her interests, hobbies, behaviour, likes and dislikes and reporting on his or her ability for independent living. The care is based on assessment of individual clients and reports on their abilities and interests by the occupational therapist. It is important to understand that people with dementia are highly sensitive to the moods of other people around them. Therefore, the carer needs to remain calm and avoid any form of criticism of the client's efforts.

The implementation requires mobilising facilities and encouraging the clients to participate in the programme according to their individual interests and abilities. The use of essential skills, eg. effective communication, handling and moving people, observation and reporting and being patient will all clients, are the main tools for this exercise. The approach to management of these activities should aim to:

- develop and maintain good interpersonal relationship skills while maintaining a flexible approach
- demonstrate an awareness of an individual client's care plan aimed at reducing dependency
- focus on the client's abilities to function as much as possible, rather than on his/her limitations. Many self-care tasks are within the capabilities of the client, even if these are performed more slowly. They will be retained longer if they are used daily
- analyse and break down each task into simple and manageable steps, eg. dressing, and accept that each daily task will gradually take more time as the problems progress
- encourage clients to perform these tasks starting with those that have little risk of failure
- give credit for trying rather than completing the task and allow plenty of time
- reduce background distractions as much as possible, such as radio or television noise, in order to promote the client's concentration and reduce anxiety level and confusion
- refrain from rushing clients as this may increase confusion, anxiety and agitation
- initiate and provide hands-on experience as dependence increases and praise the client's efforts
- encourage and help clients to express their needs, views and ideas without challenging them
- interact with clients, and always encourage them to respond; reward their efforts
- report and record any significant improvement in a client's performance
- communicate with the person all the time irrespective of whether or not there is a feedback
- encourage relatives, significant others and advocates to participate as much as possible.

## Equipment

For some residents the use of rehabilitative aids and equipment forms part of their short- or long-term care. Equipment can be used in the bathroom, bedroom, kitchen, dining room, around the home and when gardening. Specific equipment includes: Mecanaids®, Ambulift®, eating utensils, pressure reducing aids, toilet aids, walking aids, wheelchairs, beds and bedding protection.

Also, there is equipment specifically designed for the use of people with disabilities, such as speech impairment, blindness and partially sighted, deafness or hard of hearing, and disabled people. Their needs are usually reassessed periodically by the paramedical staff concerned.

## The role of care assistants

The role of care assistants is invaluable. They are front line members of the team and work in close contact with the residents 24-hours a day, probably more than any other member of the care team. In a care home where there is no provision for the services of an occupational therapist, most care assistants undertake to support their residents in the carrying out of leisure activities. Their main role is to help to restore functions of the residents by improving their concentration. They should be able to:

- develop and maintain a good relationship with clients and be aware of individual care needs as recorded in the care plan
- be aware of clients' individual interest, hobbies, likes and dislikes
- demonstrate a knowledge of simple recreational and leisure activities
- ensure that the environment is safe and control the noise so that it does not impinge on the residents. Some people like background music while they are working — but it should be maintained at a reasonable level.
- consult the residents about what they would like to do and break down the task into simple manageable steps
- show them how to do the task by following a step-by-step approach, starting with the simplest. Allow them hands-on experience, encourage and support them
- praise their efforts and reward them individually with a hug or a smile as appropriate
- allow them a rest period and offer some refreshment
- ensure everything is neatly put away at the end of the session and thank them for their co-operation
- record and report the outcome to the person-in-charge.

With the increasing diversity of skills needed in care, some care assistants have the potential to develop skills and expertise in the use of alternative therapies, such as massage and relaxation techniques. These skills are now being recognised and used, and care assistants should be encouraged and supported to develop and use them to the benefit of their residents. Moreover, it would be reassuring to individual residents and their family to know that members of the primary nursing or team nursing have close contact and rapport with specialist staff.

## Occupational therapy (X14: 1–2)

The aim is to enable clients or patients to make maximum use of their remaining skills and recover power in the activities of daily living. A variety of activities are employed to stimulate the interests of clients in learning new skills and maintaining good interpersonal relationships and interesting lifestyles. Clients are assessed and treatment is prescribed in relation to their functional abilities and needs. It is stressed that not all clients may wish to participate in these activities and their wishes must be respected. But efforts should be made to persuade and encourage them to do so, although not against their will.

### *Occupational activities*
The following activities may be used in various combinations:

***Diversional therapy*** The aim is to distract clients' attention from their disabilities and focus it towards different directions through:
- painting, drawing, sketching, flower arranging, board games, eg. draughts, skittles
- reading, listening to music on the radio
- embroidery, knitting, making soft toys, movements with music, relaxation.

***Recreational therapy*** The aim is to entertain and refresh clients by providing them with various age-related activities, such as party games, outings, visits.

**Leisure and social activities** Clients and patients are encouraged to socialise with other people including staff. The programme may include social parties especially for celebrating birthdays, community singing. Church services maybe conducted within the care establishment at any time, especially during Christmas and Easter. Some clients attend Sunday Services themselves, while others may be escorted in their wheelchairs if the local Parish Church is within walking distance.

In some cases, clients are allowed to decide and plan for their leisure activities such as coach outings, theatres, cinemas, amateur operatic society plays, concerts. Suitable arrangements are usually made in response to these needs.

**Reality orientation** This is the practice of a 24-hour real life experience involving the use of a variety of approaches to help people maintain contact with reality in order to improve the quality of their lives. It is believed that clients who are confused usually value the everyday information most of us take for granted. All staff realise the full implications of the programme and participate in it.

The programme is designed to enable clients to interact with other people in their environment, especially those involved in their care. This will enable them to be aware of everyday events, regain and maintain contact with reality and function independently as far as possible. Its success depends upon the quality of information given by the therapist and the use of various therapeutic skills, such as group dynamics, verbal and non-verbal communication in the sessions. The programme is available to anyone who needs it, but no one is forced to participate.

**Supporting facilities** Many care environments provide appropriate services which complement the principles of maintaining self-respect, dignity, privacy and individual lifestyle. These include:
- hairdresser, podiatrists (chiropodists), beautician, optician
- entertainers, shopping for personal items.

**Physiotherapy** The role is complementary to those of other professions. The aim is to encourage the movement of the body in order to strengthen the client's mobility and prevent stiffness of the joints. Gentle exercises help in 'tuning up' the muscles of the body, stimulating blood circulation and digestion of food. Heat or ice treatment may be used for the relief of pain and ultraviolet light for the management of certain conditions. In all cases, clients are assessed and treatment is prescribed by a professionally qualified physiotherapist.

**Music therapy** The aim of the therapy is to meet the emotional, social and spiritual needs of elderly people with dementia and help them to function at their best. It does not in any way improve their intellectual ability which has been damaged by the course of the disease. Music therapy involves the planned and systematic use of music specific to the individual's personal life and stage of dementia. Music preferred by the person is used in a planned music therapy session to bring about the development of feelings. Someone who has lost the ability to speak can often still sing. Research shows that people with dementia generally react to music, and aggression and agitation are often reduced by music.

**Visits to theatres** Some residents look forward to occasional trips to the theatre to enjoy drama, ie. comedies or farce or reviews, light opera and music concerts. Managers of local theatres sometimes have special nights and concessionary rates for elderly people.

# References

Central Statistics Office (1983) *Social Trends 13*. HMSO, London
Department of Health (1989) *Caring for People: Community Care in the Next Decade and Beyond*. HMSO, London
Field N (1992) *Validation. The Field method. Edward Field, Ohio, USA*
HB6 (1990) *Equipment and Services for People with Disabilities*. Health Care Publications Unit, Heywood
Loundon S, Jelier B (1993) Positively passive: activities of living, rehabilitation. *Nurs Times* **89**( 31): 71–72
Jones G, Meisen BM (eds) (1993) *Care Giving in Dementia: Research Applications*. Routledge, London
O'Donovan S (1996) A validation approach to severely demented clients. *Nurs Standard* **11**: 13–15
TVM (1985) *Rehabilitation: Medical Products Catalogue*. Thames Valley Medical, Reading
Williams J (1993) Rehabilitation Challenge. Rehabilitation of Elderly People. *Nurs Times* **89**(31): 67–70

## Audio visual aids

### Format: VHS video

GME 6637: *Physical Therapy and the Geriatric Patient*
PATUA 572 3: *Healthline: Fit for Life*
CME 6646: *Evaluating and Documenting Rehabilitation Programs for the Elderly: A Hands-on-Approach*
Oxford Educational Resources Limited

# Assignment

The purpose of this homework is to assist you in preparing for your Workbased Assessment of Competence. As there is no pressure on you, feel free to work at your own pace, but avoid the temptation to procrastinate. After you have read your notes and suggested references, submit your work for correction. The completed work becomes part of your Personal Portfolio.

# Rehabilitation (Z13: 1–2)

1. What do you understand by the term 'rehabilitation'?
2. Make a list of all the activities and equipment currently being used in rehabilitation of clients in your place of work.
3. Discuss briefly how you would help clients with the following activities:
   a) diversional therapy
   b) recreational and social therapy
   c) reality orientation.
4. There is a birthday party going on, and one of your clients suddenly withdraws and refuses to take part again. What do you think may be the cause of this, and how would you persuade him or her to join in again?
5. Discuss how you would prepare your residents for the following activities:
   a) occupational therapy
   b) a visit to the theatre.

## Personal, domestic and financial resources (Y1: 1–5, Y3: 1–3)

For many people, the decision to go into a nursing or residential care home is difficult and stressful, often arising unexpectedly. It requires a great deal of consideration which, among other things, involves making a decision on the person's life, and what to do with personal possessions. In some cases, it may mean disposing of treasured possessions because of lack of storage space in the new surroundings. Some health care homes, despite lack of reasonable space, make provisions for residents to bring a few selected and cherished possessions with them for their personal use and enjoyment according to the individual's capability. These possessions vary considerably from clothes and mementoes, to pieces of furniture, such as wardrobes, chest of drawers, arm chairs, and valuables, such as jewellery and money. However, whatever is brought in has to be secured and protected from damage, misappropriation and abuse.

### Assessment of needs

Care in the Community 1993 provides for the elderly to be cared for by carers in their own homes. The starting point is an assessment of care needs, which is the right of everyone who may need a place in a health care home. Following discussion with the general practitioner, an application is made to the local social services department. The actual assessment of needs is carried out by an officer from the local authority and the person's family practitioner, possibly with input from an occupational therapist. It is believed that if admission to a nursing home is a possibility, the care needs will be assessed by a nurse. The social services will then decide whether the person is entitled to care at home or in a home. But, whether care is to be provided at home or in a care home, a care plan will be agreed. The person has the right to appeal against the decision, if he or she believes that he or she has been wrongly assessed. The next step is a financial assessment of the person's assets if they need care in a care home.

### Personal affairs

Many elderly people and their relatives are not familiar with the system of care, especially the need to make financial decisions regarding care in nursing or residential care homes. It is important for them to explore every avenue of funding and the ability of the person to look after his or her affairs independently. Areas of personal affairs which require consideration are as follows:
- personal financial affairs
- personal affairs such as clothes, furniture
- assistance in shopping for personal goods.

### 1. Personal financial affairs

Many elderly people today do not meet the criteria for financial assistance from the local authority, because of life savings or proceeds from the sale of a former property. However, many find that their capital runs out long before the need for care ceases and with that loss goes their independence, dignity and the right of choice which they deserve at what is perhaps the most precarious time of their life. The outcome is that those still with property may be forced to sell their homes, unless a spouse is still living there, although, even then, the local authority can make a charge on it.

However, the person could discreetly rearrange his or her affairs, to ensure that the house is not possessed by the local authority by following one of a number of options, such as moving a relative in to the property as long as they are over 60 or disabled, co-owning the property or giving it away, probably to another member of the family, at least two years before the possibility of admission to a care home arises. Each authority defines the rules differently. There are new plans which will allow elderly people to keep their homes when they go into residential care if they take out an insurance policy to cover the cost of nursing.

## Sources of financial support

Anyone who uses social services support to pay care home fees will be assessed and, once the need for a home is established, a programme of care will be agreed. Residents who have been admitted to a residential care home for short periods, may need a little more help than for someone to arrange to pay their bills. For longer-stay residents, especially those on low incomes or claiming some sort of benefit, the situation may become more complicated. Listed below are some of the ways in which income could be made available to them.

### Income support
Everyone is means-tested by local authorities for care in a nursing home care, and those with £8000 or less in their savings account will not make a contribution Those with savings and other assets worth more than £16000 (including their home, unless a partner or dependant still lives there) will have to pay the full costs of their care, until the assets drop to £16000. Thereafter, fees are met pro rata by the State. Older people who remain in their own home or are cared for in a residential home have their nursing and medical care provided free. But income support will also be payable to anyone on a lower income. Claim for income support is either by completing form SP1 or by writing a letter.

### Pensions
Elderly people may derive an income from either old age and/or occupational pensions.

### Housing benefit
Home owners who go into nursing homes under local authority schemes may be able to get housing benefit (help with rates or community charges) for up to a year.

### Attendance allowance
Clients who have been receiving attendance allowance before they enter residential care homes, may be allowed to keep this allowance. But they may have this allowance taken away from their income support payment.

### Mobility allowance
Those who are already getting mobility allowance can continue to do so whether they are on income support or not. Other benefits are subject to different rules.

### Home equity plans
Residents who are home owners may receive an income from their house or flat by selling or mortgaging it, buying into an annuity or by taking out a loan secured against their home to 'top up' income support with a home equity plan. The scheme will provide a much needed extra income, perhaps by paying for nursing or residential care.

### Relatives
In many cases, relatives or close friends offer to pay all or part of the home's charges, or perhaps 'top up' any shortfall between the income support limits and actual charges.

## Claim of payment and benefits

Procedures for claiming benefits could be a source of anxiety for some patients and their families, especially long-stay residents and those on a low income. The usual requirement is either a letter or completion of appropriate eligibility forms. The nurses-in-charge should be able to provide further information and assist in the completion and submission of appropriate documents.

## Collection of payments and benefits

Residents should be encouraged to claim or collect their payments personally or be escorted to an appropriate place to do so. Following payment, they should be assisted to check the amount received against the amount due and report any discrepancies. Appropriate advice should be given on safe custody and security of their money, including reporting any loss of cash or valuables. A close relative or an advocate may be able to provide help.

## Payment of outgoing expenses

Many elderly people usually make informal arrangements for payment of their outgoing expenses and management of their property. Generally, the sources of residents' funding should be treated with confidence. Quite often, close relatives or bank managers or solicitors are assigned this responsibility. Therefore, it is not advisable for any other person, especially members of the care team to be involved with residents' financial affairs. But, there may be exceptional circumstances in which a resident may seek the help of the home with his or her financial affairs, in a limited way. The request should be reported to the person-in-charge.

It is important that sensitive help should be given to enable the individual to spend his or her money however he or she wishes. All spending in which the home is involved is accurately and legibly recorded in accordance with local policy. Receipts must be obtained and filed in the person's case notes. Under the Court of Protection Order all documents relating to residents' expenditure must be accurately maintained for inspection by authorised persons. As poverty usually brings its own feelings of dependence and lack of value, sources of residents' funding should be treated with confidence and only disclosed to entitled individuals.

## Security of personal belongings

### *Organisational policy*

Those residents who are able and capable of taking responsibility for their affairs should be encouraged to be self-sufficient as far as possible and to spend their money on personal effects and comfort items. These include: hairdressing, beautician sessions, personal shopping, private chiropody, optician, clothes, magazines, newspapers, laundry, dry cleaning, toiletries, holidays: all of which help to maintain an individual's life-style, self-respect and dignity.

A written organisational policy should be formulated indicating that care managers will not be involved in the management of a resident's financial affairs.

### *Court of Protection Order*

Under the Mental Health Act 1983, residents who are unaware or incapable of managing their own financial affairs, for reasons connected with their mental or physical disability, and where there is no suitable next of kin prepared to accept responsibility, may be referred to the Court of Protection. The Act assumes responsibility for a resident's affairs and places restrictions on access to the client, and sets out how access is monitored. It can appoint a receiver or a guardian in the case of children to carry out its instructions. An accurate record of any expenditure on the client must be maintained for the auditors' inspection and report.

## 2. Personal affairs

### Personal cleansing

Clients should be assisted and encouraged to recognise the need for personal cleansing, and to clean to an adequate standard of hygiene consistent with individual preference and culture. Quite often, and for no apparent reasons, some residents are reluctant to make use of their personal effects. They should be encouraged to do so in order to maintain their self-respect, dignity and individuality as set out in their care plan. It is also important to be aware of practices which relate to some cultural and religious groups. At times, economic factors may inhibit personal cleansing, but residents should be encouraged to buy cosmetics of their choice for personal use.

### Clothing

Clothes, especially for long-stay residents, are a great morale booster. Most people like to be well-dressed all the time, and especially on special occasions, eg. birthdays. They should be encouraged to take pride in wearing clothes in which they feel comfortable. The choice of clothing will depend, to a certain extent, on the occasion, weather and the physical condition of the individual. Colour and fashion are important to many, but they should be encouraged to choose clothes to suit their lifestyle.

Facilities should be readily available for dry cleaning, laundering, and repairing damaged clothes. Soiled or infected clothing should receive appropriate treatment. Incontinence causes staining of clothes and efforts should be made to maintain the self-respect and dignity of the person. There should be no shortage of appropriate clothing, and permission should be obtained from the individual or their relatives, should there be a need to discard worn out or damaged clothing. It is important that all residents have an adequate supply of clean and presentable clothing stored in a safe and appropriate way, to which they have unlimited access.

### Furniture

Furniture such as bookcases, wardrobes, personal mementoes may be placed in the client's room depending on available space. If an armchair is placed in the lounge, it is important to ensure that it is used exclusively by the client, and other residents should be informed in order to prevent unfortunate incidents from occurring.

## 3. Shopping expeditions

Most people enjoy shopping for retail goods or other services. Shopping expeditions should be organised to meet social needs of patients according to their individual capability, and as part of their care plan. Different age groups have likes and dislikes regarding their choice of clothing and the types of material. Shopping gives them an opportunity to make a choice which is consistent with their style and to try on the clothes before deciding.

Some care establishments have an arrangement with large department stores whereby the stores 'visit' the home at regular intervals and display their goods for residents to shop. Alternatively, a shopping expedition could be arranged by the staff. This will involve hiring a mini bus or taxi with the cost shared between the patients concerned. Patients who enjoy window shopping should be assisted to continue to do so. In all cases, an accurate record and receipts of all purchases made must be maintained. Patients' clothes and other personal belongings should be marked with their individual identification and stored appropriately. It is important that an inventory of personal belongings should be carried out periodically with the assistance of the individual concerned.

## Repairs to clients' belongings

It is important that no repairs or alterations should be undertaken without discussion with the individual. Any repairs needed must first be authorised by the owner and or his or her relative. The implication is that there may be legal action for reimbursement if belongings are lost or incorrectly used or altered in any way without the consent and permission of the owner.

## References

Department of Health and Social Security (1993) *Mental Health Act 1983*. HMSO, London.

Help the Aged (1993) *Managing a Lump Sum*. Help the Aged, London

Department of Health and Social Security (1993) *Care in the Community: Changes in Income Support and other Social Security Benefits*. HMSO, London

George M (1990) Money rights: hospital patients. *Nurs Times* **86**(5): 52–53

George M (1990) Money rights. residents in homes. *Nurs Times* **86**(6): 68–69

George M (1990) Money rights: patients at home. *Nurs Times* **86**(7): 50–51

Redfern S J (1986) *Nursing Elderly People*. Churchill Livingstone, Edinburgh

Department of Health and Social Security (1993) *Benefits after Retirement* (FB 32). BA Publications, Lancashire

Vincent M (1994) Pensions rights and wrongs. *Nurs Times* **90**(12): 45–46

## Concepts of mobility (Z5.1, Z7.1)

One of the highly valued human activities of daily living is the ability to 'move', and helping clients to move about in their care environment is vital. Everything we do involves some form of movement, most of which is under the control of the will. But, there are certain movements which are protective, and are carried out instinctively. These are known as reflex actions, eg. blinking our eyes or removing a finger from a very hot dinner plate. In any case, we all need to move in order to meet our everyday basic human needs, such as obtaining food and water, avoiding injury and reproducing.

The ability to move the whole or part of the body is controlled by the nervous system and joint movement which depends on the muscular and skeletal systems involved. In conscious people, many of the muscles attached to the bone are, at any one time, in a state of readiness for action, known as muscle tone. Those muscles which are not used, frequently become soft and flabby, and are said to have lost their muscle tone. This 'flabby' state, can be seen in some elderly people who cannot move themselves or are not encouraged to do so. Some may complain about lack of energy, and they need help. Handling and moving people or helping them to move, is a difficult and risky task, regarded as a major cause of injury. It requires skills in protecting the client and the carer doing the lifting from injury, by using good lifting techniques and appropriate lifting aids. It also involves a knowledge of positioning the body and understanding certain principles relating to movement and the structure of the human body.

### Purpose of mobilisation

The basic activity of moving from one place to another is one that lasts throughout life and well into old age, except when an accident occurs. There are, however, a wide range of reasons why we move, although the basic motivation is to explore the environment. When on holiday in a foreign country, or a new environment, the first instinct is to look around the immediate surroundings in order to orientate yourself to your new and immediate environment. The next 'move' is to venture out, to independently explore, enrich your experience and satisfy a basic curiosity. The same principles apply to a newly admitted resident into any health care home who is able to move about independently. However, in some people restraint or lack of independent movement may restrict the ability to satisfy curiosity, and may be frustrating to the individual. He or she will rely on descriptions of others in order to satisfy a personal need for knowledge of his or her new environment. The outcome, in some cases, may be a lowering of self-esteem, respect and restricted independence.

Most elderly people enjoy walking, dancing and other age-related social activities which require a reasonable amount of physical and mental energy in order to maintain good health.

Some clients may gain pleasure from watching others enjoy themselves at a party. They may at times join in by making some physical motions such as singing, clapping hands or even move their body in tune with the music. This kind of movement could be seen in some disabled people, especially those confined to wheelchairs. There are many reports of people in comas who have been helped to regain consciousness by hearing music.

## Structure of the body

The normal stucture and function of the body is complex and requires the use of energy from the muscles, the skeletal system and several principles such as leverage, contraction, relaxation and gravity to bring about physical movement. The main systems involved are:

### 1. Skeletal system
The skeletal system is the body's support system. It provides the framework for the cartilage, muscle, blood vessels, the nervous system and other organs which make up the human body. Main bones in the human body include:
- in the leg: tibia, fibia and femur
- in the arms: radius, humerus, ulna
- back: spine, pelvis, ribs
- head: skull

**Function of the skeletal system** One of its main functions is to protect delicate organs of the body such as the brain, heart, lungs. All bones where they meet, form joints with smooth surfaces to allow for easy movement. There are about 305 bones in the human body and some present uneven surfaces for the attachment of muscles.

### 2. Muscular system
The human body is capable of carrying out powerful and difficult activities with the help of its muscles, which are named and classified according to what they do. There are three types of muscles:

**Voluntary muscles** These are muscles attached to the bones of the body such as those of the legs, shoulders, thighs. They contribute to all voluntary movements we make and are controlled by the brain.

**Involuntary or plain muscles** These types of muscles are under the control of the nervous system, and are found in the walls of blood vessels, alimentary tract, the eye, uterus, and bladder. The involuntary muscles are controlled instinctively.

**Cardiac muscle** This is a unique type of muscle that resembles both the voluntary and involuntary types of muscles. It acts independently of the central nervous system and has its own rhythm. It is found exclusively in the heart.

## Functions of the muscles

The muscular system adds support to a variety of body movements. The voluntary muscles support movements, such as those used for moving the head and neck, blinking of the eyelids and the posture of the body. Muscles of the legs enable physical activities, such as walking, sitting and running by contracting and relaxing. During ill health, loss of muscle tone can cause contraction, poor nutrition, incontinence, pressure sores and painful joints which make moving and handling the person difficult. It is important to maintain good muscle tone to ensure nomal functions and movements of the limb and joints .

## Factors influencing mobilisation

A person's ability to move about can be influenced by a number of factors such as:

### 1. Physical well-being

The ability of a person to move independently may be affected by circumstances involving the muscular, skeletal and nervous systems of the body. These may include:
- prolonged bed rest due to debilitating and wasting illness, plus development of pressure sores
- fractures due to accident or disease of the bones, such as arthritis
- painful joints due to rheumatism and obesity which may make movement difficult
- paralysis or loss of muscular contraction such as hemiplegia, paraplegia.

Some of these conditions may be caused by stroke or accident which may seriously restrict movements of the individual, in some cases permanently. This type of physical impairment reduces the person's ability to enjoy freedom, and everyday activities of living to his or her optimum level.

### 2. Social and psychological well-being

There are various problems which may interfere with an individual's freedom of movement. These include:

**Confusion** This is a state in which a person's mind is clouded and the person has a diminished ability to think, act and respond to situations in the environment. Mobilising then becomes a very slow process with limited results.

**Depression** This is a mental state in which there is a general lowering of spirits and intellectual activities. The person presents a picture of great sadness with feelings of inadequacy and lack of purpose in life. The outcome of such a feeling, is that the person may present a negative attitude towards mobilising. Other factors include anxiety, fear of falling, frustration, isolation and loneliness.

### 3. Environment

The type of residence, layout and general organisation of the care environment may play an important part in handling and moving the residents. The space available within the home, type and arrangement of furniture, quality of lighting, attention to soft furnishings such as rugs and carpets, stairs, handrails for frail people may contribute to their ability to be mobile.

## Caring procedures

### Guidance

Some residents frequently associate certain discomforts and their inability to move with a variety of caring activities and procedures. Discomforts may include pain, loss of freedom, independence and dignity. Procedures associated with these problems may include:
- bed baths which require turning in bed

- the use of appliances, such as a bed cradle, splint, sand bags
- lifting which involves moving and handling, eg. in and out of baths
- carer's attitude towards the client.

## Helping clients to mobilise

### Guidance

The principles of care involve the acquisition and demonstration of knowledge, attitudes and the skills necessary for carrying out the activity of moving and handling people. As accidents or other physical and emotional disabilities may occur, it is necessary to minimise these problems by accurately assessing the individual's functional capability and habits to establish his or her ability for self-help. The information obtained will be valuable in planning care for mobile, bed-fast or chair-fast residents. It is also useful to be familiar with legislation relating to safety at work, local policies and practices. Proper training in the use of handling equipment is essential as a majority of elderly people may become dependent on others and need aids for their daily mobilisation.

## References

Downie PA, Kennedy P (1981) *Lifting, Handling and Helping Patients*. Faber, London

Roper N et al (1985) *The Elements of Nursing. Mobilising*. Churchill Livingstone, Edinburgh: ch 14

Tarling C (1992) Handling patients. *Nurs Times* **88**(43): 38–40

Write B (1981) Lifting and moving patients. An investigation and commentary. *Nurs Times* **77**(46)

### Audio visual aid

**Format: VHS video**

Ref: 417CT: *Exercise for the Elderly and/or Disabled*
Ref: CME6642: *Dysmobility of the Elderly*
Ref: CME6643: *Mobility, Spectrum and the Elderly*
Oxford Educational Resources Ltd

## Preparing clients for a journey or visit (Z5: 2–3)

Every health care home should provide opportunities for their residents to go on outings and visits outside the home and its immediate surroundings. Those who wish to leave the home briefly should be encouraged to do so and offered help with arrangements for their journey. As a result, and in keeping with the ethos of care, every resident should be assessed and an appropriate level of risk-taking agreed with all those concerned with his or her care, including volunteers. Generally, outings have a therapeutic value and provide a change of scenery which residents, especially those in long-stay care homes, appreciate and look forward to with anticipation.

### Types of journeys

Journeys may be organised for different purposes, such as going on holiday or day trips to places of interest such as the seaside. These type of outings form an integral part of social and recreational therapy activities, giving residents a chance to have a normal enjoyable day out. Everyone involved in the programme should be consulted and invited to participate in the event as far as possible, including relatives and advocates. Residents are routinely given the choice of where to go, together with an idea of what to do when they get there. The detailed arrangements for the journey involving continuing care, staff, travel, refreshments are usually carried out by all members of the care team.

A popular outing is an afternoon mini-bus trip around local places of interest. It is usually organised as a weekly event during the summer months, for either a half or a whole day, and may include a picnic.

## General preparation

The aim of the plan is to encourage clients to look after their individual personal appearance and dress according to the weather and enhance their self-respect, dignity, independence and lifestyle. Emphasis is focused on their safety and security while at the same time allowing them a degree of freedom in risk-taking. They should be encouraged to look after themselves and to take any small, personal item of comfort if they wish, eg. spending money. If the trip is to the seaside, it is always advisable to include a bucket or two for fetching sea water and sea weed, if possible, for some residents who may not be able to get down to the beach to have a 'feel of the sea water', eg. those in wheelchairs. The leader may obtain prior information about the destination, browse through it, and be able to provide residents with a commentary, highlighting any specific places of interest during the journey.

### *Guidance*
- plan for specific needs of individuals, eg. incontinence, by carrying appropriate aids and plastic bags for travel sickness
- ensure that facilities for refreshments and toilet are within reach at the destination
- encourage freedom by unobtrusively allowing a certain degree of risk-taking
- carry a list of everyone on the trip, including pre-prepared missing persons forms of those residents who are at risk of wandering. An album of recent polaroid photographs of all clients may be useful
- ensure the safety of everyone at all times; note and report any untoward incidents on return.

## Visits or journey to hospital

A visit may need to be arranged for a hospital appointment to an out-patient department of a general hospital. It may be for follow up of in-patient treatment, for further investigations or admission for treatment. The process usually relates to routine in-depth planning involving the individual resident with close attention to his or her dependency level. The general approach entails:

### *Transportation*
A number of transport modes may be used for the journey, such as staff, relatives' or friends' cars, the ambulance service, taxi, voluntary workers, public or organisational transport. But, if staff cars are used, it is important to check the insurance cover and requirements.

### *Escorts*
Some elderly clients may be anxious and apprehensive about the trip, especially if this is their first trip outside the care environment. It is essential that they are reassured by giving them explanations and information about where they are going. The escort should be someone who they know and trust, either a member of staff, volunteers, or a member of the family.

### *Guidance*
- maintain a good interpersonal relationship with clients. The day before, remind them about the visit and arrangements. Offer reassurance as necessary
- enquire about their individual disposition regarding travel sickness and make appropriate plans to cope, eg. carry plastic bags, a bowl, a box of tissues, mouthwash, receptacles

- pay attention to clients' personal appearance and cleanliness, including a change of clothes; if the journey is for an overnight stay or admission
- offer the person the use of toilet facilities before setting out
- ensure that the client wears spectacles, hearing aid as prescribed, and carries any personal walking aids as necessary
- enquire about transport arrangements for the return journey
- encourage those who are capable to carry spending money for personal things of comfort; if the journey is for a hospital admission, for newspapers, magazines
- take referral letters (doctor and nursing reports) including any current medication as instructed. Be aware of any general instructions, eg. nothing to eat or drink
- ensure that the client is accompanied with results of investigations if any, X-ray films, the hospital appointment card or letter requesting attendance
- save and present any specimen of vomit to the nurse in the out-patient department should client suffer travel sickness during the journey
- take the following personal items, if the appointment is for admission: night dress or pyjamas, dressing gown, slippers, face flannel, toothbrush and toothpaste, personal toiletries, reading material, according to client's wishes and choice.

### *An additional guidance*

- demonstrate an in-depth knowledge of the client, and be able to provide further information
- read records and be familiar with the client's treatment and care, such as diet, eg. diabetic, vegetarian, response to activities during the day
- note time of arrival at the hospital and report to a nurse in the out-patient department
- reassure the client constantly as he or she may be anxious and apprehensive during the journey
- ensure his or her safety at all times. Never let the client out of sight as he or she may wander and get lost
- accompany the client to the ward, if admitted, and help him or her to settle in before you leave
- observe and take note of any information or instructions which may be given regarding his or her care and report back to the person-in-charge. Make relevant entries in the client's care plan, and present any claims for expenses you may have incurred, in accordance with local policy and practice.

## Evaluation

It is important to ensure that following a hospital admission, a client's room in the health care home and his/her personal belongings are tidy, safe and secure. Managers of the home will make the necessary financial adjustments regarding the period of absence, in accordance with contract of care. The next of kin should be informed by the person-in-charge if the resident is admitted into the hospital as a result of the visit.

# Unit 15
# Health education and promotion (NC7)

## Health education and promotion (NC7: 1–3)

Health is a word which is difficult to define. Richman (1987) says that health is one of the most talked about topics apart from the weather. Whenever people meet, 'how are you' is a common greeting, and 'keep well' or 'take care' on departing. The *Oxford Pocket Dictionary* (1987) defines health as a, 'state of being well in body or mind; person's mental or physical condition'. The World Health Organisation (1946) also defined health as a 'state of complete physical, mental and social well-being and not merely the absence of disease or physical infirmity'. These definitions show that there is a distinction between health and illness, and by treating and preventing diseases, people would be made healthy, so reducing the cost of treatment. It was on this basis that the National Health Service was founded in 1948.

Health is influenced by many factors, ie. social, genetic, environmental, personal behaviour, lifestyle. Most people see it as a state in which one is free of pain and suffering, in which the person is not restricted from carrying out those activities of daily living. In reality, it is difficult to separate a person's healthy and diseased states because neither are static, but fluctuate at any given time, depending on how the person feels. Baxter (1987) believes that it is possible to have disease without illness, and to have illness without disease. He explains that disease without illness would be a woman with early cancer, and illness without disease could be seen in a person with physical symptoms due to AIDS. So, it is important to understand these concepts before talking about giving advice on health promotion and education.

### Health promotion

Health promotion is a wide term covering all those activities which contribute to the social, physical and psychological well-being of individuals. There is increasing evidence that early onset of disease and premature death are related to lifestyle and are preventable. The aim of health promotion is to encourage people to accept that prevention is better than cure, promoting health is better than fighting illness. The outcome is that specialist health promotion services are offering training programmes to professionals and others in the public, private and voluntary sectors of health care, in response to the Government's White Paper — *The Health of the Nation*, which sets out specific targets to be achieved for reducing illness and death in the following five key areas:

- coronary heart disease and stroke — to reduce death in people under 65 by 40% by the year 2000
- cancer — the aims are to reduce the incidence of cervical cancer by at least 20% by the year 2005, to halt the annual increase in skin cancer by the year 2005 and to reduce death from lung cancer by at least 30% in men under 75 and 15% in women under 75 by the year 2010
- mental illness — the aims are to reduce the suicide rate by 15% and the rate of severely mentally ill people by at least 30% by the year 2000
- HIV, AIDS and sexual health — to reduce the incidence of gonorrhoea in men and women
- accidents — to reduce death from accidents in children under 15 years and people aged 65 years and over by at least 33% by the year 2005, and in people aged 15–24 years by at least 25%.

## Health education

Health education offers an opportunity for individuals to learn and share information about health through the media. It places a duty on individuals to identify any risks to health at a personal level and choose to change their behaviour towards a healthier lifestyle (WHO, 1986). The concept of health promotion aims to prevent illness from occurring or to keep its effects to a minimum through the following measures:

### Primary prevention
This aims to prevent illness from occurring in the first place and includes immunisation and vaccination programmes and safety regulations against infectious diseases.

### Secondary prevention
The aims are to detect problems before signs and symptoms appear in order to take remedial action, such as screening for cervical cancer, child development.

### Tertiary prevention
The aim is to manage existing disease or disability in order to reduce any complications so that the person may enjoy a better quality of life, eg. by reducing hypertension to prevent stroke.

The whole concept of health promotion is to focus on self-empowerment by encouraging people to believe that they are in charge of their own lives, by developing self-esteem, life skills and assertiveness. The front line of health promotion is the primary health care team.

## The nurse's role in health promotion

**Qualified nurses**: should be able to provide skilled care for clients by:
1. Organisation of care, eg. team or primary nursing, partnership care.
2. Philosophy of care: individual and holistic approach to care:
   (a) assessing the need for care, teaching and learning
   (b) planning the care, teaching and learning session
   (c) implementing the care, teaching and learning session
   (e) evaluating the care, teaching and learning.
3. Setting a good example which will enable those in care to adapt their lifestyle, eg. attitudes to the effects and cessation of smoking.
4. Promoting a safe environment for care, eg. prevention of infection, safe handling of clients, effective handwashing, safe storage of food.
5. Knowledge of health education and promotion in the clinical setting, and making health literature available to clients without prejudice, eg. giving older people advice on safe sex.

## Role of care assistants

The role of care assistants is seen as assisting professionally qualified practitioners as health educators. This requires an in-depth knowledge of individual clients and the ability to help in identifying factors which may influence the performance of their individual activities of daily living, and to *treat them with dignity and respect*. The approach involves the use of specific nursing skills, eg. observation, communication, counselling to report on:

### Physical well-being
- diet: anxiety about eating enough or not eating the right type of food, obesity, anorexia or other dietary ailments, eg. hypothermia

- immobility: foot disorders and general infirmity
- loss of hearing or failing sight
- dental decay or ill fitting dentures.

### *Psychological well-being*
- confusion resulting in wandering, getting lost and getting into physical danger
- depression, loss of memory and general forgetfulness
- anti-social behaviour, general over-activity, aggression, violence
- lack of confidence and self-esteem.

### *Social well-being*
- lack of relatives' participation in care
- poverty in various aspects, to a degree which may lead to ill health
- awareness of the dangers of excessive alcohol intake, smoking, drugs which may lead to isolation, failure to look after oneself.

## Maintenance of a safe environment

### *Guidance*
- maintain good interpersonal relationships with all the residents and encourage them to ask questions about their well-being
- ensure safety of the environment by wiping wet and slippery floors, ensuring that pathways are free from ice during the winter months
- observe and report on clients at risk of abuse especially those who are suicide risks or who have attempted suicide, and those with eating disorders, perceptive disorders, eg. delusions, hallucinations
- report on obvious hazards, implications of health and safety such as outbreaks of food poisoning (*Salmonella, E. coli*)
- ensure that statutory regulations, eg. Health and Safety at Work Act 1974, Fire Prevention Act 1971, Mental Health Act 1983 and the **no smoking** policy are observed
- be aware of methods and principles of infection control and ensure that patients understand the importance of handwashing and skin care.

## Community care

Clients in the community who may experience problems, eg. in taking their medication, must be reported to responsible qualified nurses. These problems may include:
- counting tablets or forgetting to take medication as prescribed
- keeping fit in retirement, eg. diet, exercise, time and leisure activities
- keeping a healthy weight, bowels and choosing a laxative.

Although care assistants do not have a direct responsibility to provide clients with information on health education and promotion, their awareness, attitudes and skill will have an important influence on decisions relating to the general well-being of clients.

## Principles of health education and promotion

There are commonsense ideas which may be considered as contributing to good health, for example:
- the old expression 'take and do everything in moderation and all will be well with you and the world'
- maintain a state of happiness and a tolerant personal philosophy
- attempt to make a harmonious adjustment to your environment and economic implications
- develop an ability to adapt to changes without setting up conflicts or causing other people to suffer pain or feel any discomfort

- be aware of the need for continuing education, as a process of change in human behaviour.

**Factors associated with good health**

*Guidance*
- encourage people to observe and report any environmental substances that are hazardous to health, eg. notifiable diseases, infestations, noise
- help people to be aware of facilities available for detecting early signs of ill health, eg. breast and prostate screening for cancer
- encourage people to seek treatment early, to prevent complications developing, eg. stress, obesity, sexually transmitted diseases
- encourage people to participate in sports, exercises, sensible drinking of alcohol, dieting which may be beneficial to them
- encourage people to develop new hobbies and recreational activities
- encourage parents of young children to seek information on vaccination and immunisation programmes from their GP and health visitors
- encourage people to pursue any recommended routine investigations and screening programme, eg. a periodical human 'MOT'
- promote understanding of the links between cleanliness and harmful reduction strategies, eg. re-use of needles and the importance of skin care
- make use of the health education authority's posters and leaflets, eg. *Look after yourself, Stop smoking, Safe sex — use condoms*
- ensure that clients understand the boundary between legal and illegal drugs, eg. client use of drugs that are not prescribed.

# References

Baxter M (1987) Self-reported health. In: *Health and Lifestyle Survey*. Health Promotion Research Trust, London

Latter S *et al* (1993) Perceptions and practice of health education and promotion in acute ward settings. *Nurs Times* **89**(21): 51–54

Lang C (1993) Positive steps. Health promotion. *Nurs Times* **89**(11): 54–56

Strehlow MS (1983) *Education for Health*. Harper and Row, London

Richman J (1987) *Medicine and Health*. Longmans, London

Tannahill A (1985) What is health promotion? *Health Educ J* **44**(4): 167–168

Tudor-Hart J (1985) When practice is not perfect. *Nurs Times* **81**(39): 28–29

World Health Organisation (1946) *Constitution of the World Health Organisation*. WHO, Geneva

World Health Organisation (1986) *Intersectoral Action for Health*. WHO, Geneva

**Audio visual aids**

*Format: VHS video*
Ref: PAT 8438: *Come Sit by Me: AIDS Education*
Ref: PATUA 141: *Thumbs up for Kids: AIDS Education*
Ref: PAT 0607: *Nutrition and Exercise for the Elderly: Creating a Healthstyle*
Ref: PATUA 572: *Healthline: Fit for Life*
Ref: TFG 2505: *Staying Active: Wellness after Sixty*
Ref: 267 CT: *Prevent Disease — Use Latrines* (cassette tape)

Ref: GEA 8797: *Guarding Against Tuberculosis in the Health Care Environment*
Ref: CNE 4341: *Universal Precautions: AIDS and Hepatitis B Prevention for Home Health Care*
Ref: NCE 4342: *Universal Precautions: AIDS and Hepatitis B Prevention for Long-term Care*
Ref: CNE 4344: *Why Me? Dealing with an Occupational Exposure to a Blood-borne Virus*
Oxford Educational Resources Ltd
Surf: http://www.open.gov.UK/doh/target 126/cont26.htm.

# Unit 16
# Assist clients to express sexuality (W1)

## Nature and purpose of sexuality in later life (W1: 1-4)

The expression of sexuality is one of the most important aspects of activities of daily living. Human beings express themselves sexually from birth to death and the passage of time does not affect the individual's established lifestyle. Normally, a person's sex is set at conception, remains so throughout life, and becomes an important factor in the person's personality. All things being equal, a younger person, who is sexually active, will grow into a sexually active older person but may slowly decline in later adult life. In retrospect, expression of sexuality is seen as a normal part of meeting a person's basic social needs, and is no longer the taboo subject it used to be.

In health care, expressing sexuality relates to sexual health issues; better mental health, lower levels of anxiety and a generally healthier existence. The targets in the Health of the Nation includes a plan to reduce sexually transmitted diseases and conception in girls under 16 years of age.

### Sexuality

For many people, sexuality is not easy to define despite the fact that it is difficult to pick up a newspaper or to turn on the television without sex featuring prominently. Hogan (1980) believes that sexuality embodies much more than the physical act of intercourse, and that it involves biological, psychological, social and cultural aspects of our being. So, in caring for people, there is a need to be aware of their cultural differences and the ways in which sexuality can be expressed. The biological aspects include sex organs and hormones, and the actual physical expressions of sexuality, which can range from simple eye contact, smiles, kissing, holding hands, right through to sexual intercourse.

Sexuality also relates to the ways in which individuals express the idea of being a man or a women, and declare this to others through the style of their dress, the wearing of personal decoration, perfumes or cosmetics. In some parts of the world, societies are moving away from the strict interpretation of activities, attitudes, beliefs and values associated with the way people express their sexuality in terms of good, bad, normal or abnormal. However, it is increasingly being discussed and debated in the context of the prevention of sexually transmitted diseases.

### Purpose of sexuality

It is clear that the purpose of sexuality varies at different stages of a person's lifespan and lifestyle. The human sexual behaviour serves both reproductive and non-productive functions and, indeed, is much more frequently performed for non-productive reasons than for the purpose of reproduction. It is interesting that in most mammals, sexual behaviour tends to occur only when fertilisation can take place, and courting and mating activities are linked to procreation. But, in order to understand human sexuality, there is a need to consider the biological, social and psychological factors of the individual.

## Expressing sexual relationships

The expression of sexual relationships in society, although predominantly heterosexual, may be heterosexual-bisexual or homosexual. However, attitudes towards homosexuality are gradually changing, although a great deal of homophobia still exists. The nature of a relationship is of equal importance to the two partners, and whatever the feelings of carers, residents should not be judged by the carers' personal standards and values, but should be allowed privacy and self-respect without interference. The topic must be dealt with in a mature and professional way, ensuring that the people concerned are not disadvantaged in any way, and that carers remain non-judgmental in their attitude and manner.

## Inappropriate sexual activity

The most common inappropriate sexual activity is self-exposure or public masturbation. Masturbation is defined as the production of sexual excitement by friction of the genitals. It is important to remember that masturbation is a harmless sexual outlet for a sexually active person with or without a partner. Some elderly people, not only those suffering from Alzheimer's disease, do behave in this way which shows that they have normal sexual feelings. But because they express these feelings in a socially unacceptable way, it means that they have lost learned inhibitions, and so need help.

It is possible that some carers may have strong feelings about this type of behaviour, and they need to talk about it within the care team, and come to terms with their own individual values on sexuality. As they have the right and freedom to maintain these, they are expected to extend the same rights to their clients, by behaving in a professional and non-critical manner.

## Sexuality in later life

Sexuality is an integral part of an individual, and helping an elderly person to express his or her sexuality if he or she no longer feels able to do so is a basic human right. Many features of human ageing may have extensive bearings upon the expression of sexuality in later life, and these need to be looked at in some detail.

Research shows that interest in the opposite sex is natural and wholesome with the level varying between individuals. Also, sexual stimulus does not stop at 60, nor is it given up by the time the individual draws his or her pension, but remains throughout life. In fact, although the elderly are inclined to be reserved, it is claimed that about half of married couples over 60 have regular intercourse at intervals varying from once a month to three times a week. After many years, they tend to be more sophisticated and demanding, and become more easily bored and difficult to arouse.

It is believed that although most elderly in care homes prefer single sex bedrooms, they benefit by mixing with others during the day. An open show of sexuality can be seen in the way some of them maintain contact with one another. This bodily contact is more common in husbands and wives. Those who are not in close relationships, and those who no longer have intercourse, value tenderness, affection and physical closeness in old age as at any other time of life. This is normal and should be encouraged. Webb (1985) argues that if nursing is to be truly holistic, it must address the basic role of sexuality within all care planning systems.

## Benefits of expressing sexuality in later life

Through sexuality, people can express their most intimate feelings of need, individuality and emotional closeness with other human beings. It involves a continual process of recognising, accepting, and expressing self as a sexual being. These benefits allow old people to:

- establish a link with the future through children
- release physical and sexual pleasure and express love
- communicate in a gentle way or express intense feelings
- bind themselves together, maintain their identity with lots of tenderness to draw on as the result of years of companionship and build their personality
- experience feelings of self-worth when sexual experiences are positive
- discard the fear of pregnancy and the need for contraception.

**Factors influencing sexuality in later life**

The factors listed below may impede the sexuality of elderly people in any combination, especially those in residential care accommodation.

*1. Physical*
- poor physical health in people over 75 years
- physical disability such as altered body-image, mastectomy, amputation, stoma
- discomfort associated with sex, eg. soreness which makes sex uncomfortable
- pain may reduce libido, eg. muscular spasms, heart diseases, arthritis, operations
- effects of drugs such as hynoptics, hormones, diuretics, tranquillisers, alcohol, full stomach
- interference with genital organs as a result of 'plumbing faults' relating to incontinence
- direct effect of illness or disability may interfere with nerve pathways which control sexual function. Also, physiological changes, eg. menopause may affect the older person.

*2. Social factors*
- lack of partners especially for older women and permissive expression of sexuality
- code of sexual behaviour based on cultural values, norms, attitudes towards morals and laws
- a non-disabled partner adopting a caring role as well as being a lover, resulting in tiredness, difficulty in switching off the roles and guilt about having unsatisfied sexual feelings
- boredom when sex becomes routine, changes in method of expressing sexuality
- display of sexual activity, eg. exposure or public masturbation often in a confused older person.

*3. Psychological*
- fear of impotence which often interferes with erection. This can happen at any age, but elderly men may be vulnerable as a single failure can trigger the setting up of repeated failures
- mental ill health such as depression, confusion, anxiety
- attitudes relating to personal beliefs, values, culture, religious rites, sexual preferences
- lack of interest and information on the expression of sexuality and embarrassment.

*4. Environment*
In hospitals and in some nursing and residential care homes, many residents are unable to be alone with their relatives, as private rooms are rarely available and, if used, may arouse curiosity among staff, as some expect the elderly to live a life of celibacy. Other factors are:
- change of environment, eg. admission to hospital or home may diminish sexual identity
- sleeping accommodation, eg. single or twin-bedded, shared accommodation
- lack of privacy, especially fear of being overheard
- lack of opportunity to interact with those of one's own choosing
- inappropriate staff attitude — viewing their clients as asexual, teasing them about their friendships or relationships, or attempting to separate those whose pairing they feel is unsuitable.

# Helping the elderly to express sexuality

The aim is to support clients' rights to express their sexuality and self-image. Elderly people in residential care settings should be assumed to have sexual feelings and given an opportunity to express them in private. Sexual matters and problems are not easy to discuss, and require tact, sensitivity, tolerance, and an in-depth knowledge of the subject. More importantly, it requires the carers to be comfortable with their own sexuality and at ease when discussing sex-related topics with others. The starting point is to gather information about physical, social, cultural and psychological aspects of the individuals' sex lives, and plan care to meet these needs.

## 1. Assessment of needs

Assessment should address the person's attitudes towards sexual experience or what the individual expects to experience, his/her problems with sexual functioning because of his/her condition, such as pain, illnesses, disabilities. The care setting should be examined for features that may make sexual expression difficult.

## 2. Care plan

Members of the health care team, together with the individual clients, design care plans to meet the individual needs. These are reviewed from time to time.

## 3. Implementation of care

The care environment should be one that provides personal space for clients to maintain their privacy, self-respect, dignity and lifestyle. The care team should be able to identify the needs of residents, and plan care that is responsive to an individual's need for discretion and standards of sexual behaviour. The health care team should:
- issue a statement of policy for enlightened care and facilitation of expression of sexuality
- provide facilities for people to mix socially by creating a small screened off area
- offer provisions for clients to express their sexual feelings in private. This means that double rooms should be available and doors should lock from the inside
- provide information package/handouts to meet identified needs of clients on admission
- educate and induct new staff to recognise their own sexuality and those of elderly people
- provide opportunities for clients to become involved in therapeutic and diversional activities, including information, eg. leaflets on alternative ways of expressing love and affection.

## Role of care assistants

As members of the health care team, care assistants have an important and vital role to play in sexual health promotion by helping clients to express their sexuality. The starting point is knowledge, awareness of their own sexuality, without feelings of embarrassment. Once they are comfortable, it is important to develop and use caring skills, such as counselling, interpersonal relationships to make it possible to communicate effectively with residents, the basic rule of which is to be non-judgemental.

### *Guidance*
- make sure that the individual has an opportunity to masturbate in private. Explain that while he or she has the right to self-gratification, others have a right not to watch
- develop and maintain good interpersonal relationships with clients which will make it easier for them to talk about any problems and ask for help

- demonstrate a knowledge of organisational policy on clients' expression of sexuality
- show in-depth knowledge of individual client needs and sexual preferences as recorded in the care plan; show respect for their attitudes, especially when these differ from yours
- ensure that they have appropriate information to meet their identified needs, and encourage them to participate in decision-making and protect their independence
- encourage them to express their views, choices, ideas and listen to them attentively
- help them to maintain and express their lifestyles in dress and control their behaviour
- assist them to improve and maintain their physical, social and mental well-being
- knock on doors and wait for permission to enter
- show respect and regard for clients' ethnic, cultural and religious beliefs and practices
- refrain from watching or eavesdropping on residents' sexual activities
- ensure that elderly people are not 'paired off' or that elderly lovers are not separated just because you think that the relationship is unsuitable
- observe and report any unusual behaviour or any signs of sexual abuse of clients at risk
- be aware of legislation for the protection of individuals at risk of abuse, eg. the Children's Act 1989, the Mental Health Act 1983
- demonstrate skills in the use of therapeutic activities for diverting clients' sexual activities
- observe and report any complaint relating to pain in the genital area, especially women
- help clients in social behaviour, communication skills, dress and personal grooming.

### 3. Evaluation of care

Clients are able to express their sexuality in private without offending or interfering with the rights of others.

### Sexual health

Sexual health generally refers to the absence of sexually transmitted diseases or unplanned pregnancy, to which those in later life cannot personally relate. The World Health Organization defines sexual health as a capacity to enjoy and control sexual and reproductive behaviour in accordance with a social and personal ethic. It is also regarded as freedom from fear, shame, guilt, false beliefs and other psychological and social factors that inhibit sexual response and damage sexual relationships. Good sexual health is a positive entity and freedom from organic disorders, diseases and deficiencies that interfere with sexual and reproductive functions.

### Health education

The aim is to encourage positive attitudes towards sexuality and to enable people to make informed decisions based on a sense of self-esteem and respect for the rights of others.

Nurses and carers are in the front line of attempts to foster health education among the public. The issue of HIV and AIDS has forced nurses to examine many of their attitudes regarding sexuality and sexual health, and has provided a climate in which the discussion of the subject need no longer be taboo. We must take this opportunity to incorporate the promotion of sexual health in all nurse training programmes.

This is a teaching of sexual health directed at young people, perhaps in a misguided belief that elderly people do not need health education. Age Concern points out that many single elderly people take a holiday abroad and may have holiday romances. It follows that elderly travellers need to be aware of safer sex practices too — extra-marital relationships be they hetero or homosexual, as these are not only the prerogative of younger people.

# References

Archibald C (1994) *Sexuality and Dementia. A Guide*. DSDC, Stirling.

Hogan R (1980) *Human Sexuality. A Nursing Perspective*. Appleton Century Crofts, New York.

Parke F (1991) Sexuality in later life. *Nurs Times* **87**(50): 40–42

Roberts A (1989) Systems of life. No 2 172 and Senior Systems 37. *Nurs Times* **85**(24): 65–68

Roper N *et al* (1985) *The Elements of Nursing: Expressing Sexuality. Section 3:16*. Churchill Livingstone, Edinburgh

Taylor P (1994) Beating the taboo. Sexuality, patient education. *Nurs Times* **90**(13): 51–53

Webb R (ed) (1983) *Sexuality in Later Years. Roles and Behaviours*. Academic Press, New York

Webb initials??(1985) *Sexuality, Nursing and Health*. John Wiley & Sons, Chichester

## Audio visual aids

### *Format: VHS Video*

Ref: *Am I Normal?*
Concord Films Council

Ref: PATUA 668: *Sexuality and Ageing, Part 1*

Ref: PATUA 669: *Sexuality in Ageing, Part 2*

Ref. PATUA 670: *Sexuality and Ageing, Part 3*

Oxford Educational Resources Ltd

# Unit 17
# Community care (W4, Y2)

## National Health Service and Community Care Act 1993 (W4: 1-2, Y2: 1-2)

The National Health Service and Community Care Act, 1993 has brought many changes to the provision of care to people in their local community. The service is developed around the needs of clients and their family, to enable them to live as independently as possible in their own homes or in a homely setting in the community. Hospitals have to ensure that appropriate services are in place to support and help individual clients to live as independently as possible, before they are discharged home. These changes are meant to give the consumer choice, value for money service by effective management, and good quality service by the continuous review of services being offered.

### Assessment of clients' needs

Social services departments are responsible for assessing individual clients' special care needs, and describing what services will be provided to meet those needs. The nature of assessment carried out is widespread, and relates to anyone with social care needs for home help or meals-on-wheels. Assessment should also include those who have been discharged from hospital, and their needs are referred to the local social services department. Following assessment, those with health care needs are referred to the district nursing team and other community staff.

After assessment, those people who may be in need of nursing or residential home care and assistance with fees, will be further assessed. Depending on their earnings and savings, the social services department may be able help pay their fees but the person will be asked to contribute towards the cost. People who enter residential or nursing homes can generally claim income support in the same way as people living in their own home.

### Care plans

As from April 1993, social services are responsible for assessing most people needing nursing or residential care to ensure that the individual's needs are fully considered and appropriate care plans formulated for their areas. The service covers the needs of the elderly, mentally ill, those with learning difficulties, ethnic groups, those suffering from disabilities or the disabled, people with drug and alcohol problems, as well as dealing with problems of employment, housing and hazards in the environment.

If the social services departments think that people need help from the National Health Service, they will be able to make appropriate arrangements. Also, within the Patient's Charter (1990), everybody has the right to be registered with a general practitioner working in a primary health care team.

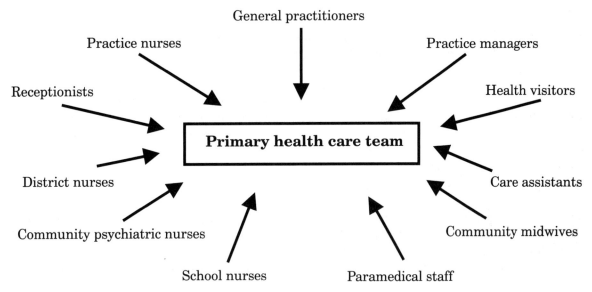

Diagram showing the members of the primary health care team

## Primary health care team

Health promotion and care is the responsibility of a team that requires strong leadership. Every member of the team works together to provide a service assigned to a local community. It is made up of all those people based within the practice, most of whom are either partners, or directly employed by the general practitioner.

### The practice nurse

This is a qualified nurse employed by the general practitioner.

### The practice manager

He/she is responsible for the smooth running of the practice. Practice managers are members of the Association of Health Centre and Practice Administrations. Fund holding practices may also employ separate business managers to deal with placing contracts, management of the budget and monitoring the services provided.

### Receptionists/medical secretary

They are the first point of contact with the public and responsible for controlling the number of telephone calls put through to the practice. They are often called the 'gate-keepers' to the doctor by prioritising appointments. In smaller practices, secretarial duties may be combined with reception work, but larger practices employ medical secretaries to deal with referral letters.

### Paramedical staff

Larger practices may employ other professional staff such as dieticians, physiotherapists, counsellors and chiropodists to increase the range of services available to patients. Pharmacists are joining some practices to help with more effective prescribing. Alternative therapists, eg. aromatherapists and masseuses are also being welcomed and form part of an integrated practice.

## District nurses

A district nurse is responsible for providing skilled nursing services within the community by:
- assessing the care needs of patients and their families
- formulating individualised care plans and revising them as necessary
- implementing the care or delegating to other members of the district nursing team
- monitoring the patients' or clients' progress and reassessing their needs for care

Liaison with other primary health care team members, social services and voluntary agencies is often as important as direct care-giving. The role also includes teaching other nurses, medical students and general practice trainees. District nursing teams work in a similar way to hospital ward teams, with mixed skills.

## Health visitors

Their role is concerned with public health, maternal and child welfare. The role can encompass health promotion with people of all ages. Teaching and liaising with other agencies is an important aspect of the role of health visitors. They can help to compile profiles of individual practice populations, so that the primary health care team can target services to the groups with particular health needs locally.

## Community psychiatric nurses (CPNs)

They are registered as mental health nurses, most of whom have completed a post-registration course. The service developed out of hospital-based psychiatric nursing and most CPNs continue to be based in hospitals. CPNs carry out mental health assessments with patients and their families within the community, and offer a range of therapeutic strategies.

## Community midwives

They have statutory responsibilities for the care of women during pregnancy, confinement and the puerperium. Community midwives organise antenatal and postnatal care in health centres and general practices, and run antenatal and parentcraft classes. A community midwife must provide a home confinement, and be responsible for a domino scheme or delivery within a general practice hospital maternity unit.

## Care assistants

The role of care assistants is a flexible one which combines the skills of a home help and those of caring acquired in hospitals or residential care homes. The specific care that they give is under the supervision of registered nurses.

## Other nurses

Other nurses can be considered as outside members of the primary health care team. Each has a specific contribution to make.

## School nurses

They have a major role in health promotion for school children, as well as in dealing with their health problems at school. Practice nurses may have most contact with school nurses through the care of children with asthma.

## Social services

Referrals can be made on behalf of patients who require home care, 'meals on wheels' or other social service support. However, few practices have a social worker attached and referrals for social services are usually made by telephone or letter. Social workers are required to make a full needs assessment of the patients referred to them.

## Voluntary services

A number of voluntary services, self-help groups and charities exist. They provide financial and practical assistance, as well as offering information, advice and research funding. Some are organised locally to help people in need in the community, while others help sufferers of a specific illness or disability. Patients and their carers can benefit from the knowledge of a practice nurse who can tell them who to approach for help. A database of contact addresses can be built up, either in a manual file or on the computer.

## League of friends

Some practices have a league of friends who organise transport for disabled and immobile patients, arrange prescription collections and sometimes raise funds to buy extra medical equipment for the practice. This type of voluntary work can offer significant help in both urban and rural communities.

# Services and facilities in the community for the elderly

After a period of illness patients are not able to carry out some of the activities of every day living that we take for granted when well, and appreciate extra help and supporting services to alleviate some of the problems associated with independent living. There are a range of social measures which are available to support individual clients to live independently in the community. Some of these include:

- day care and day hospital facilities
- community services and home care service, eg. counselling, housework
- night sitting and visiting service
- appliances and aids to daily living
- home adaptation facilities
- specialist advice in the medicine of the elderly
- promotion of aids and laundry
- community physiotherapist, podiatrist (chiropodist), opticians and speech therapists
- carer support groups
- bathing service
- monitoring system for people who live alone
- user friendly information service on care available in the locality and how it is accessed.

Other social services include:

- borough councils which provide for home improvement schemes
- home care services, eg. home case assistants, meals-on-wheels
- Red Cross Society — they may organise loans of a practical nature, eg. wheelchairs, walking aids
- sheltered accommodation, registered care establishments, warden-controlled flats
- Community Health Council

- members of parliament, local county councillors
- religious bodies and clergy, eg. street warden schemes exist in some parishes of the Church of England
- Health Education Council
- disablement resettlement officers
- police, Citizen's Advice Bureau
- libraries services
- relatives, neighbours, milkman, newspaper boy
- DHS benefits agency, financial facilities
- ambulance service
- voluntary organisations such as: MIND, Schizophrenia Association, Samaritans, RWVS (Royal Women's Voluntary Service), Age Concern, Alzheimer's Association, Royal National Institute for the Blind
- neighbourhood watch and street warden scheme.

# References

Barefoot P, Cunningham PJ (1977) *Community Services*. Faber and Faber, London
Department of Health (1991) *The Patient's Charter*. HMSO, London
Department of Health and Social Security (1990) *The National Health Service and Community Care Act*. HMSO, London
Lamb A (1977) *Primary Health Nursing*. Bailliere Tindall, London
Lubbock G (ed) (1983) *Stroke Care: An Interdisciplinary Approach*. Faber and Faber, London
Mellor HW (1985) *The Role of Voluntary Organisations in Social Welfare*. Croom Helm, London
Office of Population Concensuses and Surveys (1990) *General Household Survey*. HMSO, London
Royal College of Nursing (1993) T*he GP Practice Population Profile*. RCN, London
Royal College of Nursing (1994) *Public Health: Nursing Rises to the Challenge*. RCN, London
Smith S (1993) All change: Community Care Act. *Nurs Times* **89**(3): 24–26
Sterenborg Y (1982) Home to home. *Nurs Times* **78**(22): 2191–2193
Teasdale K (1983) Reality orientation. A programme for the elderly. *Nurs Times* **79**(9): 49–52

## Audio visual aids

### Format: VHS video

Ref: CEA 6049: *Hospital Sponsored Community Care for the Elderly*
Ref: CME 6646: *Evaluating and Documenting Rehabilitation Programs for the Elderly: A Hands-on-approach.*
Ref: CME 6643: *Mobility Spectrum and the Elderly*
Ref: 225/and 3: *Voluntary Service in Hospitals*
Ref: 329/1-2 CT: *Social Services for Older People*
Ref: OUE 1013: *Rehabilitation Unit*
Ref: 334/1–2: *Aids and Adaptation in the Home*
Ref: CNE348: *Safety in Home Care*
Ref: CMEUA 830: *Treating the Elderly: Physician Home Visits for the Frail Elder*
Ref: 387/1– 2 CT: *The Home Care Service*

Ref: 292CT: *Nursing in the Community*
Oxford Educational Resources Ltd
SURF: http://www.open.gov.UK/doh/newnhs.htm

# Assignment

The purpose of this homework is to assist you in preparing for your Workbased Assessment of Competence. As there is no pressure on you, feel free to work at your own pace, but avoid the temptation to procrastinate. After you have read your notes and suggested references, submit your work for correction. The completed work becomes part of your Personal Portfolio.

## Community care (W4: 1-2, Y2: 1-2)

1. What do you understand by the terms 'community care' and 'primary health care team'?
2. The National Health Service and Community Care Act came into being in 1993. Discuss briefly what you understand by this Act, and how it affects you personally.
3. List members of the primary health care team and briefly describe the role of care assistants in the team.
4. An elderly resident in your area of work is being discharged home:
    a) discuss arrangements that may be made for the person's discharge
    b) list facilities and services that will be available to support and help the person to live as independently as possible in the community
    c) describe the role of care assistants in the person's care in the community.
5. List other services available in the community. In what circumstance would you recommend one of these services to one of your clients?
6. Discuss how and where you could contact the local continence advisor.
7. What do you understand by health education and promotion?
    a) list aspects of health education that you have seen promoted in the national media
    b) discuss your role as a member of the health education and promotion team
    c) in what aspect would you introduce the concept of health education in your work area?

# Unit 18
# Support clients in the activity of dying (NC1, NC3, Z15)

## Nature and purpose of dying

Dying is the final activity of daily living which signifies the end of life just as birth marks the beginning. For some, life is short and for others it may cover many years. It is, however, true to say that all of us will die one day, but what is uncertain is where, when, why and how. The topic of death is surrounded by many taboos which seems to influence the way people see and value their lives. It is sensible to talk about death, for it is probably these doubts that provoke uneasy feelings when people think about the prospect of their own death. But life would not be worth living if people ignored the mystery of death.

Death determines the length of an individual's life-span and can occur at any age. It is believed that about 50% of all deaths in the United Kingdom occur in those over the age of 75 years, and a similar percentage of the elderly die in hospital even though many express a wish to die at home. Dealing with death is not easy, and coming to terms with someone who is dying or terminally ill is particularly difficult.

### Nature of dying

Death is seen as the sudden removal of people in the midst of their life or as an unnatural intrusion into someone's life. Quite often, and in some cultures, death is known as 'good death' when the person who has died is in his 80s, has not suffered loss of dignity and has pursued a successful career well into old age. But, should it occur earlier, it is seen as cruel, especially if the person has left young children. In the past health care professionals — doctors, nurses — regarded death as a failure of their skills.

### Causes of death

Death may result from illness. The most common causes are drug overdose, AIDS, cardiac failure, infection, eg. pneumonia. It may also occur suddenly following a massive cerebral haemorrhage or heart attack, trauma, haemorrhage, respiratory arrest. The suffering in these cases is by the relatives rather than the person dying. Many old people, especially those with extensive brain damage, may fade away gradually with an increasing cloudiness of consciousness and all concerned may feel that death, when it comes, is merciful. Some people's minds may remain clear until the end.

### Forms of death

Some people die suddenly from natural disasters, such as accidents, earthquakes, floods, acts of war in defence of one's country. The incidence of death is rising, but murder is not common, although during the 1970s the act of terrorism was prevalent as a means of achieving some form of political objective. The majority of people do not want to die but there are those who for reasons of their own, commit suicide. In the United Kingdom, the most common method is poisoning, and the rate of suicides and parasuicides rise as age increases. This is more common with professionals and executives, rather than manual workers. Attempted suicide was a criminal offence until the law was changed in 1962. Deliberate ending of a dying person's life is known as euthanasia or mercy killing. The debate persists on its ethical issues.

### Purpose of death

Many people have personal beliefs about the meaning of death. A majority base their idea on the philosophy of a particular religion with reference to the fate of a man's spirit and soul after death. Christians believe that, although death marks the end of life on earth, there is an afterlife, and that death is in fact the beginning of an eternal life with God. In this respect, they believe that the purpose of death is to allow for a religious progression from life on earth to an afterlife with God. But others, with no religious background, hold the view that life is full of 'letting go and moving on', and that death is the final stage of the journey which, in essence, is an inevitable end of living.

## Bereavement and grieving (NC1.1)

The death of someone with whom you share your life is known to be the severest form of stress. It is an experience that everyone will have to cope with at some time in their lives, particularly as people grow older. Bereavement can mean the end of a loving relationship which has lasted for many years. It is highly personal and everyone will experience it in his or her own way. In most cases it is not only the close relatives, eg. spouses or children that will be affected by the death of someone who is significant to them. Many other people may be affected and suffer great distress and a deep sense of desolation at the loss of the person, eg. friends, colleagues, neighbours, doctors, nurses, pets, teachers, and fellow patients alike.

### Grief

This is a deep or violent sorrow at the loss of a loved one. It is an emotional response which follows death and is one of the most intense human experiences. Culturally, different societies mourn the departed loved ones according to their customs. In times gone by, there was more formality in mourning, and ritual expressions of grief were part of the lifestyle of our great grandparents. Nowadays, with the passing of time some people have overlooked the need to mourn which is essential to our well-being and recovery. However, many find additional comfort through religion and this is not only regular church goers. The aim of grief is to enable one to come to terms with the loss. It is also seen as the cost of commitment in our lives.

### Stages of grief

The feelings of loss and grief are almost universal responses to loss and many other reactions can occur, such as shock, disbelief, denial, guilt, resentment, anxiety, anger, shame, depression, despair and signs of recovery.

Each stage will vary from person to person and one does not necessarily progress through each stage in a logical fashion nor, indeed, through all of them. Your own personality, inner strength and experience might help you to cope with one stage better than another. In most cases, it is believed that the sharing of grief with members of the family and close friends provides one with an emotional support that enables the person to readjust to the demands of everyday life.

### Shock
The initial shock at the loss is often described as a numbness, a sense of disbelief, sometimes the fact and meaning of the loss may be denied by the bereaved. 'No not me' is a natural reaction that tends to cushion one against the loss and allows one to feel it more slowly. An attempt to suppress this feeling can delay the healing process.

### Guilt
The dying person feels guilty about the emotional pain caused to others, broken promises or family feuds which may weigh on the dying person's conscience. There is often a great desire to 'make up and put things right' before they die.

### Anger
Many people, even those in their nineties, experience great anger at having their lives cut off before they are ready. 'Why me?' may be expressed as a resentment that others will remain alive while they must die. It can also be directed at those people with whom the dying person feels safest — usually close relatives, who will feel hurt and confused. They need a great deal of support to help them understand this type of behaviour, so that they do not retaliate or withdraw from the dying person when they are most needed.

### Fear
This is a reaction to any illness but is particularly intense in terminal illness, where there is no prospect of recovery. There is great apprehension about death, pain and the process of dying, the loss of control and dignity and, more importantly, being alone and rejected.

### Depression
The knowledge that death will mean parting from family and friends is obviously a source of great sadness and despair. People tend to reflect critically over their lives as they approach death, examining their family life, friendships, marriages and the contributions they have made to society. Some feel disappointed and depressed by what they discover, but others may gain strength and courage to face death, and find their religious beliefs an invaluable resource.

### Loneliness
People who die in hospitals or nursing homes, sometimes experience an overwhelming sense of loneliness. Although they are not 'alone' they are, in retrospect, without the close companionship of members of their family. The contact which the carer has with the dying person, if allowed, can become the basis of a trusting relationship which will prevent loneliness and isolation.

### Relief
Many elderly people will feel great relief to know that the end of their suffering is in sight. Those with a firm religious faith in a life after death may anticipate their reunion with God and their loved ones with nothing but joy. The most important role of caring is to allow all these feelings to be shared. And, to make this possible, a trusting relationship should be developed and maintained throughout, so by the time they die, many seem to have reached a state of tranquillity and acceptance.

## References

Carthcart F (1989) Death: coping with distress. *Nurs Times* **85**(42): 33–35
Lamberton R (1980) *Care of the Dying*. Penguin Books, London
Richardson R (1980) *Talking about Bereavement*. Open Books, Somerset

Trevelyan J (1990) A Matter of Life and Death. *Nurs Times* **85**(9): 35–37
Parkes MC (1972) *Bereavement. Studies of Grief in Adult Life*. Penguin Books, London
Tom-Johnson C (1990) Talking through grief. *Nurs Times* **86**(1): 44–46
Saunders C, Baines A (1983) *Living and Dying*. Oxford University Press, Oxford
Woods RT (1989) *Alzheimer's Disease. Coping with a Living Death*. Souvenir Press, London

## Management of problems (NC1.2, NC3.3)

Caring for the dying is never easy and is laden with emotional demands of a highly complex nature on everyone, the dying person, his family and the staff. As dying is the final activity of daily living everything should be done, as far as possible, to meet the wishes of the dying person and their relatives. The person should be able to die peacefully with dignity and composure, in keeping with the wishes of his or her family. The majority of dying people slip out of this life with little pain or suffering. This is usually seen when a previously healthy person suffers a massive heart attack and dies suddenly as a result. In others, especially those with long-term serious illnesses, death does not come easily, but is accompanied by pain, distress and disability which may last for many weeks or even months.

### Principles of care

The framework of care is based on a care plan designed to make the dying person as comfortable as possible, and to enable the person to participate if he or she wishes. A flexible routine is necessary to allow family and friends to participate in the care if they want to. But, emphasis is placed on providing the dying person with the best quality of care, comfort and freedom from unpleasant symptoms with an opportunity to maintain his or her lifestyle and pursue social and recreational activities until a peaceful and dignified death. He or she is helped to cope with activities of living and grow in the process of dying within an atmosphere of 'unhurried care'. This idea is a continuation of holistic care based on a recognition of the dying person's beliefs, values and spiritual needs, and those of his or her family. Management of the problem is based on assessment of the total care needs, based on Roper *et al* (1983), *Model of Care*.

### Role of carers

The process of caring for the dying requires carers to have certain skills, knowledge and attitudes to enable them to give a high standard and quality of care to the dying patient and his or her family. These skills include knowledge of the dying patient with special consideration to what is happening to the person and the changes in his or her behaviour because of the dying process. Emphasis is placed upon helping the person to perform activities of daily living, being with the client, and encouraging him or her to express and maintain his or her beliefs. The process is enhanced by:

- a good and trusting interpersonal relationship based on effective communication with an attitude of openness motivated by genuine compassion
- the use of counselling skills and a good doctor/nurse or carer partnership and expert symptom control, eg. of pain
- an ability to create an environment in which residents can live their lives as fully as possible. Helping residents to pursue their religious beliefs, by maintaining contact with the appropriate priest as desired
- ensuring that everything is carried out as reverently as possible.

## Implementation of care

### Physical needs

### Pain
This is probably what many people fear most about the process of dying. It is more than a physical experience, it is always constant and can be particularly distressing to the dying.

*Intervention*
Pain is usually relieved through a recognised strategy in an individual client's care programme and is kept under control, generally every four hours. It may be possible to alter the cause of pain by a change of position.

### Mouth care
The mouth should receive frequent attention especially before and after feeds.

*Intervention*
- give frequent sips from a beaker
- moisten lips regularly with a foamstick (relatives can do this)
- give crushed ice to suck
- appy Vaseline to prevent cracked lips.

### Anorexia
It is helpful if carers pay special attention to a client's intake of nourishment and fluids.

*Intervention*
- identify client's preference for food and drink, offer small amounts of easily digestible and appetising meals at regular intervals
- encourage and, if necessary, help the client to clean his/her mouth and teeth
- maintain a fluid balance chart.

### Nausea and vomiting
Where vomiting is persistent, it can lead to dehydration.

*Intervention*
- remove the vomit and any soiled clothing and linen immediately from the vicinity
- save a specimen of the vomit for inspection
- provide facilities for sponging the face and hands, and rinsing the mouth
- give a refreshing mouthwash and keep the tongue and lips moist
- allow him or her to lie in a semi-prone position, turn the head to one side and support with pillows. Change pyjamas and bed linen if these are soiled.

It is possible that anti-emetic drugs may be prescribed to relieve persistent nausea. A nasogastric tube may be passed to prevent constant retching.

### Dehydration
Terminally ill patients frequently become dehydrated, but the only symptom of any consequence is a dry and uncomfortable mouth. Dry mouths rapidly become furred and dirty, and may become infected especially with thrush.

*Intervention*
- give frequent, small quantities of a drink of choice and maintain a fluid balance chart
- clean the teeth frequently followed by a mouth wash. If the tongue is furred, a little bicarbonate of soda dissolved in warm water may be used in cleaning the tongue.

### Dyspnoea (difficult in breathing)
The client and his or her visitors may be very distressed by extreme breathlessness. The very noisy breathing known as the 'death rattle' may be present and is a terrible experience that haunts many relatives long after the patient has died.

*Intervention*
- sit the person in an upright position to allow for maximum expansion of the lungs
- encourage the client to sit in a chair or lie in the most comfortable position even at night
- ventilate the room by providing a cool, circulating atmosphere and in warm weather air conditioning and fans are a great help
- place the bed near a window even if only for its psychological effect and being with the patient may ease the sense of panic and fear
- place a foot-board or bolster at the bottom of the bed to prevent the client slipping down
- talk to the person and encourage him or her to express personal feelings.

### Incontinence
The dying person can be very distressed by incontinence. It is necessary for the problem to be approached with tact and sympathy. Observe for retention of urine. Despite its hazards, catherisation may be ordered to deal with the problem.

### Dysphasia (difficult in swallowing)
Eating and drinking become very difficult and uncomfortable.

*Intervention*
- identify the patient's preference for food and drink
- give tiny amounts of food very slowly to ease his or her difficulty
- offer liquidated food or products, such as Complan, Clinifeed
- show understanding, reassurance and practical caring skills, eg. communication.

### Constipation
This may be due to lack of exercise and inadequate intake of nourishment.

*Intervention*
- offer food with high fibre content, such as whole grain cereals, bread, fruit
- encourage adequate fluid intake
- mild aperients may be given to soften and increase the bulk of the bowel contents
- support the client if suppositories or enemas are given
- encourage gentle exercise.

### Personal hygiene
Pay meticulous attention to care of the mouth, skin, eyes and nails.

### Pressure sores
General debility, reduced movement and food intake including impaired sensation may cause pressure sores to develop more easily in the dying person.

*Intervention*
- ensure that the person is turned regularly to relieve prolonged pressure on any one part
- use bed appliances to take the weight of bed clothes as the dying person often seems to become very sensitive to pressure
- make and help the dying person to remain comfortable in bed.

## 3. Psychological needs

The dying person and his or her family will react to the approaching death in a very individual way. These reactions may take the form of:

### *Fear and anxiety*
This is due to an awareness of impending death accompanied by intense fear. The intensity is marked in terminal illness as there is no prospect of recovery. The apprehension relates to fear of death, pain and the process of dying, loss of control and dignity, and of being alone or rejected.

> *Intervention*
> - maintain a good interpersonal relationship with the dying person
> - identify the problem by encouraging the client to express his or her feelings
> - reassure and encourage the maintenance of self-esteem to cover the symptoms
> - stop for a moment and share your presence with the dying person and his or her family, if they are present.

### *Depression*
This is almost a universal feature of the dying process. The individual will express profound regret over missed opportunities and failures of the past, and is overwhelmed with sadness. At times, he or she may feel rejection and despair.

> *Intervention*
> - re-establish and maintain a good interpersonal relationship with the dying person
> - find out and remind the person of his or her personal achievements by showing that he or she is well-respected and loved by everyone around
> - offer friendship, make time to sit, talk and give an opportunity for the person to express him or herself. Listen attentively and solemnly
> - allow the client to vent personal feelings and offer reassurance and appropriate counselling. Encourage social and gentle exercise and recreational activities of choice
> - reassure the client that he or she will be looked after to the end and that what is important is for him or her to cope with each day at a time, and make the most of what is left.

### *Confusion*
In the dying person, confusion may result from many situations, such as delirium or as part of acute organic brain disease. There may also be muddled thoughts arising out of weakness, fear and anxiety.

> *Intervention*
> - provide a calm and reassuring environment
> - reassure the person that he or she is safe and that the people around are trying to understand and to help
> - assist the dying person to realise and rationalise any underlying anxieties
> - co-operate with others to provide a peaceful yet cheerful environment.

## 4. Social problems

### *Loneliness*
One of the greatest concerns of dying people is that they will be left alone. Those who die in institutions sometimes experience an overwhelming sense of loneliness, even if they are not really 'alone', but are in the close companionship of the nursing and other care staff.

*Intervention*
- make frequent contact with the dying person
- develop a trusting relationship which inwardly will prevent loneliness and isolation
- accept that reactions, such as anger and depression are 'normal' in the dying process
- answer questions posed to you truthfully and refer difficult ones to the person-in-charge
- show sympathy and compassion to help with the many psychological problems.

**Rest and sleep**

Encourage the person to have maximum bodily comfort and peace of mind, and to rest and sleep as necessary. The person should not be disturbed except for medical treatment.

**Care environment**

Unpleasant odours can be related to caring activities such as incontinence or discharging wounds. The resident will appreciate any attempts to minimise what is a distressing problem. Good ventilation of the room and discreet use of aerosol sprays can be helpful.

**Spiritual needs**

Great attention should be paid to the spiritual needs and religious practices of dying people and their family. Some people may make requests themselves to be visited by their priests. In some cases, requests may be made by members of their family. At times it may be necessary to inquire of the relatives whether they would wish for the services of a priest or minister. If so, whether they would like to send for one they know or permit the services of local clergy, before proceeding further. It is useful to have a knowledge of some religious rites during and following death.

**Christians**

Dying residents usually ask for Holy Communion. It is important to make the individual presentable with clean clothes and bed linen before the priest arrives. The bed should be screened and the person left alone. There are, at times, objections to post mortem or cremation.

**Jews**

When death occurs the body should not be touched. The Rabbi should be informed. Burial arrangements are normally made by relatives for burial on Saturdays or Sundays.

**Muslims**

The body should be left untouched until washed by another Muslim of the same sex. If possible, the body should be left in a position facing south east (Mecca).

**Sikhs**

Most wear turbans which, if possible, should not be removed even after death. Hair, beards and other body hair should not be cut.

# References

Help the Aged (1989) *Bereavement*. Sponsored by Dignity in Destiny Ltd, London
Charles-Edwards A (1983) *The Nursing Care of the Dying Patient*. Beaconsfield Publishers Ltd, Bucks
Robbins J (1989) *Care of the Dying Patient and the Family*. Harper and Row, London

Williams J (1980) Appetite in the terminally ill patient. *Nurs Times* **76**(20): 875–876

Wright S (1987) Patient centred practice. Primary nursing. *Nurs Times* **83**(38): 87–89

# Last offices (Z15: 1–2)

The laying out of the dead should be reverently and quietly carried out; all unnecessary talking must be avoided. As soon as the person has breathed his or her last, the carer should gently close the eyes, if they are not already closed. Loved ones, if they are present at the time of death are allowed to see the body before further procedures are carried out. The carer must be accessible during this time as quite often the relatives grief is close to unbearable. After they have seen the body, they are then led from the room to speak to the person-in-charge or the doctor. If possible, the carer should have help, as the body can be more easily and reverently handled by two as it is now a very heavy weight to move.

## After death

The following observations should be maintained:
- note the time of death
- notify the person-in-charge who will in turn inform the doctor and relatives
- assist in completing routine documentation for notification of death
- be aware of the cultural wishes of the family
- screen off the bed unless in a single room already.

## Last offices

This is the laying out of the dead, performed about an hour following death. The person-in-charge will ensure that the routine procedures are carried out with respect and dignity. The procedure is usually carried out by experienced/qualified staff with the help of care assistants. Therefore, it is important that care assistants let experienced staff know if they have ever seen a dead person before, so that they can be gradually introduced to the procedures of the last offices — known as 'laying out' of the dead person.

### *Guidance*

The practice may differ slightly in each care establishment. But the general principle is, as far as possible, to carry out the procedure in a dignified and reverent manner.

### *Procedure*

- remove pillows, bedclothes and personal clothes
- close the eyes with small pledgets of damp cotton wool placed on the eyelids
- express and empty the bladder if necessary
- remove jewellery unless relatives have expressed a wish that an article, eg. wedding ring should remain, also, ascertain their wishes regarding dentures
- clean the mouth. A thick pad or a small pillow may be placed under the jaw to keep the mouth closed
- lay the body straight with the arms at the sides and leave a pillow under the head
- cover the body with a clean sheet and leave for an hour
- make a list of the deceased's personal belongings and get them ready for the relatives to collect. If rings are left on the body, a record should be made to that effect. It is important to obtain a receipt for every item taken home by the relatives
- leave the body for an hour and prepare equipment for completion of the procedure.

## Equipment

The following materials will be required to complete the procedure:
- Princess Alice Hospice Last Offices box, if available. Some care establishments use these arrangements
- clean nightwear or clothing as may be requested by the family
- bowl of warm water, soap, flannel and towels
- pad and pants
- hairbrush and comb, shaving tackle if necessary
- a bowl of cotton wool and gauze swabs
- a receiver for soiled dressings and instruments
- clean sheets and a shroud
- a carrier for soiled linen and blankets.

### *Guidance*
- give a full blanket bath and wash the body all over, trim and clean nails and dry the body thoroughly
- renew dressings if any and seal the wound with clean dressings and strapping
- ensure that the rectum and other orifices are packed in accordance with local policy to prevent leakage
- men may have a 'wet' shave and face moisturised to prevent shadows forming
- brush and arrange the hair neatly as worn by the deceased, if long plaits tie with a white tape or ribbon
- spigot any catheter but do not remove. Put on pads and 'Nestalast' pants to reduce the risk of leakage after the body has been removed by the funeral parlour attendants
- dress the deceased in nightwear or clothes as requested by the family
- cover the body with a small sheet specially designed for this purpose, and attach an identification label. The use of shroud is no longer current in some places
- wrap the body in a sheet, attach a second identification label and arrange for the body to be removed to the mortuary as soon as possible
- strip the bed and place linen and blankets in water-soluble bags for laundry
- wash bedstead and locker with disinfectant in accordance with local policy
- everything used for the last offices should be removed from the room as quickly as possible and care should be taken to make the room neat, and pleasant.

## Infectious diseases

In the case of infectious disease, the carer must wear disposable gloves and a plastic apron when carrying out the last offices. Once the body has been placed in a body bag, no further intensive care precautions are required.

## Notification of death

Generally, when death has occured, the doctor who attended the deceased during the final illness will visit to certify the cause of death. He or she will issue a Medical Certificate which should be placed in a sealed envelope, and addressed to the Registrar of Death. A formal notice will be issued at the same time for registration of death. The next of kin should be informed if he or she was not present at the time of death. Arrangements for removal of the body from the premises are usually made with local funeral directors unless the relatives arrange for it to be taken away.

## Support for relatives (NC1: 2-3, NC3: 1-3)

Caring for the bereaved relatives is as demanding as caring for the departed relative. It is about life after death and must be handled with skill and sensitivity. On their arrival in the home, they are met by the person-in-charge, as their need for psychological support is great. They are equally entitled to counselling, honest interaction and an essential information-giving process. All efforts should be made to help them cope with the loss, and the daunting administrative work involved with the registration of death. Some homes maintain information packs for staff and relatives.

Under the Births and Deaths Registration Acts 1947, relatives are the people required to report a death. They are given information about registration of death. Payment of a fee would be necessary for the certificate which they will need for other transactions such as insurance policy, pension claims, will. Once a death certificate has been issued, the death must be registered within five days at the Registrar's office in the district where the death took place. They will need the deceased's medical NHS card, medical certificate and the Pink Form if applicable.

After registration, they will be issued with a document allowing arrangements to be made for the funeral. The deceased's property and valuables should be checked and returned to the family in accordance with local policy.

Some relatives may feel guilty that the deceased has had to spend the last period of his or her life in hospital or a nursing home, and blame themselves for failing those whom they love. At times, these guilt feelings show themselves in unjustified complaints about the care previously given. Occasionally, some may find the situation confusing, especially when they reflect on the deceased's feelings of anger towards them. It is important for carers to recognise that this type of behaviour and reaction are normal. Therefore, an attempt should be made to discuss observations of these feelings with the person-in-charge.

Apart from emotional problems of grief, social adjustment and sometimes economic strains present problems. This means that they must be given time to grieve, talk, reminisce and express openly their fears and worries and begin to plan for a new future. Showing compassion to the bereaved will be a reminder that despite their loss, they are not entirely alone and that there is a reason to renew their sources of faith and hope, and have courage to begin a new life again.

### Recovery

In some cultures, bereavement can be a long and painful process, in which relatives may experience intense anxiety for the future. They may feel completely incapable of taking decisions and coping with everyday demands. In some cases, the dead person may appear in their dreams and hallucinations, which tends to present a comforting experience and makes up for the reality of the loss and loneliness they feel. However, a bereaved person should try and give up the old life and develop a new one. Quite often the new life is moulded gradually to embrace some events such as returning to work, moving house and making new friends. It is true to say that, 'time heals'.

## References

Costello J (1990) Dying at home. *Nurs Times* **86**(8): 49–51

Department of Health and Social Security (1995) *What to Do after a Death*. Leaflet D49S. HMSO, Oldham.

Gooch J (1988) Dying in the ward. *Nurs Times* **84**(21): 38

Hinton J (1975) *Dying*. Penguin Books, London

Kubler-Ross E (1970) *On Death and Dying*. Routledge, London

Parkes MC (1986) *Bereavement. Studies of Grief in Adult Life*. Penguin Books, London

Wiseman C (1992) Bereavement care in an acute ward. *Nurs Times* **88**(20): 34–35

## Audio visual aid

***Format: VHS video***

Ref: 371CT: *Care of the Dying Person and their Families*

Oxford Educational Resources Ltd

# Unit 19
# Special care needs (mental health)
# (CL7, NC10, W2, X1, X2, X16, Z8)

## Mental health problems in the elderly

The concept of mental health and mental illness is difficult to define or explain as we cannot with any degree of certainty draw a simple dividing line, and say that the features of mental health are on one side and those of mental disorder on the other side. This is due to the numerous problems which result when physical, psychological, social and environmental factors interrelate with each other. The person is an individual entity and responds to stress in an individual way. At any given moment, the individual's mental health may be affected by the way he or she happens to be thinking, behaving and feeling. It is correct to say that at times we feel as if we have 'just got out of bed on the wrong side' or just recovered from a very bad dose of flu. At other times we 'feel on top of the world'. All these feelings are not static. They change and tend to affect the way we behave towards our friends, spouses, pets, colleagues, residents and how we respond to difficult situations in the environment.

As can be seen, no single characteristic of the personality is by itself positive evidence of mental health, as extremes may make the person unable to cope with his or her actions, thoughts and feelings. Everyone has strengths as well as weaknesses, and the way we behave tends to relate to the predisposing and precipitating stresses involved. It follows that things that influence behavioural disruptions affect the whole person. But, to a much greater extent, what is happening to a person at any particular moment may be the outcome of things which have happened in earlier life, influencing his/her ability to cope with stress in later life.

The World Health Organization (WHO) (1987) defines health as, 'ideal physical, psychological and social well-being and not merely the absence of disease'. It looks at mental health as 'the full harmonious functioning of the whole personality'. These definitions focus on an ideal state of health, and exclude disease as an aspect of health. Health and ill health are something that we all experience.

### Predisposing factors

Mental health is not a static condition because of the way it fluctuates. It is influenced by a variety of factors in different combinations, eg. biological, psychological, social, economical interacting with situations in the physical environment. In most cases, evidence of mental health problems are shown by the individual's ability to:

- develop and maintain a good and harmonious relationship with themselves and others
- contribute to changes in their social and physical environment
- balance their own conflicting drives in a socially acceptable and realistic way
- cope effectively with both expected and unexpected life events
- integrate his/her own personality with a sense of freedom from conflict
- recognise and respond to certain situations in life in order to avoid stress and anxiety, and develop a coping strategy.

Hereditary factors seem to play a part in severe mental health problems, such as schizophrenia, which may be triggered off by interaction with events in the environment.

## Classification

This relates to the degree of insight and symptoms presented by the person. The main types are:

### Neurosis
This is an abnormal emotional reaction to disturbing situations. The person retains insight into his or her condition and maintains contact with reality. Although crippling and always unpleasant, it does not lead to disintegration of personality and the person may be able to continue functioning normally, although in a restricted way. But, its nature may make the person attempt suicide.

### Psychosis
This is a serious mental illness in which the person has little or no insight into his or her condition, and has restricted contact with reality. If untreated, or sometimes despite treatment, it may lead to disintegration of the personality, usually accompanied by symptoms of delusions and hallucinations which affect the person's ability to make adjustments in life. Psychosis is divided into two parts:

1. **Functional illness** — the name suggests a disorder of performance rather than changes in the physical structure of the brain. It may mean that this type of illness will always have been present even until old age, eg. schizophrenia. Depression has a high suicide rate. There are other diagnoses, eg. psychopathy, alcohol and drug dependency, sexual disorders, mania.
2. **Organic states** — these result from some physical change in the brain and where there is visible cerebral pathology, eg. dementia.

## Ageing process and mental health

Age is not a cause of mental health problems. It is claimed that changes in the tissues affecting certain endocrine glands and the brain are of great importance when considering causes of mental health problems in the elderly. It may also be indirectly related to changes in experience, mental outlook and especially, in the tissues of the body over the passage of years.

## Effects of ageing

Many signs and symptoms of mental health problems may be viewed as the person's inability to cope with particular situations. This may be the result of diminished ability to maintain good interpersonal relationships with other people, and to cope with everyday activities of living. The outcome is that the person concerned will have other significant problems with which he or she may require help and assistance. Some may suffer from instability or intellectual impairment and incontinence which is often a feature of mental health problems in the elderly.

## The study of elderly people

Geriatrics is a branch of medicine covering old age and the problems arising from it. At times, one comes across the term 'psychogeriatrics' which is the study and treatment of the elderly with psychological problems. Some people may develop mental health problems usually classified as organic or functional. These are a group of serious mental health disorders associated with changes in the brain tissues, resulting in emotional and behavioural disturbances, leading to the condition known as dementia.

## Parkinson's disease

This is a degenerative disease of the nervous system. The individual looks rather lethargic with a blank facial or mask-like expression. Its main features are a shuffling gait with tremor of the hands. The person may become irritable, fault-finding and difficult to please. Dementia is not present, but the person is easily depressed and may attempt suicide.

## Dementia

This is a serious and progressive intellectual impairment caused by organic brain disease. It is a degenerative condition which results in a permanent mental deterioration affecting memory, judgment, behaviour and orientation. In most cases there is a gross personality change. There are different types but the most common is Alzheimer's disease.

## Alzheimer's disease

This is an organic disease of unknown causes which affects the brain tissues. It occurs between the ages of 40 to 60 years, affecting more women than men, and is the most common form of senile dementia. The disease is marked by a progressive and irreversible condition that involves the death of brain cells. It has an insidious onset followed by disintegration of the personality. Memory speech and judgment are affected leading to severe social and behavioural changes. The majority of elderly people in nursing homes seem to suffer from this condition.

### *Aetiology*

People with Alzheimer's disease often show evidence of delusions, hallucinations, memory impairment and confabulation. These are usually severe and orientation is affected first, then place, and finally, person.

### *Diagnosis*

Although this has not been possible except by post-mortem, recent research advances show some promising results. Observation of the brain under a microscope reveals a generalised cerebral atrophy with shrunken gyri and widened sulic. In the early stages of the disease, muscle tone often increases with rigidity and awkward and unsteady movements. It is claimed that epilepsy may occur in about 25% of the cases.

### *Clinical features*

The course of the disease progresses to a change in the personality. During this stage there is cognitive impairment, followed by speech disorder in the terminal stage. Mood changes may occur causing the person to isolate him/herself as a result of inappropriate social behaviour. The person may show repetitive and stereotyped behaviour including forgetfulness and fearfulness.

There may be evidence of delusions, misidentification of people and carers and visual and auditory hallucinations. Other features include:

#### *Judgment*
- This is severely impaired in advanced cases with an inability to plan and carry out activities of daily living. At times the person may behave in a childish, impulsive and erratic way.

#### *Memory*
- In the early stages, distant events may be recalled with great clarity, and memory of recent events starts to fade. As a result of memory failure, the individual may speak of people long dead as though they are still alive.

### Mood
- There may be an increased anxiety with loss of emotional stability. The person may be easily moved to anger or tears with emotional outbursts for trivial reasons, eg. difficulty in fastening a button.

### Confusion and disorientation
- These disorders tend to become steadily worse as the disease advances. In some cases, orientation in time, place and person are completely lost and the individual wears a certain expression of querulous perplexity. He or she may turn day into night and will often get dressed in the middle of the night, announcing when asked that he/she is getting ready to go to work, go shopping or take children to school.

### Social behaviour
- A person suffering from chronic brain dysfunction, usually tends to be uninterested in things around him or her. This attitude may show itself in various types of behavioural disturbances such as aggression, wandering, lack of sexual inhibitions or promiscuous activities. Personal hygiene deteriorates, obscene language may be freely used including random sexual advances to complete strangers. This personal behaviour may become a travesty of the person's former self. Clothing tends to become food stained and the person may carry out excretory functions in a random, careless way, often urinating in corners of rooms.

### Prognosis
There is as yet no known cure for Alzheimer's disease and the severe intellectual and behavioural deterioration persists until death. In the terminal stage, the person may show profound dementia, with a tendency to live a stuporous and vegetable existence, with legs usually drawn under him/her. In spite of precautions, the individual suffers from sores and ulcers, and quite often death occurs from infection within two to ten years.

## Admission for care

The NHS and Community Act 1993 requires each local authority to provide a cost effective service for keeping elderly people in the community and in their homes. The aim is to ensure that there are sufficient resources to target all those who are in greatest need. In some cases, this is not possible and the person is admitted to hospital or a nursing home. The illness may have an acute or insidious onset, or may be chronic — which is progressively slow, forcing the person to suffer from progressive lack of the ability to move. Consideration should be given to the effects of ageing because of the complexity of the elderly person's needs.

## Factors leading to admission

A significant number of elderly people are likely to have been frail prior to admission or suffer from disabling conditions. Some may live alone with limited means and capabilities for self-care. When an elderly person becomes ill, the problem may present itself in a number of ways, but quite often brings about deterioration in physical, psychological and social well-being. Any one of these conditions and, in any combination, may lead to admission, about 80% being emergency admissions.

### Immobility and falls
Falls and immobility are among the common reasons for admission to a nursing home or hospital.

### Dehydration
Some elderly people have an impaired sense of thirst and become too weak and apathetic to drink. Those who are confused may refuse nourishment, although they may continue to lose fluid in urine and sweat and become dehydrated.

## Confusion

The function of the brain is readily upset by any form of bodily disturbance, and a sudden onset of confusion is one indication of physical illness in old age. It may also be due to the side-effects of drugs, such as hypnotics, tranquillisers and anti-depressants.

## Temperature regulation

The rise in body temperature in response to infection is frequently less severe. Rigors, which is a shivering attack, may be an indication of a urinary or gall bladder infection. If the elderly person seems unwell, the fact that his or her temperature is normal cannot be used as an indicator. The pulse and respiration will often be a better guide to the person's condition. In fact, faulty temperature regulation may also be seen in his or her reaction to cold and the body temperature may fall below normal as in hypothermia.

## Reaction to drugs

The older person is very sensitive to drugs and harmful side-effects are common. Drugs are metabolised more slowly in the liver and excreted more slowly by the kidneys. Therefore, it is necessary for medicines to be given in small doses.

## Loss of pain and sensation

Pain in the elderly person may be less severe and, although it may make life less uncomfortable, it increases the risk that he or she might injure him/herself. For example, he or she may have been burnt by sitting too close to the fire, or may have bruised his or her leg against a bed cradle. Even serious injuries like fractures may not be obvious and, for the majority of elderly people, are painless.

## Inability to cope

Quite often, elderly people are presented by relatives, friends, neighbours or even by themselves in the following terms: 'it takes him more than two hours just to get dressed'; 'he does not know day from night'; 'he cannot recognise me any more'; 'his room smells of gas and I am afraid he cannot look after himself and can put other people at risk of explosion'. The elderly person may also suffer from incontinence.

### The framework of psychiatry

Generally, psychiatry deals with people who have common disturbances affecting their behaviour, emotions, thinking and insight. The most important of all is the recognition that 'psychiatric illness' occurs when these disturbances are real changes which persist and exceed the limits of normality. He or she may complain, be bothered and puzzled about these changes. At times, the person may not be able to complain. But, it is said that the face is the mirror of emotions, so that in general the face will show how the person feels and if he or she is in need of help.

# References

Burns A *et al* (1990) Psychiatric phenomena in Alzheimer's disease. *Brit J Psych* **157:I** (iv): 72–94

Ironbar NO, Harper A (1989) *Self-instruction in Mental Health Nursing*, 2nd edn. Bailliere Tindall, London

Lyttele J (1986) *Mental Disorders. Its Care and Treatment*. Bailliere Tindall, London

Kasner K, Tindall D (1984) *Bailliere's Nurses Dictionary,* 20th edn. Bailliere Tindall, London

Tollis D (1991) Who was Alzheimer? *Nurs Times* **90**(34): 49

Pitt B (1988) *Dementia. Psychogeriatrics. An Introduction to the Psychiatry of Old Age*. Churchill Livingstone, Edinburgh

## Audio visual aids

**Format: VHS video**

Ref: *Mental Confusion in the Elderly: Management and Diagnosis*
The Scottish Central Film Library
Ref: CME6640: *Introduction to Dementia and Alzheimer's Disease*
Ref: CME6641: *Developing a Program of Alzheimer's Disease Care for Family and Patient*
Ref: CNE 7604: *Functional Assessment of the Elderly Part 1: Cognitive and Special Senses*
Ref: CNE 4331: *Physical Assessment of the Frail Elderly*
Ref: CNE7605: *Functional Assessment of the Elderly Part 2: Activities of Daily Living*
Ref: CME7717: *Geropsychiatric Nursing*
Oxford Educational Resources Ltd

# Assessment of functional abilities (X2: 1–3)

The care of the elderly, mentally infirm is a composite and challenging undertaking. Its aim is to restore some measures of self-control and independence for the individual to enjoy a good quality of life. A multidisciplinary approach is essential — comprising doctors, nurses, paramedical staff in consultation with members of the client's family and advocates. It is not always possible for members of the multidisciplinary team to work together in nursing homes, and nurses being at the front line of care are responsible for assessing, planning and the implementation of total care needs, using their knowledge of behavioural, physical and social sciences, including research findings. The approach used has been discussed in Models of Care and is based on Nursing Process — Individualised Nursing Care.

Assessment of functional abilities is an important stage of this care and lays the foundation for all subsequent care. It is a complex, time-consuming and demanding procedure in which functional abilities are assessed to enable a care plan to be devised. The process always poses a challenge and tests the skills of all those involved.

As part of the admission procedure, initial assessment is usually carried out in the client's home in the community before he or she is admitted, and is continued by a detailed assessment following admission into the care establishment. It involves continuous *observation of* the person and analysis of information over a period of time. The method used has been described under Nursing Process and involves the following four stages:

***Assessment*** — information for identification of nursing problems or clients' needs. The aim is to collect and analyse information relating to the physical, social and psychological well-being of the individual. Information may be obtained from individuals themselves, their family, their general practitioners' letters, nurses in the care establishments and those professionals who looked after the individuals in the community, such as community psychiatric nurses and social workers. Assessment has three important aspects: functional or existing disabilities of the individual; of the services which need to be provided in order to make up for such disabilities; and of the existing services. The outcome of this assessment establishes the need to plan care to make up for specialist services, the individual needs such as occupational therapists, physiotherapists and speech therapists.

***Planning*** — formulating a care plan to meet these needs.

***Implementation*** — carrying out or putting the care plan into practice.

***Evaluation*** — judging the effectiveness of the care given.

The whole process of assessment embraces the individual's holistic concept of health and his/her interaction with others in the care environment. The use of specific monitoring tools, such as the assessment of functional ability form is essential and must be reviewed at regular intervals. It is also important that risk assessment should form part of the overall assessment process with guidelines on how to manage any risk-taking problem.

## Assessment of functional ability

Name: ................................................... Date of birth: ...................................

Date of admission: ...................................

Care establishment: ...................................

**Physical assessment**

| Functional ability | With or without assistance | With or without supervision | Date review | Outcome | Assessor's signature |
|---|---|---|---|---|---|
| Dresses self regulary | | | | | |
| Eats and drinks regularly | | | | | |
| Grooms self regularly | | | | | |
| Dresses suitably for weather | | | | | |
| Uses bathroom as necessary | | | | | |
| Walks and manages stairs | | | | | |
| Remains fully continent and uses lavatory regulary | | | | | |
| Sleeps well at night | | | | | |

## Sociological assessment

| Functional ability | With support | Without support | Date review | Outcome | Assessor's signature |
|---|---|---|---|---|---|
| Awareness of environment | | | | | |
| Socialises with other people | | | | | |
| Demonstrates interest in reading, outings | | | | | |
| Works and plays | | | | | |

## Psychological assessment

| | Low dependency | Medium dependency | High dependency | Review date | Outcome | Assessor's signature |
|---|---|---|---|---|---|---|
| **Communication**<br>— understands personal needs<br>— speaks clearly | | | | | | |
| **Orientation**<br>— identifies people correctly<br>— completely lost | | | | | | |
| **Mood**<br>— stable<br>— depressed<br>— anxious, suspicious | | | | | | |
| **Behaviour**<br>— well behaved<br>— anti-social | | | | | | |
| **Memory**<br>— recalls with clarity<br>— confused | | | | | | |
| **Social behaviour**<br>— expresses sexual needs<br>— disinhibition or promiscuous | | | | | | |

# References

Howard G (1992) *Alzheimer's: A Care Giver's Guide and Source Book Sheet.* John Wiley & Sons, Chichester

Jacques A (1988) *Understanding Dementia.* Churchill Livingstone, Edinburgh

## Audio visual aids

### Format: VHS video

Ref: CEAHIN827: *EMS Vitals: Patient Assessment*
Ref: CEA6292: *Treating the Elderly: Treating Dementia*
Ref: CNE4331: *Physical Assessment of the Elderly Frail*
Ref: CNE 7604: *Functional Assessment of the Elderly Part 1: Cognitive and Special Senses*
Ref: CNE 7605: *Functional Assessment of the Elderly Part 2: Activities of Daily living*
Oxford Educational Resources Ltd

## Management of mental health problems (X1: 2–3, X2: 2–4, X16: 1–2)

The provision of care is based on identifying total care needs of individual residents, the nature and extent of their abilities and interest in performing their activities of daily living. These needs are at times diverse and widespread, requiring specialised skill and a sound knowledge of the individual and team work. The aim is to help the residents to use their remaining skills to carry out their individual activities of daily living. It is complex and demanding work and, at times, stressful, especially when caring for them for the rest of their lives. It is essential to be aware of your own ability to cope with stress within your personal network system. Refer constantly to individual clients' care plans. Think through what you are going to do in a realistic way, and develop your own role and skills in order to grow as a valuable member of the caring team.

### Guidelines

It is true to say that caring is easier when one is well informed. So having identified the needs, the next thing is to implement them. This requires the use of various schemes, notably helping or 'teaching' the residents how to use their remaining skills and to try to do things for themselves, allowing them to take reasonable risks, which develops in them a sense of achievement with improved self-esteem and companionship.

#### *Guidance*

- think of what you want to do, analyse and break down the task into simple steps
- set a *goal* for each step, ie. what you hope the client should be able to achieve
- take each step at a time, starting with simple activities that have little risk of failure
- allow plenty of time to perform the task and do not rush the client as this often increases confusion, anxiety and agitation
- give credit for trying, rather than completing the task
- promote friendship with occasional hugs and smiles and invite evaluation on what is being done, ie. 'is that all right?'
- encourage the client to express personal needs, views, ideas and wishes
- try to improve concentration by reducing distractions, eg. background noise of radio or television.

### 1. Physical well-being

#### *Personal grooming and dressing: bathing*

- demonstrate knowledge of agreed procedures for bathing clients
- assemble equipment for bathing, eg. towel, soap, face cloths, clean clothes
- fill the bath and test the temperature of the water before the client goes to the bathroom
- explain procedures to the client. Do not add hot or cold water once bathing has begun

- prevent slipping and falling by using a non-slip rubber mat in the bath
- ensure that adequate and suitable equipment is available, eg. bath seat and handles, stool, hoist, provide warmth, privacy and seek help if he or she resists bathing
- assist the client into the bath/shower if necessary, but encourage independence
- **never leave a client alone in the bath or shower.**

## Dressing

- assist the client to select clothes and allow time for him/her to decide what he/she would like to wear
- provide verbal clues, eg. 'the blue shirt would look nice with those trousers'. Lay clothes out in the order of his or her personal preference for dressing, eg. stockings or socks on top or if necessary hand over individual items one at a time
- prevent the client from putting on too many clothes by laying them out in advance, or give him or her clues, 'you already have your shirt or dress on'
- lay out pyjamas or a night-gown as a trigger, if he or she refuses to undress for bed at night
- reinforce required actions with verbal cues and prompting.

## Eating and drinking

- maintain a relaxed atmosphere and reduce distractions at meal times
- encourage clients to be independent as far as possible
- serve meals in an area which can be cleaned easily if a client has poor eating habits
- use a disposable apron to protect clothing, and allow plenty of time for eating
- cut food into small pieces, or puree food if client has a particular problem with chewing or swallowing. Watch for hoarding of food in the mouth
- monitor the client's weight regularly and report any weight loss
- watch for and report any signs of dehydration and malnutrition
- observe and report on suspected pain or discomfort due to ill fitting dentures, or poor eyesight which may affect the client's ability to see food.

## 2. Psychological well-being

### Aggressive behaviour

The aim is not to arrest the course of the illness but to manage behaviour so that it causes the least possible distress to the client and to other people.

- look for a trigger event, eg. distractions in the care area
- seek help to remove the client to his/her room and remain with the client until he/she is settled
- divert the client's attention and encourage him/her to express his/her views
- explain and reassure other clients that this behaviour is a symptom of the client's illness and not a deliberate action
- keep a log of the behaviour in accordance with the client's care plan.

### Confusion

This may be due to a limited concentration span and disorientation in which the client is unaware of what is going on around him or her. The person may have difficulty in finding the right words and to correctly name people he or she recognises. Quite often, the individual may become agitated, restless, aggressive and suspicious of others, and may even accuse them of stealing.

- be familiar with the reality-orientation programme and validation therapy
- establish trust and a good interpersonal relationship with the client
- address the individual by his or her preferred name
- provide him or her with everyday information, using a variety of approaches, eg. cue cards, colourful pictures, personal mementoes
- avoid arguments, disagree tactfully if necessary and correct misunderstanding

- maintain the individual's self-respect, dignity and independence by praising and rewarding his or her efforts when appropriate.

## Suspicion

A client may accuse someone of stealing his or her belongings. This may be a way of preserving his or her self-esteem in order to maintain some control of his or her life.
- assess environment for factors of excessive stimulation which may lead to misinterpretation, eg. loud noise from radio or television, whispering in the vicinity
- refrain from using the word 'why' which may give the impression that you are arguing or engaging in a confrontation with the client
- try and divert the person's attention with some diversional activities
- reassure the client regarding any underlying fear or anxiety
- explain to those involved that any accusations are the result of the illness and not a deliberate act of malice on the part of the client.

## Social behaviour

Inappropriate behaviour is common and can be extremely embarrassing and upsetting to other residents and staff. This type of behaviour may include forgetting to dress and at times undressing in the lounge area, or urinating in unacceptable places. It may also include sexual behaviour or remarks of a sexual nature to other people accompanied by a lack of inhibition.
- promote and maintain a good interpersonal relationship with the client
- try and divert his/her attention to something else but maintain his or her self-respect and dignity
- encourage the use of the toilet in accordance with his or her care plan
- reassure and orientate your client regarding the importance of acceptable social behaviour.

## Promotion of independence

Alzheimer's disease does not necessarily deprive the individual of all independence. So, it is necessary to assess the functional capabilities of clients to enable them to use their remaining skills to carry out activities of daily living as independently as possible. If expectations are too low, they will be denied the chance to succeed and will be unable to perform given tasks.
- develop and maintain a good interpersonal relationship with the client
- analyse each task in accordance with the guidelines given above
- try and reduce any distractions in an attempt to improve the client's concentration
- stand back at times and allow the person to try and carry out the task
- intervene as gently and tactfully as possible and only when it becomes clear that he or she is not able to complete the particular task
- give plenty of support and help, and allow an opportunity for him/her to use his/her remaining skills and independence without exposure to failure or undue stress
- reward his or her efforts with praise, a smile, touch, or a hug.

## Communication

Failure of memory is one of the many barriers which may prevent effective communication. Therefore, it is important to try and keep the lines of communication open at all times to avoid frustration, anxiety, aggressive outbursts and behaviour.
- develop and maintain a good interpersonal relationship with the client
- reduce the background distractions as a means of increasing concentration, eg. noise
- find out and address the individual with his or her preferred name
- ensure that a client who has sensory deprivation uses appropriate aids, eg. spectacles and that these are kept clean and worn for particular tasks

- ensure that the person wears his or her hearing aid with a working battery, dentures and spectacles as prescribed
- address him or her as an adult and speak slowly, clearly and distinctly
- use simple words and short sentences and avoid interrupting
- ask one question at a time and allow time for a response
- use the same words when repeating statements
- encourage the person to talk and express personal views, rights, needs and fears without causing distress to other people
- avoid correcting his or her mistakes or arguing and do not use the word 'why' as this may give the impression that he or she is being challenged or confronted
- initiate contact by holding the person's hands and looking at his/her face
- maintain eye contact and communication through occasional hugs and cuddles
- use posture, facial expressions and a modified tone of voice as much as possible to pick up additional clues to help you understand what the person is saying, and assess whether what you are saying is being understood.

## Wandering

Restlessness may be the result of too much stimulation, the effects of medication, fear or anxiety. Boredom, delusions, hallucinations, effects of hunger or the need to use the toilet may cause the individual to wander. Also, disorientation and, more importantly, the inability to communicate his or her wishes and needs.

### During the day:
- observe and determine if the person is restless or wandering and try to determine the reason. It may be that the person wants food or a drink, or he/she may feel that there is too much noise from radio or television
- ensure that the care environment is safe and maintain constant but discrete observation
- protect the individual from harm or abuse by others
- remove him or her from a noisy room to a less stimulating environment, such as his or her own room
- divert attention by providing the individual with something to do, such as simple age-related activities which may include reading, painting or a walk in the grounds
- ensure regular use of the lavatory in accordance with his or her care plan
- reassure and orientate him or her regarding socially acceptable behaviour
- be aware of local practice and procedures for reporting missing persons.

### During the night:
- try to find out the nature and extent of the problem of wandering
- leave a light on in the client's room, preferably dimmed according to his or her wishes
- leave the door to the toilet open so that the person does not get lost on his or her way back from using the toilet
- occupy the person with simple diversional therapy of his or her choice, eg. a card game
- provide hot drinks of choice and companionship until he or she is settled
- reassure and re-orientate the individual with respect to time, place and person
- offer hot drinks of choice to other clients who may be disturbed by the wandering and reassure them that the behaviour is a symptom of the person's illness.

# References

Carroll M et al (1993) *Caring for Older People: A Nurse's Guide*. Macmillan, London
Jorm AF (1987) *Understanding Senile Dementia*. Croom Helm, London
Mace NL (1993) *36 Hour Day*. Edward Arnold, London
Woods RT (1989) *Alzheimer's Disease. Coping with a Living Death*. Souvenir, London

## Audio visual aids

### Format: VHS video

Ref: CMEUA835: *Treating the Elderly: Cognitive Impairment of Special Deprivation in the Elderly*
Ref: NCE4331: *Physical Assessment of the Frail Elderly*
Oxford Educational Resources Ltd

# Specific treatment programme (X2: 2-4, X16: 1-3, NC10.3)

People suffering from dementia, especially those with severe forms, may exhibit signs and symptoms which are similar to those experienced by a visitor lost in a foreign city, ie. they do not know the way back to their hotel. Also, because they do not understand the language they are unable to communicate their needs to strangers and they become frustrated. In other words, the person feels confused and disorientated which leads to anxiety, fear and irrational behaviour. In this situation, clients require help, just as the visitor in a foreign city needs help to find his or her 'bearings'. The aim is constantly to remind the individual of reality and how to make maximum use of his or her remaining skills to maintain his or her lifestyle, self-respect, dignity and independence. First, it requires knowledge of the person's background and needs, and should include the use of various therapeutic skills to help restore the individual's self-esteem. There are many approaches. The following are the most commonly used:

## Reality-orientation

As the name suggests this involves the use of approaches which help people maintain contact with reality to improve their quality of life. It is believed that clients who are confused usually value the everyday information that most of us take for granted. The programme is designed to enable clients to interact with their environment and people involved in their care so that they become aware of everyday events, regain and maintain contact with the environment, and function independently as far as possible. The success depends upon the quality of information given by the therapist and the use of therapeutic skills such as group dynamics and verbal and non-verbal communication in the sessions.

Relatives should be made aware of the basic principles of reality-orientation to maintain continuity of this method of care. Sometimes they may remember trivial objects and practices which may be part of the client's personality and so be useful to his or her care.

### Individual reality orientation

A programme is designed as part of a total care plan for a confused client. It may be given on a continuous and informal 24-hour basis. Activities relate to clients' needs, abilities, interests and hobbies, eg. gardening, cooking, pets, reflections on old films, ornaments, pictures, sports and games, special events.

## Structure of the session

The session should be able to provide information about:
- the person — his or her name, who he or she is
- the location — where this is, what is the function of this place
- date and time of the day, year, day of the week, seasons, weather
- activities on a particular day, menu for the day, religious events
- local and national events and names of famous people; for example, the Prime Minister.

Most homes practising this approach, display information on a reality orientation board and place it in a strategic position where everyone can see it. Also clocks with large dials and calendars are kept accurate for those with visual impairment. A client is usually assigned this responsibility. Doors can be marked with appropriate descriptions, eg. the lavatory and footprints on the floor guide residents to various destinations in the home. The only reservation is, that after a period of time, people become complacent and the programme is taken for granted. Without a positive attitude and reinforcement, the board becomes a white elephant and the programme fails in its objectives.

## Social group setting

The aim is to enable clients to socialise with each other and develop communication skills within the group setting.

### Guidance

- sit where everyone will see you. Speak briefly but clearly
- use short sentences to maintain interest and promote conversation
- promote discussion and repeat information as necessary to reinforce the message
- use clients' past experiences as a bridge to the present
- avoid argument but disagree tactfully with those who are confused, and correct any misunderstanding without causing loss of face or dignity to the person
- be able to change the direction of discussion with tact and in confident terms
- target recent events except for those with strong emotional overtones
- encourage a sense of humour in the group
- provide positive reinforcement, eg. a nod, a smile or touch to correct responses
- provide a running commentary of some events taking place in the care environment
- develop skill in correcting inappropriate responses and behaviour in the group.

## Environmental stimulation

The care environment should be modified to reinforce reality with:
- signs with different colours on the floor indicating specific places such as bedroom, lounge, toilets, kitchen, bathroom
- cue cards and colourful pictures
- clocks with large numerals
- pictures and photographs, personal belongings, eg. ornaments, mementoes
- supply of daily newspapers, magazines
- seasonal flowers, calendars with as large a print as possible.

### Guidance

The exercise should:
- encourage clients to find their way round the care environment
- help them to identify their rooms, beds, chairs and clothes
- use routine to provide a sense of security, self-respect and dignity
- use contact with clients to reinforce the time, day, place and individual identity.

## Reminiscence therapy

This is generally known as 'recall group' in which various items are used, relating to the era of the group, eg. clothing, films, books, newspapers, pictures and various artefacts belonging to that period. The main aim is to use past events to stimulate long-term memories so that they remain accessible. In some places, rooms may be set aside, decorated and furnished in the style of a period relevant to the group. The most important desirable goal is for the elderly person to continue experiencing normal reminiscing, while maintaining the ability to return and participate, voluntarily in reality.

## Validation therapy

This is an attempt to promote healing by acknowledging that a 'real person' exists inside a confused client, to accept that his or her feelings are true, and to respect the individual as an individual. The assumption is that all behaviour has meaning, and validation therapy is a method used to interact verbally and non-verbally with those clients who are disorientated and suffering from dementia, eg. Alzheimer's disease. It is believed that people affected by this illness lose certain aspects of their former personality, and their memory of self may vanish. The person can still be content and express pleasure — he or she can smile and laugh, express sadness, frown or cry. He or she should not be treated as though he or she is unconscious.

### *Aim of the therapy*

The purpose is to help to restore a sense of emotional well-being in their present 'here and now' reality through the use of verbal techniques of discovery and spending time in their company. The starting point is to review the client's life, observing behaviour and talking to the client's relatives and friends to 'discover' the hidden meaning behind his or her behaviour and the feelings which are aroused by remembering and re-enacting these actions. The rule is 'to try it, if it works, use it'.

#### *Guidance*

Seek and try to understand that all the behaviour of the confused older person has meaning and aim to make sense of it. For example, a client may wander aimlessly asking a repetitive question, 'where is Rose' (being his deceased wife). The process, therefore, is to use an open-ended questioning technique, asking questions by beginning with the words who, what, when and how, avoiding the word 'why' which gives the impression that the person is being criticised or challenged. The procedure should be non-threatening, or judgmental, and last for a few minutes and continue later in the day:

- ensure that the person is happy and is given the chance to express him or herself
- approach the person in a calm and reassuring manner with a welcoming smile
- assess the situation and remove any barrier to effective communication which may exist by allowing the individual to wear his or her hearing aids or spectacles if he/she has any
- encourage him or her to have any significant personal mementoes, eg. a watch or photograph, during the session and allow the person to speak while you listen attentively for cues about his or her feelings
- be able to interrupt, eg. if he or she is talking about a spouse and wanders away from the point
- be able to paraphrase, eg. his statement by saying 'Mr Jones, I follow what you are saying, but you seem to be missing your wife — Alice. Is that right? Tell me what she was like as a person? How long were you married to her?'
- help him to look at a photograph of his wife and talk about his memory of her. This may validate his feeling of longing to see her in a 'here and now' situation
- help him to maintain contact with his family and those significant to him by phone, writing and visiting old friends.

# References

Field N (1992) *Validation. The Field Method.* Edward Field, Cleveland, Ohio, USA

Jones G, Miesen BML (1993) *Care — Giving in Dementia: Research and Applications.* Routledge, London

O'Donovan S (1996) A validation approach to severely demented clients. *Nurs Standard* **11**(13–15): 48–52

Novis A (1988) *A Reminiscence with Elderly People.* Winslow Press, Bicester

## The depressed elderly person (W2:1, Z8: 1–2)

Depression is a feeling resembling sadness or grief, that many people experience in response to the different types of stress that they have been exposed to in everyday life. It is a serious mental health problem in which the person may attempt suicide. It relates to excessive mood changes that exceed those experienced in ordinary everyday situations, both in duration and quality. With elderly people, it may be accompanied by complaints of bodily disturbances and the individual may have difficulty in carrying out activities of daily living.

The general feeling is that of worthlessness and disappointment, coupled with an inability to cope with life, possibly leading the person to react or behave in a peculiar way. Some elderly people may feel uneasy about admitting that they have a mental health problem, a loss of insight and mental faculty. Depression may be regarded as morbid in terms of intensity and duration of mood disturbance, especially when it develops 'out of the blue' and without any apparent cause. It is intensified if the thoughts, feelings and behaviour are life threatening, and the person may not recover if left untreated. But, despite these unpleasant feelings, most people are usually able to continue to cope with their daily lives. It is believed that depression is more common in women than men.

### Causes

Quite often bereavement and the loss of a partner may produce a feeling of inability to cope with life. For those who have been admitted into health care homes long-term, the thought of losing the family home and personal possessions, may predispose them to feelings of inadequacy and rejection. A lack of interest in life and boredom, loss of self-respect, rights and dignity may, in any combination, lead to depression. More importantly, a reduction in the amount of social contact, income and a reminiscence of one's life and lost opportunities as a result of retirement may lead to mental health problems.

It is believed that clinical depression is common and may co-exist with dementia in elderly people living in nursing homes. This situation makes it difficult to assess the total care needs, and start treatment early. It can also be linked with certain conditions such as Parkinson's disease, cancer and strokes. The outcome is that care is directed to these illnesses rather than depression. This may be due to a lack of recognition of the mental health problems of depression in elderly or physically ill people.

### Symptoms of depression

These can be seen in the way that elderly people usually present the signs and symptoms, in terms of complaints about bodily symptoms, memory problems and anxiety. Some will not admit that they have mental health problems, and it is essential to observe and report on:

- poor appetite, weight and energy loss, loss of libido, lack of interest and fatigue
- sleep disturbance, inability to think or concentrate

- spontaneous onset with loss of insight
- severe mood change, agitation, aggression and violent behaviour
- feelings of worthlessness and guilt resulting in isolation
- psychotic symptoms may be present, eg. hallucinations, delusions
- the presence of bodily disturbances, eg. retardation, constipation.

## Effects of depression

In the depths of their despair, guilt and hopelessness, the depressed person may feel that the only way out of their misery is to kill or harm themselves. It is frequently assumed that although their attempts at self-harm appear to be counter-productive, most depressed people are too stressed and confused to undertake logically, an act of self-destruction.

*Be warned — take all suicide threats seriously.*

## Common symptoms with depressive illnesses

### Delusion

This is a false idea or belief held by a person which cannot be corrected by logical reasoning. For example, the individual may claim to be of a royal descent or that 'they are trying to kill me'. He or she may express guilt, hopelessness, worthlessness, poverty or hypochondriasis (bodily complaints). On investigation, none of these things exist. Quite often in the elderly, if delusion is present, it is associated with consciousness and bodily changes.

### Hallucinations

These are false perceptions in which the person believes that he or she sees, hears, tastes or feels things crawling over him, or a person giving him commands where there is no basis for this belief. Hallucinations usually affect the sense organs of the body. In extreme cases, voices may condemn the person, accuse him of crimes and wickedness. Usually, these changes are due to dementia and may result in:

- lack of insight into behaviour with limited concentration
- irritability, agitation, irrational behaviour with difficulty in relating to others
- extreme preoccupation with hallucinatory and delusional problems.

## Care and treatment

The general approach is activation of a readily accessible service to support the person and their family in residential care or the community.

## Assessment

The initial observation may report on difficulties the person is having in communication, social skills and the ability to express feelings. Information obtained should form the basis on which the care plan is formulated for the care of the individual. It should include assessing the risk of suicide and agreeing ways in which the problems should be managed.

## Implementation of care

- be aware of information on the care plan, especially relating to suicidal intentions and ways of managing the problem
- initiate, promote and maintain a good interpersonal relationship. Listen to and accept the person's ideas in a non-critical way, but avoid expressing your disbelief in the client's presence

- encourage the person to reminisce about his or her life, to express personal feelings, beliefs and needs in a way that will not affect other people's views. Respect and do not disagree with any of these views
- identify interests, hobbies and encourage the pursuit of personal interests, such as reading, board games. Reinforce reality orientation, spend time with the person, promote self-esteem and independence as far as possible
- use a non-verbal form of communication such as touch to demonstrate your sincerity
- ensure that the person uses his or her hearing aid and/or spectacles during conversation to ensure that he or she understands and sees you
- observe the person unobtrusively, and report any statements of suicidal intent, guilt and hopelessness to the person-in-charge and ensure that all potentially harmful substances are discretely removed. If possible, try and make a verbal contract with the person not to harm him or herself
- spend time with and reassure the person using counselling skills
- help the person to maintain contact with people who are significant to them, eg. spouses, friends in an attempt to maintain orientation and keep in touch with the outside world
- make sure that the person takes medicine when given and that he or she makes no attempt to hoard it
- try and encourage diversional activities to help the person's concentration
- find out reasons for the person's criticism by other people if this happens
- organise experiential exercises, eg. drama, games, music, social and recreational activities and encourage the person to participate. Respect personal wishes if he or she refuses to participate
- promote and reinforce self-respect, rights, identity and dignity of the person by encouraging attention to an individual's personal hygiene and cleanliness
- do not encourage or reinforce hallucinations and delusions, do not collude with the person.

*Be warned — take all suicide threats seriously.*

## Evaluation

When the individual is able to cope better with the problems identified and gives accurate and reasonable information about his/her health.

## References

Beck AT et al (1979) *Cognitive Therapy of Depression*. The Guildford Press, New York.

George M (1997) Depression in older people. *Nurs Times* **11**(28): 26–27

Ironbar NO, Hooper A (1998) *Self-Instruction in Mental Health Nursing,* 2nd edn. Bailliere Tindall, London: unit 7.4, unit 10.4

Royal College of Nursing (1996) *Guidelines for Assessing Mental Health Needs in Old Age*. RCN, London.

Warrington J (1996) *Depression and Dementia. Coexistence and Differentiation*. University of Stirling Dementia Services Department, Stirling.

## Audio visual aids

### Format: VHS video
Ref: 177 *CT: Recognising Depression* (tape slides)
Ref: CNE 4261: *Caring for Psychiatric Patient Part 1 — The Suicidal Patient*
Ref: CNE 4263: *Caring for Psychiatric Patient Part 2: The Inebriated Patient*
Ref CNE 4396 : *Depression in the Long-term care*
Oxford Educational Resources Ltd

## The confused elderly person (CL7: 1-2, Z8: 1-2)

Confusion is a term used to describe a mental condition in which the person's thoughts are mixed up, and he/she is puzzled and perplexed. The person appears to have 'lost his bearings' and is unable to identify who he or she is, to whom he or she is talking and, in its most serious form, cannot recognise his or her relatives. The individual may also experience difficulty in telling the time of day, day of the week, month of the year or the year itself. During this period, the person may loose insight into his/her behaviour and environment. If these difficulties are present, then the person is said to be disorientated in time, person and place. Confusion is not a disease, but a symptom or side-effect of other problems. The experience of disorientation and lapse of memory may interfere with the person's ability to cope with his or her needs during the everyday activities of living and he/she may be at risk of abuse.

### Causes

It is believed that the condition may be due to a temporary decrease in blood supply to the brain cells, during an acute confusional state as a result of:
- chest and urinary infection, dehydration and malnutrition
- congestive cardiac failure, profound exhaustion, toxins
- alcohol withdrawal, drugs (night sedation in the elderly, other chemical agents, vitamin deficiency).

Other causes include dementia, trauma, cerebrovascular accident (stroke), brain tumour, damage due to deprivation of oxygen (anoxic damage). Changes in the environment, such as an admission from home or hospital to unfamiliar surroundings, new routines and procedures, and changes in staff could confuse the person.

### Effects of confusion

During this period, the person may lose insight into personal behaviour, lack awareness of immediate surroundings, and suffer the following outcomes:
- reduced ability to form and maintain meaningful relationships and communicate with others
- loss of self-respect and dignity, and exposure to abuse by others
- reduced ability to meet his or her daily physical, social and emotional needs
- absence of awareness on risks arising from personal behaviour or in the environment where he or she lives
- hallucinations — usually of moving objects; includes delusions
- deterioration of memory especially for recent events with a tendency to confabulate
- restlessness, agitation, wandering and getting lost.

### Management of care

This is usually based on an assessment of the person and information which has been collected in order to formulate the individual care plan. It also includes information on taking risks and ways in which these should be managed.

#### *Implementation of care*

##### *Guidance*

- develop and maintain a good interpersonal relationship, adopting a non-judgmental or non-critical attitude to care; be approachable and available
- recognise and safeguard the rights and interests of the individual from abuse and possible harm in the environment

- ensure that his or her basic physical, social and emotional needs are met
- identify the interests of the individual and provide activities which foster and support these interests
- use approaches identified in the care plan with due regard to your competence, eg. validation therapy
- organise age-related social and recreational activities and encourage individuals to participate
- encourage the person to join in any daily recall or reminiscence group activities
- do not whisper to others or giggle in the vicinity of the person
- use touch and other non-verbal signals to demonstrate your affection to the individual
- provide an opportunity for the person to express him or herself openly
- act as advocate by seeking the person's best interests at all times.

## Evaluation

When the person is able to find his or her way around the care environment, to identify self and members of his or her family, including carers. It is also important that the person is able to make a choice, assume responsibility for independent judgement, and maintain a personal lifestyle without involving other people.

## Reference

Ironbar NO, Hooper A (1989) *Self-instruction in Mental Health Nursing. Topic 13: Confusion in Later Life.* Bailliere Tindall, London

### Audio visual aid

*Format: VHS video:*
CNE 7501: *Alzheimer's Disease 1: Coping with Confusion*
Oxford Educational Resources Ltd

## The overactive elderly person (NC10: 2–3, NC11: 1–3)

The process of caring for people involves dealing with behavioural problems, and relates equally to any care setting. It is believed that aggressive behaviour can nearly always be traced to disturbances in relationships between people, and so it can be a means of communication. At times the elderly find it difficult to get on with other people, and have a tendency to behave and overreact in an anti-social way. This may be due to the fact that, as people advance in age, they experience a decline of mental functions associated with memory, relationships and intelligence. This can lead to the development of a full range of mental health problems. The outcome may be abusive and disruptive actions, the degree and level of which may interfere with the rights of others and cause distress to the staff who have to cope with the situation. In some cases, it may be seen as out of character.

### Behaviour

This refers to those activities which can be observed, such as crying, wandering and getting lost, restlessness, destructiveness, obstinacy, nocturnal confusion, lack of concentration and making threats to other people. These may take the form of:
- difficulty in communicating or socialising with other people, leading to conflict
- an inability to meet personal physical, social, spiritual, psychological needs
- being at risk of harm or abuse
- overactivity combined with impulsive acts of violence.

### Causes of behavioural problems
These problems may be influenced by thought disorders, denial of needs, misunderstandings, but are more often due to:
- fear of being hurt, anxiety, frustration, boredom, discrimination
- provocation, taunting, teasing, threats, abuse, restraint, constraints
- an unsatisfactory care environment, substance abuse, rejection resulting in attention seeking syndrome, psychiatric conditions, eg. hallucinations.

### Forms of behavioural problems
The forms may take any of the following:
- overactivity which may lead to potential self-harm, threatening and disturbing other residents confusion, response to delusions and hallucinations
- physical, sexual, discriminatory, exploitative, self-inflicted.

### Direction of behavioural problems
This may be directed at people at risk of abuse such as the confused, frail and elderly mentally infirm, children, people with learning difficulties, unconscious, confused and disorientated people. It may take the form of both verbal and physical threats. It may also relate to potential self-harm involving mutilation of various parts of the body, eg. hair pulling, slashing of wrists, unexplained cuts.

### Management of behavioural problems
The aim of care is to change the individual's behaviour within the framework of local policy and the assessment of an individual client's total care needs. Therefore, on admission or following the first episode of over-activity, a detailed plan on management of the problem is agreed by everyone involved in the care. This information is recorded in the care plan including the use of any restraint, which should be contemplated only as a last resort after exhausting all other options. The care plan is reviewed at a specified time, but the actual management of the problem should be directed by the person-in-charge. Care assistants will be required to assist.

## Implementation of care

The suggestions given below relate to a skirmish between two residents in the lounge in which you were summoned to intervene. There is, however, no magic formula, but local guidelines on approaches to care should be followed.

### Guidance
- demonstrate good interpersonal relationship skills; a non-judgmental or critical attitude; trust and anti-discriminatory approach to care
- be familiar with guidelines in the care plan and local policy on management of the person's problem, eg. eliminating unwanted behaviour (modification programme)
- sound the alarm, summon help on discovering any act of violence. Do not attempt to restrain an overactive person single-handed
- be aware of circumstances which may lead to an outburst of abusive behaviour and be able to locate those at risk. This must be consistent with the care plan
- show knowledge of dealing with the problem, the rights of the person with reference to legal requirements, eg. Mental Health Act 1983
- use appropriate relationship skills by seeking support in handling the situation
- help the disturbed individual to a less stimulating room using minimal force. Use a non-verbal method of communication to calm the client, eg. touch

- spend some time with the person until settled. Encourage his or her orientation and a sense of belonging. Make a record of the frequency of the problem
- be aware of your own feelings and always seek guidance if you are unsure of your role
- encourage the person to express any feelings, needs and beliefs
- try to find out the cause of the problem and explain the effects of the action to the person in a calm way, offering appropriate reassurance
- assist in giving medication (PRN) as ordered by the doctor
- protect and reassure other residents
- demonstrate knowledge in the use of behaviour modification approaches for preventing abusive situations, based on an individual care plan
- maintain accurate records and submit a report on actual or potential abuse.

In any disturbed situation, do not attempt to save the furniture. Focus on protecting the residents and yourself, as furniture can always be replaced.

## Evaluation of care

When the individual is able to moderate the extent of his or her behaviour so that it does not put others at risk.

## Prevention

These are legal guidelines designed to protect specific client groups, eg. the Mental Health Act 1983, the Children's Act (1989). Organisations are required to provide local policy relating to risk-taking for all individuals in their care.

Staff training to make them competent at seeing and interpreting residents' wishes from their behaviour rather than spoken words. As a starting point, assume that residents are trying to find some way of communicating their wishes rather than presuming that they cannot.

## Report of injuries

Any injuries to residents and staff must be fully reported and documented in accordance with local policy. In all cases the people involved must be examined by a medical officer and entries made in appropriate records.

## References

Altschul A (1985) *Psychiatric Nursing*, 6th edn. Bailliere Tindall, London

Ironbar NO, Hooper A (1989) *Self-instruction in Mental Health Nursing*. Bailliere Tindall, London: unit 11.3

Poster E , Ryan J (1993) Violence at work. *Nurs Times* **89**(23): 30–35

Ramprogus V, Gibson J (1991) Assessing restraints. *Nurs Times* **87**(26): 45–47

Royal College of Nursing (1988) *Focus on Restraint: Guidelines on the Use of Restraints in the Care of Elderly People*. Scutari Press, Harrow

## Audio visual aids

*Format: VHS video*

Ref: CNE6522: *Violence in the Emergency Room*
Ref: CEN7348: *Managing Assaultive Behaviour*
Ref CEAU377: *Mind and Body: Calming the Elderly*
Oxford Educational Resources Ltd

# Mental Health Act 1983

The care of people with mental health problems is historically linked with ill-treatment, neglect and indifference. Treatment was mainly custodial in nature and provided by institutions under various legislative control. Admission was compulsory since voluntary admission was impossible. Moreover, if a person entered an institution, he/she stood only a small chance of returning to the outside world, especially as society did not welcome his/her return, believing him/her to be dangerous and beyond hope of improvement.

However, during the last 100 years, legislation has been in place to improve the conditions and quality of care. A great deal was achieved, mainly by finding people useful occupations and removing restraint. The most important breakthrough in legislation was the Mental Health Treatment Act 1930, which enabled people to enter hospital voluntarily. Due to legal and administrative problems, this Act was revoked and replaced by the 1959 Act.

### The Mental Health Act 1959

The Act brought further changes which made it possible to treat and help people with mental health problems in an atmosphere free from legal control on their liberty. It also placed the care of people with mental health problems and of physical illness on the same basis, and removed the stigma attached to mental disorder. But it still allowed for the use of compulsory procedures when necessary for unco-operative people to receive treatment, and prevented the misuse of these powers. It was claimed that there were many reasons why this Act did not work as well as it should, and so it was repealed following the passing of the 1983 Act.

### Mental Health Act 1983

This Act did not alter the basic idea of the 1959 Act, but updated and improved it by making a requirement for a second opinion for certain treatments compulsory with emphasis on consent for treatment, and it established a Mental Health Act Commission.

Most people agree to come into hospital when the need arises, but a minority refuse. They are entitled to do so, unless there is good reason to believe that the refusal is the outcome of mental health problems, and that there is a serious risk to the person's health and the safety of others. In these circumstances, compulsory admission becomes necessary. This means that the person is compelled to go into hospital, but not that the hospital is obliged to take him or her. An agreement with the hospital will be necessary for compulsory admission just as for informal patients. But efforts are always made to safeguard the civil liberties of the individuals admitted under compulsory powers.

### Presentation

It is presented in ten major parts, and it is difficult to deal with its provisions in detail. A few of its various sections are presented below.

## Admission procedures

### Section 2: Admission for assessment
Admission for assessment allows for detention of the person for assessment or to be followed by treatment for up to 28 days.
     Application may be made by the nearest relatives or an approved social worker but must be supported by written recommendations from two medical practitioners.

### Discharge
The patient can be discharged by the responsible medical officer or by three members of the hospital management or by the nearest relative who must give 72 hours notice.

### Section 3: Admission for treatment
The patient is detained for his or her safety and the protection of others. He or she is detained for six months during which period he or she should receive treatment. The application can be made by the nearest relative or an approved social worker supported by two written medical recommendations.

### Discharge
The patient can be discharged by a responsible medical officer, three members of the hospital management, the Mental Review Tribunal or after 28 days of absence without leave or by the nearest relative or after six months continuous absence.

### Section 4: Admission for assessment in cases of emergency
An emergency application for admission for 72 hours may be made by the nearest relative or an approved social worker, supported by one doctor, preferably the patient's family practitioner.

### Section 5(4): Nurse's holding power
An informal patient suffering from a mental disorder may be restrained from leaving the hospital by a nurse for his/her own safety or for the protection of others. The duration is six hours.

### Section 26: Nearest relatives
Husband or wife, son or daughter, father or mother, brother or sister, grandparent or grandchild, uncle or aunt, nephew or niece are recognised.

## Powers of the courts

### Section 37: Hospital or guardianship order
The courts can order hospital admission or guardianship of a prisoner without restriction. The person can be discharged by the responsible medical officer, but the nearest relative has no power to discharge.

### Section 41. Restriction order
A restriction order is made only by the Crown Court and not a Magistrate's Court, for various reasons, eg. protection of the public from serious harm. The order is supported by written recommendations of two medical practitioners.
     Discharge is only by the Home Secretary and Mental Health Review Tribunal.

## Consent to treatment

### Section 57:
This relates to treatment requiring consent and a second opinion, eg. surgical operations for destroying brain tissue or its function, specific treatments, implantation of hormones to reduce male sexual drive. It applies to both informal and detained patients.

These treatments require: the patient's consent, three people appointed by the Mental Health Act Commission. An appointed independent doctor must consult a nurse and one other person but not a nurse or doctor, who have been concerned with the patient's treatment.

### Section 58: Treatment requiring a second opinion
This applies to any specific treatment, eg. electroconvulsive therapy and the continued administration of drug treatment three months after initial administration. No detained patient may be given treatment unless he or she has consented and the responsible doctor has certified the validity of the consent or a second independent doctor certifies that the treatment should be given. Second opinion as for Section 57.

### Management of affairs and property

### Court of Protection
The Act assumes that all detained people are incapable of managing their own affairs. The Court of Protection exists to take responsibility for these people. But anyone can apply to the Court of Protection which asks for medical evidence. Once under its authority, the Court has control over all the person's property and affairs. It can appoint a receiver, often a family member to carry out its directions.

### Offences under the Act

**Section 127**: This deals with ill-treatment or neglect of patients, which are offences.

**Section 128**: Relates to Sexual Offences Act 1967. It is an offence for: a man to have sexual intercourse with a woman who is severely mentally handicapped; a man to commit 'buggery' or an act of gross indecency with another man, knowing him to be a severely mentally handicapped patient; a male guardian to have sexual intercourse with a woman subjected to his guardianship; a man on the staff of a hospital to have sexual intercourse with a woman patient.

**Section 129**: States that it is an offence to assist a detained patient to escape or go absent without leave, or to harbour or hinder the return of the patient to hospital.

### Miscellaneous and supplementary provisions

### Section 131(5): Informal admission
This section allows for admission of patients to any hospital or nursing home informally for observation or treatment of their own free will.

### Section 136: Power of the police
Police officers can remove to a place of safety, a person whom they find in a public place, and who appears to be suffering from mental disorder; and to be in need of immediate care and control. A patient cannot be detained for longer than 72 hours.

### Section 139: Protection of staff
Staff are not protected against civil or criminal proceedings if they do not carry out their work in good faith. But any proceedings will require the consent of the Director of Public Prosecutions and the High Court.

## Role of care assistants

### *Guidance*

As members of the health care team, care assistants should aim to:
- demonstrate knowledge of the Mental Health Act 1983 and local policies on equal opportunities and anti-discriminatory practices
- be aware of your role and right to information regarding care plans
- be aware of clients' rights and needs under the Mental Health Act 1983
- display in-depth knowledge of all clients, eg. those detained under the act
- observe and report changes in client's condition to the person-in-charge
- support and encourage individual clients to express rights, choices
- ensure that clients have individual privacy without unnecessary intrusion
- show sensitivity to the client's needs, and be aware of the effects of denial of those needs; eg. crying, isolation, resentment, anti-social behaviour
- address individuals by and refer to them using their preferred names
- note and report to the person in charge any suspected breach of the Mental Health Act 1983, which deals with equal opportunities and anti-discriminatory practice
- listen to clients, support and encourage them to express their views
- keep accurate and concise records on clients in relation to care plans
- maintain the confidentiality of information in care
- ensure that the client's right of expression does not distress others.

## Community care

Some care assistants may undertake home visits as members of the primary health care team, and should take certain precautions to safeguard their interests and well-being.
- demonstrate in-depth knowledge of clients within your case load
- be familiar with the primary health care team's policy on reporting on any untoward incidents; for example, by contacting colleagues, police and your team leader in case of an emergency
- let everyone know your whereabouts at any given time, including the expected time of return; report back after completing your visits or any delay, before going off duty
- be alert to danger signs of anti-social behaviour, abusive comments or language, display of potentially dangerous instruments, such as kitchen knives
- carry a personal alarm system to attract attention if attacked
- avoid any confrontation and being injured.

## References

Bluglas RA (1983) *A Guide to the Mental Health Act 1983*. Churchill Livingstone, London.
Brooking J (1985) Mental health forum. *Nurs Times* **159**(10): ii–vii
Department of Health and Welsh Office (1993) *Code of Practice. Mental Health Act 1983*. HMSO, London
Jones R (ed) (1983) *Mental Health Act 1983*. Sweet and Maxwell, London
Leopoldt H (1985) The act translated. *Nurs Times* **81**(42): 42–43

# Section VI: Personal development

At the end of this section, candidates should be able to understand the basic principles and process of personal development in relation to the following unit.

*Units and elements of learning*

| | | |
|---|---|---|
| **Unit 20: Vocational qualifications** | **CU7, CU10** | 377 |
| o Concepts of human needs and motivation | CU7: 1–2 | 377 |
| o Personal portfolio | CU7.1, CU10.2 | 384 |
| o Adult as a learner | CU7.1 | 387 |
| o Resources and opportunities for learning | | 391 |
| o Vocational preparation for adults | CU7.2 | 392 |
| o National vocational qualifications | | 394 |
| o Preparation for Workbased Assessment of Competence | CU7.2, CU10.2 | 398 |

# Unit 20
# Vocational qualifications (CU7, CU10)

## Concepts of human needs and motivation (CU7: 1–2)

Needs are what any person lacks, wants or requires in order to make optimum adjustment to the environment and society in which he or she lives or works. Maslow (1954) identifies needs in order of their importance, such as basic-order and higher-order needs. He believes that unless man satisfies basic needs, eg. air, food and warmth there will be no drive to meet higher-order needs. It follows that all human activities are directed towards meeting the person's physical, social and psychological needs. If there is a deficiency in any of these needs, the person is motivated to take action to restore this lack.

In the context of holistic care, needs are nursing problems associated with any deficiency of physical, psychological, social or environmental well-being of the person, which must be fulfilled for the individual to enjoy a reasonable good health. Therefore, every effort is aimed at assisting the individual to meet his or her own needs as independently as possible. But, in life threatening situations, where the person cannot correct the deficits personally, it is vital that the carers try using various approaches to correct these deficits on behalf of the client.

### Factors which influence needs

The following factors define and direct our individual needs.

*Behaviour*
This refers to the way we respond to a situation which confronts us. The intensity of our needs drives us to behave either appropriately or inappropriately.

*Drive*
This is an impulse or force which arouses the individual to take action by doing some tasks, at times, without thought or deliberation to achieve an end. It is difficult to define precisely what *drives* us to take such a course of action. However, it is said that often anxiety generated by fear of failure, can act as a spur to work harder and increase the level of performance. This is the way learning takes place.

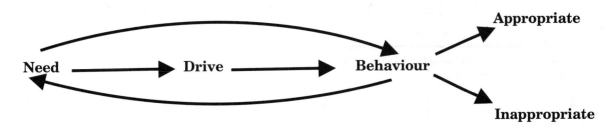

**An illustration showing how needs influence behaviour**

## Culture
A pattern of behaviour associated with social customs. It is often acquired within the family, passed on and preserved in a number of ways. It assists in shaping ideas, attitudes, beliefs, morals and religion.

## Upbringing
Relates to association with parents, peers, personal experiences, education, colleagues, and other interactions with the physical environment.

## Religion
The belief in higher powers, provides a sense of symbolic religious belief, shaping and providing the person with a purpose in life.

## Fear of failure
This can cause a loss of self-esteem and may be regarded as a punishment for poor work. High achievement encourages and builds self-confidence, diligence and satisfaction. For learners, past failures need to be seen in perspective as a natural part of human learning. Failure can enlarge a person's experience and be an incentive to change.

## Attitude
This expresses our responses to people and situations and governs and shapes our views. They may include a caring attitude, gratitude, discrimination and prejudice. Attitudes which define what kind of person we are may be acquired from our parents or peers. It is often difficult to influence or change attitudes despite appropriate education and logical reasoning.

## Values
These are the measure, worth and qualities with which we regard ourselves and others. They are the dreams which shape our lives, eg. self-respect, memories.

### Hierarchy of human needs

Maslow's theory (1970) of personality and motivation classifies human goals according to what he calls a hierarchy of needs. He believes that when a lower need is satisfied, the next need is aroused. But, in extreme cases, there may be difficulty in meeting the higher-order needs such as self-esteem, and he points out that this failure can lead to feelings of weakness, helplessness and inferiority. The levels of hierarchy needs are as shown.

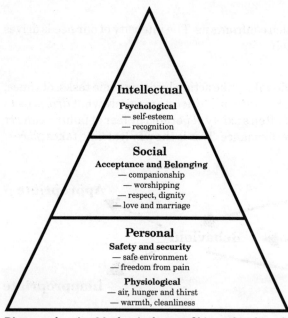

**Diagram showing Maslow's theory of hierarchical needs**

## Physiological needs (personal)

| Needs or problems | Action of intervention |
|---|---|
| Cleanliness | Assist clients to maintain their personal cleanliness and grooming to prevent the development of pressure sores and maintain personal confidence and self esteem. |
| Hunger and thirst | Ensure that clients have a well-balanced diet and plenty of fluids as prescribed to prevent malnutrition and dehydration. |
| Elimination | Observe and report on clients' daily bowel and bladder movements to prevent constipation and incontinence of faeces and urine. |
| Air | Ensure that rooms and care environment are well-ventilated. Help clients to exercise and breathe properly to prevent lack of oxygen and respiratory problems, eg. dyspnoea. |
| Warmth | Check that the heating in the care environment remains always at the correct room temperature. Ensure that clients at risk are adequately dressed according to the weather to prevent hypothermia. |
| Safety and security | Maintain a safe environment to prevent falls and accidents. Be aware of the whereabouts of clients at risk of wandering and ensure that the security system is working properly. Protect those clients at risk of abuse, eg. the frail with a history of falls, the confused and disorientated. Talk to them and provide information about their care and of the care environment. Reassure them at all times about their fears and anxiety. |
| Pain and discomfort | Arrange furniture to help clients with painful feet, arthritis to walk about freely. Encourage them to have adequate rest whenever necessary. Report any discomfort and pain that clients may complain of. |

## Social needs

| Needs or problems | Action or intervention |
|---|---|
| Acceptance and belonging | Maintain a good interpersonal relationship. Reassure but do not patronise clients. Counsel as necessary. |
| Worship | Encourage clients to worship in accordance with their faith and culture. |

## Psychological needs (intellectual)

| Needs or problems | Action or intervention |
|---|---|
| Self-esteem | Maintain good interpersonal relationship skills with clients. Address clients by their preferred names and encourage the use of personal items such as clothing. Praise and reward efforts with a genuine smile. Provide relevant information and suggestions. Encourage self-reliance and the ability to express themselves and make their own decisions. But do not patronise them. Help them to take reasonable risks to maintain their self-respect, dignity, privacy and independence. |
| Recognition | Address clients by their preferred name. Praise and reward any achievement. Introduce them to other residents as appropriate. Encourage and allow clients the opportunity to express themselves. Show respect and appreciate client's cultural, religious, racial background, beliefs, values, ethnic origins. |

## Effects of deprivation of needs

### Clients

The effects of deprivation of needs can be devastating to the individual. For example, a male resident who was in bed asked for a urinal. A considerable time elapsed before his request was met. During the intervening period, he had an accident and wet his bed. In another situation an elderly lady lost her favourite doll which provided her with some emotional comfort during routine bedmaking. A search was unsuccessful. It is likely that both these distressing situations may be responsible for causing the following problems:
- anxiety, frustration
- sulkiness, depression, crying
- temper tantrums, moodiness
- withdrawal and isolation.

The reasons for the lack of proper care could be attributed to pressure of work. While this may be true, it should be weighed against the amount of specialised skills and time spent trying to 'mend fences' and restore the trust, good relationship, self-esteem, dignity and confidence which residents had previously enjoyed. It is important that carers should have in-depth knowledge of individual clients, develop and use their caring skills to report on any signs of reactions they may see, no matter how trivial these may seem.

> *Guidance*
> - refrain from making promises to clients which you cannot fulfil
> - explain any delay you may anticipate and offer reason(s) for the delay
> - reassure the individual concerned but do not patronise the person
> - ask somebody else to take over and fulfil the need after prior explanation if it is not possible for you to do so personally
> - remind the person of his or her right to complain in accordance with local policy.

### Staff

Deprivation of needs may have a similar effect to those described above and lead to:
- poor job performance, sickness and absence record
- resentment and anti-social behaviour. Lack of job satisfaction, complaints from clients, visitors, colleagues. These may lead to disciplinary action, dismissal or resignation and other consequences.

> *Guidance*
> - develop and maintain good interpersonal working relationships with everyone
> - be aware of local policy on complaints and grievance procedures
> - be assertive and exercise your right within the principles of equal opportunity and anti-discriminatory practices.

### Motivation

The term generally refers to the drive or force which gives direction or causes someone to behave in a certain way in order to achieve his or her *needs*. It provides an incentive, together with a feeling of satisfaction when the goal is achieved. With motivation, the person is fully aware of what needs doing, and the reasons for doing it. For example, a hungry person eats food believing that this will relieve his or her feeling of hunger. Motivation is not always that simple. Sometimes it needs self-sacrifice, hard work and persistance to achieve the goals you have set yourself. However, when these goals are achieved, there is a sense of satisfaction that stems from the knowledge that you have done what you set out to do.

## Theories of motivation

The instinct for survival is one basic motivation and reproduction of the species is another. The 'fight or flight' mechanism could be considered a third. However, much of human behaviour is a 'learned response'; eg. babies learn to walk and talk, and people continually learn from life experiences. We are also taught to question, form opinions and look for reasons for behaviour patterns. A person may be aware of the *need* to improve him/herself and be directed by a drive strong enough to persuade him/her to enrol on a course of study or even change his/her job. The action is a conscious one and may be influenced by curiosity, a desire for adventure and self-esteem as a result of support and informed knowledge from a teacher, manager or peer.

## Motivation for work

There are many theories regarding motivation in general, and work in particular. Some of these theories have become very popular with managers, eg. Maslow (1970) and Herzberg (1960). These theories have formed various aspects of social skill training, such as flexibility, decision-making and problem-solving.

Employment is necessary, whether it is enjoyable or not. It is necessary to provide food, shelter, clothes, education for children and the social entertainment to which we have become accustomed. As well as being goal-directed, it affects the workers' physical, social and psychological health, and many suffer from work-related illnesses, eg. stress, hypertension because of the type of work they do. Herzberg (1960) was interested in the effect that work and working conditions had on the lives of workers. He concluded by saying that things which gave people satisfaction were related to job contentment. He called them *motivators*. He called bad feelings about work *hygiene factors*.

### *Motivators*
Factors which lead to extreme satisfaction are:
- recognition, achievement, reward (praise)
- responsibility, growth, advancement
- work itself and the environment in which it is performed.

### *Hygiene factors*
Factors which lead to extreme dissatisfaction are:
- administration and policies, supervision, salary and security
- working conditions, personal lifestyle, status, values and beliefs
- relationship with peers and supervisors.

Herzberg's theory can be compared to Maslow's need hierarchy. The hygiene factors are similar to Maslow's lower level needs. It is said that hygiene factors can prevent dissatisfaction, but do not always lead to job satisfaction. The workers do not necessarily become satisfied with their jobs just because policies, pay, conditions, supervision and benefits are improved. Like primary needs, these can be satisfied and, after a certain point, will no longer motivate.

## Promoting quality of care

Reference has been made to quality of care in *Section II*, 'Appendages for care'. But in this section, we explore ways in which carers can assist in bringing about acceptable standards of care, within the concept of motivation. The approach involves creating the necessary climate in the care environment which encourages risk-taking, and where mistakes or failures are seen as positive learning. It is based on mutual respect and shared values, openness and trust between all involved in a flexible and responsive way.

### *Guidance*

- develop and maintain good interpersonal relationships with your colleagues, patients or clients and everyone that you come into contact with at work or in your social life. Endeavour to master and use basic caring skills, eg. social, assertiveness, counselling
- assist in identifying the needs and interests of individual clients, which could be used to bring about high standards and quality of care
- be sensitive to clients' needs, and encourage them to express their feelings, wishes, problems and respond to them with respect for the right of the person concerned
- identify their own development needs and set goals to achieve them. Use your personal portfolio
- promote effective communication in ways which are consistent with your role
- assist in identifying and promoting individual client's beliefs, interests, choices
- encourage and support clients to have and share their interests and experiences in social and recreational activities with others, and praise their efforts
- explore ways in which personal beliefs and preferences may have an effect on the interests of individual clients
- promote the individual's rights and choice which are consistent with your own role and relevant legislation and local policies.

## Personal development

The general view is that our personal and social values cannot be separated from our professional or vocational values, so development is an individual's affairs and responsibility. If we require something, we need to get up and do something positive about it, in order to promote our own self-esteem, values and beliefs. First we have to set goals, and then address the following points:

- what was the reason or motive for our choice?
- what keeps us where we are today?
- what personal or vocational value do we recognise as motivating us, eg. money, security, need for change, promotion, role model?
- how much are we influenced by other people, eg. colleagues, family, policies, those in charge. In all cases we need to re-examine our goals and objectives and where necessary seek guidance.

It must be remembered that with every good intention mistakes are made, no matter how experienced and skilled people are, they may still fail. Failure is not based on a particular mistake, but rather on a series of events which have a negative influence on the person. Past failures need to be seen in perspective, as a natural part of human learning and an incentive to change and learn from experience. Change cannot happen on its own; therefore, we have to take and accept personal responsibility for bringing about a change.

There is no magic formula which will bring about personal growth and job satisfaction, other than by developing and maintaining good interpersonal relationships, making your own needs known, setting personal goals and working towards achieving them. At work, immediate feedback on performance, a 'pat on the back' with a smile for a job well done, can be positive motivators.

# References

Argyle M (1987) *The Psychology of Interpersonal Behaviour*, 4th edn. Penguin Books, London

Argyle M (1972) *The Social Psychology for Work*. Allen Lane, Penguin Books, London

Burns R (1982) *Self-concept Development and Education*. Holt, London

Cooper L, Makin P (1963) *Psychology for Managers*. Macmillan, Basingstoke

Child D (1978) *Psychology and the Teacher*. Rinehart and Winston, London

Herzberg F (1960) *Work and the Nature of Man*. World Publishing, Cleveland

Locke EA. (1976) The nature and causes of job satisfaction. In: *Handbook of Industry and Organisational Psychology*. Rand McNally, Chicago

Payne R (1983) *Organisational Behaviour*. Macmillan, Basingstoke

Maslow AH (1954) *Motivation and Personality*. Harper and Row, New York

Maslow AH (1970) *Motivation and Personality*, 2nd edn. Harper and Row, London

## Audio visual aids

### Format: VHS video

Ref: CEM 6312: *Communication: Motivating People*

Ref: CEM 6533: *Understanding People at Work*

Oxford Educational Resources Ltd

# Assignment

## A motivational exercise

This assignment is to help you explore what motivates you and others to work, and gives you an idea about your own future direction. Be free to discuss your observations with a trusted friend, assessor or course tutor. It forms part of your Personal Portfolio.

### Guidance

In completing the sentences below, please insert words and phrases that first come into your mind. In this way you will generate a spontaneous reaction and an insight into your own individual motivation. Remember that there is no right or wrong answer.

**Time allowed:** Ten minutes

1. I go to work because _____
2. Work means to me _____
3. My job is _____
4. I choose to do this job because _____
5. I remain in my present role/job because _____
6. The best part of my job is _____
7. The worst part of my job is _____
8. My motivation for work will improve if _____
9. If I could have one change to make my work more interesting, it would be _____
10. If I could have one thing to do to improve myself, it would be _____

## Personal portfolio (CU7.1, CU10.2)

Much of what we do is the result of formal training and experience gained during and throughout our lives. As a result, we develop knowledge, skills and other attributes that make us what we are now. Learning, especially from experience, is very important to everyone, although quite often it is unrecognised or undervalued. Nevertheless, we have this knowledge and it is unique to us as we use it in our work and personal life.

There is now a general awareness for recognising the worth of the learning and experience people gain from formal education and training, such as in schools, colleges, professional, vocational and occupational settings. All learning will help the individual with his or her future development. First, we have to record such learning and experience in a formal and sensible way, just like any other historical document. A few years ago, a curriculum vitae (CV) was recognised as an acceptable way of presenting credentials, especially for interviews, but writing them was regarded as a bore and a chore. Nowadays, emphasis is placed on maintaining a personal portfolio system which helps us to relate learning to learning goals, to explore, develop, and set realistic targets for our own vocational growth.

### Portfolios

These are a means of collecting and presenting evidence of personal learning and achievements from a variety of sources, about competence to practice. It describes what we have learned, identifies what we need to know now, where we might be heading and what we need for the future. It forms the basis of planning for further development. It is unique to the person and supports the picture of the individual's personal development.

It should incorporate learning experiences and provide a profile for employers and other professionals to assess the individual's strengths and weaknesses. The individual can use it as a basis for reviewing and planning the next stage in his/her development. Its main aim is to make us more responsible for our own decisions about future career developments, focus on ourselves, identify our strengths and develop them actively, in the hope that those areas which need developing can be identified and a development programme adopted.

#### *Organising the portfolio*

The process of building a portfolio can be daunting. A portfolio in a flexible form is a folder, file, a portmanteau or similar collection of information stored in an orderly manner. Its development is an ongoing process which needs thought and planning. It involves you in a process of self-evaluation, reflection on your life experience and action. In most cases, it requires keeping a *reflective diary* of events as they happen in your life, critical incidents at work that are unusual, challenging and that influence your actions.

#### *Parts of a portfolio*

A portfolio is in four parts. It is about you, so take all the time you need to develop it. The starting point is:

#### *1. Personal and life history (private)*

Developing a personal profile is a useful exercise in self-awareness which allows you to recognise and examine your attitudes, beliefs and skills and how they affect your life and practice. It is an autobiography, or a picture of yourself, so you need to find ways of exploring your personal skills to develop potential. Start by sitting down and writing, eg. 'I am 25 years old', then ask yourself:

- who am I?

- what are my needs, strengths and weaknesses?
- what is my plan for the future?
- where am I going?
- what equipment will I need for the journey?
- how will I know when I get there?

Include areas, such as:
- your education and the school you attended
- where you lived, what you did since leaving school
- close friends and associates, beginning and ending of friendships
- significant events and changes in your life, eg. passing a driving test, membership of a youth organisation, eg. scouting movement, athletic achievements.

It is important to remove the *private section* should you want to present your portfolio to anyone, because details of your private life should not be given to possible employers etc.

## 2. Record of employment and general education
This section relates to your practical skills, competencies and achievements to date, and acts as a curriculum vitae. It will assist with the process of recording workbased assessment, including recognition of your prior learning and achievements which may be judged as possibly current and valid for accreditation.

It should provide the following evidence:
- education and training history, eg. schools, colleges, qualifications, ie. GCSEs
- past employment up to the point you became a care assistant
- type of work experience, dates, duration
- references from an employer
- informal learning at work, eg. observation, working with other people, feedback
- involvement in any new system of care
- prior learning, interests and achievements, eg. certificates, prizes.

As this self-awareness exercise progresses, it should be possible for you to note down what you have learned about your working life.

## 3. Record of training and development
This section may highlight those areas that you find problematical, together with attempts to plan how best to deal with current and similar situations in the future. It should contain information on:
- personal assessment record showing strengths and areas of knowledge and skills you wish to develop
- current development programme, eg. courses attended, study days including course information, eg. handouts, notes, course work, assignments
- information on any in-house induction and orientation programme received
- assessment of needs and plans for future development, eg. further training, open learning.

## 4. Record of vocational achievements
This section should contain information relating to your workbased assessment of competence, eg.
- initial candidate assessment record
- personal goal and action plans
- assessment plan
- evidence log sheet
- assessment summary sheet.

## Advantages of maintaining a personal portfolio
The portfolio can be used as a framework for evidence during ward-based assessment of competence. During ward-based assessment the assessor may look for, collect, and use evidence which is current

and reliable within the system of accreditation of prior learning or achievement. It provides prospective employers with evidence of your practical skills, competencies and achievements to date, in support of your application at job interviews. Other uses include:
- information on prior learning and achievement readily available for accreditation towards a national vocational qualification
- it is job-related and linked with current opportunities at work for personal and vocational development
- a personal audit, looking back to past achievement, and ahead to plans for the future
- evidence of competence to practise.

## References

Bond C (1993) *Using Portfolios for CPD*. Training and Development TRACE, London

Gartside G, McGough S (1991) High profiles. *Nurs Times* **87**(4): 40–42

Rogers C (1986) *Becoming a Person*. Constable, London.

Klob D (1987) *Experiential Learning: Experience as a Source of Learning and Development*. Englewood Heights, Prentice Hall, London.

Mangan P (1995) PREP School. *Nurs Times* **91**(3): 16

Skelton G (1987) Student profiling. *Nurs Times* **83**(11): 62–63

United Kingdom Central Council for Nursing, Midwifery and Health Visiting (1994) *What PREP will Mean for You*. Register No. 15. UKCC, London

United Kingdom Central Council for Nursing, Midwifery and Health Visiting (1997) *PREP and You*. UKCC, London

### Audio visual aids

***Format: VHS video***
*Profile and Portfolio*
*Nursing Times Update Series*
RCN Education Unit, London

## Assignment

The purpose of this homework is to assist you in preparing for your Workbased Assessment of Competence. There is no pressure, and you are expected to work at your own pace, but avoid the temptation to procrastinate. After you have read your notes and suggested references, submit your work for correction. The completed work becomes part of your Personal Portfolio.

1. Describe a 'portfolio'?
2. Discuss how you would create your own personal portfolio.
3. List six uses of a personal portfolio.
4. What aspects of your portfolio would you be prepared to share with the Workbased Assessor?

## Adult as a learner (CU7.1)

Learning is not an easy word to define because of the different views about its process. Almost everything we do in our daily lives is the outcome of learning, whether riding a bicycle, making a bed or solving complex problems. Learning is, therefore, a hidden mental process since we cannot observe what actually takes place when a person learns something. The only way we know that a change has taken place is by observing the individual's behaviour after the event or instruction. Gagne (1970) defines learning as 'a change in human disposition or capability which can be retained, and which is not simply ascribed to the process of growth'.

In more simple terms, it is a more or less permanent change in a person's behaviour following education and training. This change, therefore, involves acquisition of knowledge, skill and attitude. It is effective when the learner is able to do something, which he or she was not able to do safely before the instruction.

An adult learner is a person with a background in learning, who sees learning as a means to an end, although what he or she learns depends upon what is available to learn. For those returning to study after a considerable break, it is a major step and an active commitment to learning is necessary. An adult learner's school experiences and experiences of life after leaving school, enriches his/her understanding by relating to these past experiences. In this respect, learning involves adjusting behaviour through experience to bring about a permanent change in skills, knowledge and attitude. An adult learner usually adapts better to demanding situations. He or she often prefers courses where the subject matter relates to learning by problem-solving. Although the old adage 'you cannot teach an old dog a new trick' may often be quoted, it should be discounted. People never stop learning, and so we can learn new things, although it takes longer for some people than others.

## Forms of learning

There are various forms of learning such as *cognitive* change relating to acquisition of some new knowledge, eg. understanding the constituent of a balanced diet or a change in attitude, motivation and belief — for example, helping a confused elderly person to smile and say 'thank you' — something he or she had not previously been able to do.

*Experience* is the sum of knowledge gained in life through travel, work, marriage, parenthood etc. However, experiential learning is another type of learning. It relates to the ability to organise new thoughts and events in such a way as to increase our knowledge. It is how we shape our knowledge, behaviour and, subsequently, competence and make the most of our experience in a systematic way

The most common type of learning is the ability to achieve control and skill in carrying *psychomotor skills*, such as learning to ride a bicycle safely. At work, it is the ability to carry out practical procedures safely and competently.

*Vocational preparation* provides an opportunity to learn for those faced with a new learning situation. Their vocabulary of responses may be restricted to or by previously acquired knowledge and skills, but appropriate support and training will remedy the situation.

## Factors which may influence adult learning

There are many factors which may affect one's ability to pursue active learning. The most common ones relate to:

### *Habits and set*
Habits are a set of everyday routine activities generally acquired by repeating a sequence of activities until they become spontaneous. Many of the activities of daily living are formed by habit, eg. washing, dressing, eating which are carried out in a regular pattern without any conscious effort. Apart from habits, as people grow older, they identify events in accordance with past experience. This can lead to a person becoming 'set in his ways'. It is said that as a result, the person would resist change and reject unfamiliar ideas. Learning new things then becomes difficult, making an extra demand on the

person's attention span. He/she may become sensitive to distractions, which may also make learning impossible. But he or she may be forced by contradictory evidence to relinquish this 'set'.

### *Age and feelings*
Being old is quite often used as an excuse not to learn. Some older people may claim to learn from living and experience but, at the same time, say that they are too old to learn. However, in reality, people never stop learning, although some may need more time, especially in planned learning situations, in order to keep abreast of new ideas. An article by Stephen Castle, educational correspondent, *The Sunday Times,* January 15, 1989 gives an example 'Pensioners Top of GCSE class'.

### *Motivation*
The term 'motivation' relates to a desire or a yearning to learn or show interest in learning something and working to achieve it. But, it is not quite clear whether the action of the adult learner in being present for a learning experience is due to a basic drive or goal-directed behaviour. In any case, some form of incentive may be necessary.

### *Changes in lifestyle*
Changes in the individual's lifestyle such as professional, family, social, responsibilities may affect his or her ability to pursue any planned learning activity. The 'load' is always given as a reason for resisting any attempt at learning because of its increasing demand on the person's time.

### Reasons for learning

The following are common rationale given in pursuance of adult learning:
- self-direction and improvement
- professional or statutory requirement
- professional or vocational advancement
- personal challenge to prove that 'I can do it'
- for pleasure.

### Reasons for rejecting learning

There are many reasons but the most common are:
- older people may need to overcome guilt, fear or lack of self-confidence before committing themselves to learning
- changing social roles in which people commit themselves to social and civic activities, eg. starting and bringing up a family, being a local county councillor
- lack of opportunity: in some care environments there is no in-service education and training, and learning takes place by trial and error
- lack of motivation, interest, self-confidence and positive commitment to a course of study
- a belief that the time spent away from work, loved ones, family, housework, in pursuit of further learning is wasted time
- fear of failing to meet certain expectations
- a negative attitude and bias about learning because of the absence of immediate reward and recognition
- self-imposed limitations as a result of lack of interest
- fear of making errors or failing or being called stupid. When this happens some people tend to take it personally, and it can result in damaging self-esteem and confidence.

## How adults learn

People learn in different ways, and the 'you do it your own way, and I'll do it mine' idea is a principle to be encouraged. The following approaches are commonly used by care assistants in the care setting:

### *Supervision*
Learners should be supervised and procedures explained to them prior to demonstration. Skill and competence should develop as a result of continuous hands-on-practice. Learners should be encouraged to develop an ability to criticise their own work. It is important to ask questions during this process to demonstrate understanding.

### *Role model*
The 'role model' has been found to be a powerful influence in learning caring skills. A great deal of learning takes place by watching others 'do it', and we tend to emulate those who possess the skills and qualities that we admire or a status we aspire to. What we *are* sometimes speaks louder than what we say. Therefore, what a learner sees being done may be a more powerful influence than what he or she is told to do. In fact, social learning has invariably taken place and all qualified nurses become role models.

### *Demonstration*
It is believed that 'what we hear we forget, what we see we remember, what we do we *know*'. Practical demonstration is a repetition of responses and practical routine work activities such as, moving and handling clients. Adult learners need opportunity to practice as, 'practice makes perfect'.

Learning is meaningful and more effective when conditions for it are right and learners are given an opportunity to have hands-on-experience and experiment with their newly acquired knowledge and skills. First hand experience and participation enhance learning. Also, an abundance of realistic practical demonstrations followed by hands-on-experiences contribute to learning. They should be combined with a positive feedback which reinforces learning

### *Feedback*
Information about what constitutes a good performance and knowledge of our strengths and weaknesses reinforces learning. To be effective, feedback should be timely, that is, given when an individual is ready for it. The aim is to fulfil the needs of the learner not only in doing the given task, but to achieve the desired level of competent behaviour. Feedback should be clear, concise and straight to the point focusing on observed behaviour and not on the motivation behind the behaviour.

### *Problem-solving*
This involves the ability to define the problem and devising ways that can help to overcome it. In most cases, it depends to some extent on how the person feels and his or her ability to communicate effectively with other people.

### *Taking notes*
In a learning situation, such as a classroom, taking notes in a precise and concise way of what the teacher says or projects on the chalkboard or overhead projector, has the potential to help you to remember and thus reinforces learning.

### *Personal attitude*
Generally, attitude or emotional feelings tend to influence choices for personal action by the individual. These are acquired by socialising with other people and are likely to affect the way the

individual behaves in certain situations. However, learning which involves feelings as well as the intellect are the most lasting, although too much emotional tension and stress may decrease efficiency in learning. It is important to seek support by discussing any emotional problems with a trusted colleague or a teacher. Therefore, there is a need for care assistants to feel supported and valued as members of the team.

**General guidance on approaches to:**

### 1. Effective learning

The following approach may be helpful, when pursuing any vocational preparation programme. The learner should be able to:

- set clear and realistic goals, both long- and short-term
- seek support from those close to him/her. This can be helped by being part of a good study group. Support can also be gained from family, friends, supervisors and colleagues
- plan what he or she wants to achieve in the next day, week, month
- stick to such plans, or modify them only for good reason
- learn to make the best use of time and be prepared to make sacrifices
- open his or her mind to new ideas and experiences, and be able to develop a high tolerance to ambiguity
- establish links between a new subject and his or her own practical experience of the world, and motivate him/herself
- find a place or corner in the home for his or her own use, free from distractions and interruptions, with good ventilation and lighting
- form a habit of studying and stick to it
- tackle written assignments.

### 2. When to study

- make a personal timetable for the week
- study sessions should be from one to three hours long, no longer
- take regular breaks — about five to ten minutes every hour
- plan recreation and relaxation into your timetable
- accept responsibility for your learning
- learn at your own pace and ability, avoiding late hours
- do not procrastinate.

### 3. How to study

- concentrate your attention on the subject to be studied
- remove irrelevant and unwanted stimuli, eg. noise, hunger, cold
- put aside other pressing matters by listing or timetabling them
- suppress unwanted thoughts by quickly switching to the topic under study
- read the piece once or twice, understand what you have read and make notes
- review what you have read and check that your recall was accurate
- take a lively interest in the subject outside study hours
- discuss with fellow students, friends, family and others who are interested
- seek help and support from assessors/trainers and others with experience
- submit your work or assignment on time for correction
- visit and use your local library and talk to librarians about any of your worries, especially which books to borrow.

Generally, if your interest is high in a particular subject area, so too will be your *motivation* and concentration. Consequently, you are likely to spend longer on the topic than planned. However, it is important to remember that 'no teacher, however brilliant, can learn for his students; true learning is that which you do for yourself' (Betty Issacs, 1983). Therefore, allow yourself a treat and reward.

# References

Beard R (1976) *Teaching and Learning, the Psychology of Learning*. Penguin Books Ltd, London

Child D (1977) *Psychology and the Teacher. Learning Theory and Practice*. Holt, Rinehart and Winston Ltd, London

Cooper S, Hornback MA (1973) *Continuing Nursing Education. Principles of Adult Education*. McGraw-Hill Book Company, London

Gibbs G (1981) *Teaching Students How to Learn: A Student-centred Approach*. Open University Press, Milton Keynes

Gagne RM (1970) *The Conditions of Learning*. Holt, Rinehart and Winston Ltd, London

Honey P, Mumford A. (1982) *The Manual of Learning Styles*. Peter Honey, Maidenhead

James D (1978) *Adults in Education, Learning*. BBC Publications, London

Knowles M (1990) *The Adult Learner: Neglected Species*. Houston Gulf Publications, Houston, USA

Rowntree D (1988) *Learn how to Study. A Guide for Students of all Ages*. Macdonald Orbis, London

Rogers C (1978) *Adult Learning*. Open University Press, Milton Keynes

The Further Education Unit (1987) *Supporting Adult Learning*. FEU, London

# Resources and opportunities for learning

Learning involves the use of a vast array of materials, equipment (hard and software) and valuable learning resources. The resources and opportunities to learn vary considerably from one care home to another. However, some care establishments subscribe to and carry a reasonable number of the following.

### Learning resources

- textbooks
- journals such as; *Caring Times, Nursing Times, This is Caring Business, Nursing the Elderly, Care Concern, Caring UK*
- research documents
- television, video tape recorders, radios and cassettes, projectors and other audio visual aids.

### Human

- patients or residents, their relatives, family and friends
- tutors, assessors, internal verifiers, matrons and trained staff. Also, doctors and all members of the health care team, including advocates and visitors
- colleagues and peer groups
- qualified staff directing carers to seek information and by sharing their experiences.

### Learning opportunities

These vary depending upon the type of care environment. They may include the opportunity to:
- observe clinical practice and share experiences with qualified staff
- use life experiences, previous learning, training, qualifications
- apply general experiences to develop understanding
- participate in giving and receiving reports at the beginning and end of shifts, and staff meetings
- seek information and ask the question 'why'

- read daily reports and case notes on residents.

### How to use the library

A library may be a room or a building containing a collection of books for use by the general public. A list of resources and suggested reading is provided at the end of each 'Unit of Learning'. Some care homes carry textbooks and a few professional journals. It is, however, important that carers should seek the services of their local public lending libraries as an additional source of references. They should be able to:
- register as a member of their local county library
- obtain information from the reception desk on how to search in the library catalogue
- borrow books in accordance with the short loan collections scheme, ie. a week or normal three week loan period including reservations on some titles
- reserve a book by providing the librarian with information. See 'How to write a reference' see *Section II*: Research appreciation. Some librarians may require the ISBN or other control number.

*Information contact:*
Adult Learners Week, NIACE
21 de Montfort Street, Leicester LE1 7GE
Tel: 0116 204 4200
Fax: 0116 223 0050
Free helpline tel: 0800 100 900

## Vocational preparation for adults (CU7:2)

The purpose of vocational preparation is to make a plan for supporting anyone, especially adults, who are passing from one job to another, from unemployment to employment and from home to college. It is a scheme aimed at offering access and an opportunity for personal growth of the person, to support any change that may occur in his or her life, irrespective of age, gender, ability and race. Therefore, it is available to everyone who requires it, and remains so throughout active life.

### The need for the programme

The people who need it most are those who require new skills as a result of redundancy, change of job or unemployment, especially if they have a family to support. Some people may be pressed into retraining as a result of the changing nature of their job. Although the attributes, including prior knowledge, experience and skills, they brought with them may be adequate to meet challenges posed by the new situation, a retraining programme may become necessary to support and develop them.

### Vocational training programme

The agenda is learner-centred, relevant, flexible to support the needs and potential of individuals. The aim is to enable them to develop confidence in their ability to cope with the change and their individual circumstances. The process is based on identifying a person's needs for the type of training they require, with the opportunity of gaining credits for prior learning. In some cases, distance learning may be recommended, although the option is the individual's. In the caring situation, the need for training and development is recognised together with those of the organisation and service being provided. The outcome is that the organisation will devise *a competence-based programme* to prepare and develop skills, knowledge and attitudes to enable individuals to carry out their roles successfully with regards to the service being provided.

In all circumstances, adults need support to prepare and realise their goals, preferably by profiling. For those who have difficulty in retaining previously acquired skills and knowledge the pace of learning may be slower and they, therefore, require additional, long-term support; while those with special needs are likely to require other forms of support to integrate into the care team, in order to express and value themselves, and to be valued for their contributions to the delivery of care.

The hallmark of Inservice Education (Nursing) Consultancy Service (IECS) is based on providing employers with **on-site** staff training and a development programme to meet the needs of their staff and that of the service they provide. It is a flexible 'rolling' scheme of training provided on a day suitable for the individual care establishments. The scheme is augmented by an adequate mentorship system, with supervised hands-on-experience for candidates.

## Workbased training

Training is the recognised means by which staff acquire the necessary information, knowledge and skills to become competent. It is by no means the only, or the best way of helping people to learn, but it has to be kept in mind that care staff are a very mixed group of people from a wide range of educational and social backgrounds. There cannot be a simple solution to the array of training needs which this represents. What is required is a means whereby people are able to learn continuously from the point of entry to a job.

Towards this end, Inservice Education (Nursing) Consultancy Service (IECS) was established with the aim of taking training to nurses and carers wherever they may be in the private sector of health care. The catalyst depends largely upon an overall willingness of all personnel, at all levels, to participate and support this innovative scheme of on-site staff training.

The process usually involves assessment of the training needs of individual candidates, recognition and accreditation of prior experience and skills, including achievements brought into the care team. The existing and experienced staff do not necessarily need to be taught what they already know, but will be able to gain access to work place assessment immediately, and start building up credits towards an NVQ. However, they often use the development course as a refresher and updating course, especially those working in isolated care establishments.

Although attendance at a course of preparation is not a pre-requisite, NVQs emphasise the assessment of performance and accumulation of credits, and that any training for a particular area of work should be provided by qualified practitioners. This is based on supervision of defined activities, leading to the accumulation of credits towards an NVQ. This is similar to a 'block building' approach whereby candidates work to build up an aggregate of units in their personal portfolio of credits. No doubt qualified practitioners have much to offer by way of their expertise and specialised knowledge and skill within this approach, but some proprietors believe in a realistic framework of staff training, and make appropriate financial arrangements. Others believe that training is a luxury and an optional extra.

## References

The Further Education Unit (1986) *Preparing for Change: Management of Curriculum-led Institutional Development*. Longmans, for FEU, London

The Further Education Unit (1987) *Supporting Adult Learning*. FEU, London

The Further Education Unit (1982) *Progressing from Vocational Preparation — Towards a Solution*. FEU, London

# National vocational qualifications (NVQs)

During the early 1980s, the idea of a large number of staff caring for people in a variety of settings, eg. hospital wards, nursing homes and in people's homes in the community, without recognised qualifications, became a national concern. It was regarded as a waste of potential as they had no opportunity to progress within their chosen vocation, and obviously they were in a 'dead end job'. The need for job training towards a nationally recognised award became a concern for everyone and, in 1986, the government set up targets for training the whole workforce, leading to the introduction of NVQs with different levels of attainment of skills.

National vocational qualifications in care (NVQs) are new types of qualifications which relate to a person's ability to do a job competently and safely, based on nationally agreed standards expected from the worker. The particular job area should offer an opportunity for assessment of candidates in terms of their performance and application of knowledge, skills and attitudes in the work setting. NVQs are not courses, and differ from academic qualifications in that, while they are likely to involve some general learning and theory, they also involve practical elements which are relevant to a particular area of work. Therefore, training for these qualifications is workbased and employer led.

Accordingly, NVQs are a statement of competence of the actual practice of caring, in which everyone is entitled to be assessed and accredited by the NCVQ. In the health sector, they offer the opportunity for progression into professional and nursing training, although the UKCC stipulates that entry should be above that of Level 5.

## The National Council for Vocational Qualification (NCVQ)

The council was established in 1986 to oversee the introduction of NVQs. It is an independent body which provides a framework through which everyone moves towards assessment by agreed national standards. It works through established joint awarding bodies to provide a single system for registration, collection of fees and certification of NVQs. In October 1997 NCVQ ceased to exist and its duties were taken over by the new Qualifications and Curriculum Authority (QCA) and the Scottish Qualifications Authority in Scotland.

## Joint awarding bodies (JAB)

These are relevant bodies approved by the new Qualifications and Curriculum Authority to award NVQs and unit certificates. They are responsible for approval of centres who wish to offer assessment services. They also ensure that the assessment process is carried out fairly and consistently.

## Care Sector Consortium (CSC)

The consortium was established in 1988 to develop nationally agreed standards and qualifications for care. In 1992, it published *National Occupational Standards* for the new national vocational qualifications (NVQs) and Scottish vocational qualifications (SVQs) in care, based on the work of an integrated project. In March 1998 CSC was closed and its duties were taken over by the new Health Care National Training Organisation (NTO).

## Approved assessment centres

These are establishments such as colleges, training agencies or nursing homes, wishing to offer candidates access to workbased asessment of competence based on nationally agreed standards.

They should be able to provide a structure for the overall control and management of assessment arrangements approved by the joint awarding bodies. These arrangements should include:
- registration of candidates
- training of candidates and assessors
- equal opportunities and anti-discriminatory policies
- appeals procedures
- assessment methods conforming to the requirements of the awarding body
- maintenance of an internal verification and self-monitoring system.

## Framework and levels of competence for NVQs

The main aim of NVQs is to provide a meaningful classification of the qualification to smooth progression within the areas of competence by analysing different work roles. There are currently about twenty NVQs in care. In the hospital and nursing homes setting, the role of care assistants is to assist professionally qualified practitioners who have direct control and responsibility for the standards and quality of total patient or client care. It is understood that the levels of NVQs do not relate to any time period or years of experience, but to the achievement of levels of competence. The levels are therefore assigned in relation to a variety of features, such as breadth, range, complexity of competence, and includes the ability to organise and supervise others.

The Beaumont Review (1997) defines competence as, 'the ability to apply knowledge, understanding and skills in performing to the standard required in employment. This includes solving problems and meeting changing demands'.

The following definitions have been produced by QCA as a general guide to the levels for care assistants, and are not expected to be prescriptive:

### *Level 1: Foundation and basic work activities*
'Competence is in the performance of work activities which are in the main routine and predictable or provide a broad foundation, primarily as a basis for progression.'

### *Level 2: A broad range of skills and responsibilities*
'Competence in a broad and more demanding range of work activities, some complex and non-routine. It requires the ability to accept responsibility and to work in collaboration with others, especially as members of the health care team, and in different settings.'

### *Summary of awards at level 2:*
- awards in care
- community work
- special needs housing
- operating department practice (health care)
- child care and education
- blood donor support
- early years and education
- physiological measurement.

### *Level 3: Complex or skilled and supervisory work*
'Competence in skilled areas that involve performance of a broad range of work activities, including many that are complex and non-routine. In some areas, supervisory competence may be a requirement at this level.'

### Level 4: First line managerial

'Competence in the performance of complex, technical, specialised and professional work activities, including those involving decision-making, planning and problem-solving, with a significant degree of personal accountability. In many areas competence in supervision or management will be a requirement at this level.'

### Summary of awards at levels 3 and 4

- caring for children and young people (levels 3 and 4)
- dialysis support (level 3)
- community work
- special needs housing
- operating department practice (health care)
- diagnostic and therapeutic support (level 3)
- promoting independence (level 3).

### Level 5: Professional and senior managerial

'Competence in the application of fundamental principles and complex techniques in a wide range of unpredictable work situations, commonly associated with professional people at middle management level. Quite often with responsibility for the work of other people and the allocation of substantial resources.'

### New awards

The Institute of Health Care Development (IHCD) is currently working with the Open University in reviewing plans for introducing new awards for the care sector, such as a certificate in care delivery, a certificate in clinical supervision, a skill mix award and continuing professional development.

### Benefits of NVQs

Generally, it is a way of realising equal opportunities, but its introduction in a care environment may bring about any or all of the following benefits to the following groups.

### The service users: NVQs

- combine the values and attitudes expected in care, including the right to privacy, choice, self-respect dignity within the principles of equal opportunities and anti-discriminatory practice
- provide improved standards and quality of care or service provision
- assure the delivery of care in relation to the agreed national standards.

### The employers: NVQs provide opportunity to:

- employ a more efficient workforce
- ability to identify the training needs of employees and plan for the development and training of target groups, especially unskilled workers
- recruit and retain staff through an effective staff development scheme
- recognise staff achievements and reward them accordingly
- facilitate investment in people with increased staff motivation
- assist in meeting statutory requirements of registering authorities
- ensure a commitment to high standards and quality of service
- monitor the standards and quality of service being given
- help to meet the skill mix requirements of new and developing roles.

### The employees: NVQs offer:

- recognition of past learning, skills, experience and achievements

- a flexible system to self-directed learning and development through continuous assessment of competence in the workplace and a credit accumulation system
- an opportunity to obtain nationally recognised qualifications by working in your own time, and at your own ability
- a scope for progression within the vocational areas with entry to professional training and qualifications
- an opportunity which facilitates good working relationships.

## How to become a candidate

The policy of the Qualifications and Curriculum Authority is that every employee should have access to NVQs at a level appropriate to his or her role within the Equal Opportunities Act. It is, therefore, expected that employers will have a procedure for recruitment and selection of candidates and offer their workforce access to NVQs assessment, although this may be influenced by resource implications.

It is not a requirement to have training before becoming a candidate. However, in order to have the necessary knowledge requirements, and prepare adequately for assessment of competence, it is essential to attend a prescribed course of preparation.

Registration with an awarding body such as the Edexcel BTEC, City and Guilds and CCETSW through an approved assessment centre is a pre-requisite.

## Isolated candidates

People working in isolated situations on their own as self-employed, or those who are not in full-time employment, may seek access to NVQs workbased assessment in conjunction with an approved assessment centre.

### Tax relief

Candidates may get relief if they are paying for their own vocational training. NVQs and SVQs are made up of units of competence, and candidates may get tax relief for any unit or part of a NVQ or SVQ even if they are not studying for the full qualification.

## Award of qualifications

There is no restriction on access to assessment of competence as candidates can choose their own level and work in their own time and at their own pace and ability. But, emphasis is on accumulation of credits. This self-directed approach, together with other contributing factors, may undoubtedly influence the duration of training. Contributory factors may include:

- the range of competence required and arrangements for the delivery of underpinning knowledge
- an opportunity for supervised practice and hands-on experience
- the pace at which the candidate is capable of learning, including the ability to prepare for a workbased assessment of competence
- availability of workbased assessors within assessment arrangements.

# References

Institute of Health and Care Development (1996) *25 Questions & Answers on National Vocational Qualifications*. IHCD, Bristol

Institute of Health and Care Development (1996) *A Candidate's Guide to the NVQs in Care*. IHCD, Bristol

Care Sector Consortium (1992) *National Occupational Standards fo Care, Based on the Work of the Integration Project*. CSC, HMSO, London

Inland Revenue (1992) *Personal Taxpayers Series IRI 19*. Tax Relief for Vocational Training, HMSO, London

Joint Awarding Bodies (1997) *Newsletter No 3. Revision of NVQs in the Care Sector*. Update. JAB, London

NVQ Update 18 (1998) *Standards and NVQs*. Jo Frisby Publications, Sheffield

## Audio visual aids

### Format: VHS video

*Pathways to Care Learning Themes* (VHS video)

*Pathways to Care*. PO Box 3077, London NW18

SURF: http://www.open.gov.UK/qca/

# Preparation for Workbased Assessment of Competence (CU7.2, CU10.2)

## Guidance for candidates

The framework for workbased assessments is based on the principle of continuous assessment and involves gathering and judging evidence against performance criteria set out in the *National Occupational Standards*. It is a planned process in which emphasis is placed on close working relationships, so that both the assessor and candidate are clear about their individual roles and responsibilities. The process is candidate-centred, initiated and controlled. But, it is important to realise that the ethos of equal opportunity and anti-discriminatory practice prevails, and is fully addressed throughout the process.

### Purpose of assessment

This is to:
- assess the competency of candidates based on the evidence they present to the assessor, who will then judge whether it is sufficient to merit accreditation in relation to the core national performance criteria
- provide a feedback
- identify candidate's needs, make suggestions and provide guidance on remedial action as may be necessary.

### Procedures for assessment

In order to carry out an adequate and objective assessment, both the assessor and candidate should meet, plan and formulate a *contract*.

### 1. Contract of assessment

There is a need to set out the 'ground rules' for assessment. For example:
- what is to be assessed, how, and if any other person may be involved, eg. the patient
- when the assessment will start and finish
- evidence which will be sought and methods for gathering it
- who will have access to the recorded information and documentation
- the uses to which assessment information may be put
- arrangements for feedback, resolving any associated problems.

It is important that the candidate should be aware of procedures and feel able to raise the matter with the internal verifier if agreement cannot be reached.

## 2. Day and time of assessment

It is essential that the assessment takes place as part of a normal working shift, and as near as possible to an ordinary period of care, so that patients or clients are not aware that assessment is in progress. It could be undertaken either on day or night shifts of duty, merging into the background of care, but not part of the care itself.

## 3. Sources and gathering of evidence

Evidence may be obtained from historical events, such as prior achievement or learning, performance at work or specially set tasks, and by questioning. The candidate's handiwork may provide a direct source of evidence, eg. a project report. Indirect evidence may be a reference from a previous employer, certificates of competence, photographs and prizes.

Normally, in a work setting, the assessor may naturally observe a candidate's behaviour in carrying out routine work activities, question the candidate and examine records maintained by the candidate (*primary method*). Both the assessor and candidate may look at a project which the candidate has produced or performed, check its quality and judge the outcome; whether it was carried out properly in accordance with established practice, eg. bed-making.

There may be circumstances where the use of the primary method is not possible, then other methods (*secondary*) may be used in any of the following combinations.

### *Testimony of others*
Other people involved in the work may be asked to provide comments on what was done and how well it was carried out. This may include clients or patients, colleagues and co-carers.

### *Projects or assignments*
Candidates may be asked to undertake a special project, assignment or look at an individual case which is then used as evidence of competence in a particular area.

### *Direct or oral questioning*
Specific questions may be asked on a particular piece of work the candidate has undertaken. This may require the assessor to experience the work of the candidate without any variation, and ask questions on the reasons for doing the task in a particular way and its possible outcome. The candidate's response is written down on a special oral questioning form.

### *Review or reflect on work*
The candidate may be asked to talk through an activity, eg. a project, record or assignment internally set which he or she has personally undertaken and presented for assessment. He or she may be asked to reflect on work already carried out.

### *Written questioning*
This method is used to find out more about a candidate's in-depth knowledge and competence in a particular area.

### *Prior achievement*
This relates to evidence of what the candidate has done or achieved in the past, which has been previously assessed. He or she may be credited with this, if it is current, sufficient and appropriate to the element of competence.

### Role play or simulations
This method involves setting up specific situations to gather evidence. This may involve simulation of the work environment with the necessary equipment or work situation using other people to play the necessary roles, eg. in emergency situations.

### Audio visual recordings
Video camera and tape cassette recordings may be used to provide evidence of the candidate's performance, where there is a communication problem. Assessor and candidate should agree the format before assessment starts.

## Candidates' responsibilities

### Guidance
Assessment should take place after a candidate has been able to:
- value and demonstrate work experience carried out in the clinical area to be assessed
- be aware of opportunities to gain underpinning knowledge, practical skills and attitudes related to the units of competence; if possible attend a course of preparation
- accept personal responsibility for preparation for assessment
- have access to and understand requirements as contained in the record of assessment expressed in units of competence for NVQs
- appreciate methods of gathering evidence
- make requests, and arrange the date and time with the assessor
- spend time with the assessor to identify the units and elements of learning he or she wishes to be assessed upon
- submit a portfolio of evidence of prior learning and/or achievement as may be necessary
- attend for assessment as arranged with the relevant document; be punctual
- be friendly and demonstrate communication and interpersonal relationship skills
- inform the assessor of any factors which may influence assessment eg. ill health
- undertake the assessment in the time scale set
- be well-prepared and take each working day, shift, duties as an assessment rehearsal
- practice and be familiar with any equipment to be used before the actual assessment
- be aware of the appeal procedures and what to do if something goes wrong with the assessment.

## Presentation of project works, assignments

To present any project or assignment the candidate needs to:
- organise his or her work, ideas and notes in a logical order
- be confident in the presentation — use his or her voice appropriately by speaking clearly and positively
- be aware of the importance of body language (non-verbal communication) and his or her appearance
- be assertive by asking questions — if you do not understand say so as the question should be repeated
- have a sense of humour, learn from and enjoy the presentation.

## References

City & Guilds (1992) *3033 Care NVQ Level 2 . Record of Assessment 1992 Onwards*. City and Guilds Institute of London, London

Meteyard B (1992) *Getting Started with NVQ: Tackling the Integrated Care Awards*. Longman Group Publications, Essex

Messenger K (1990) The NVQ pilot programme. *Journal of Training and Development* **1**(2). PEPAR Publications Ltd, Birmingham: 7–16

**Audio visual aid**

***Format: VHS video***
Ref: *Pathways to Care Texts : NVQs/SVQs Project*
Pathway to Care, London

# Section VII: Appendices

# Appendix A — Flow chart a pathway to NVQs in care

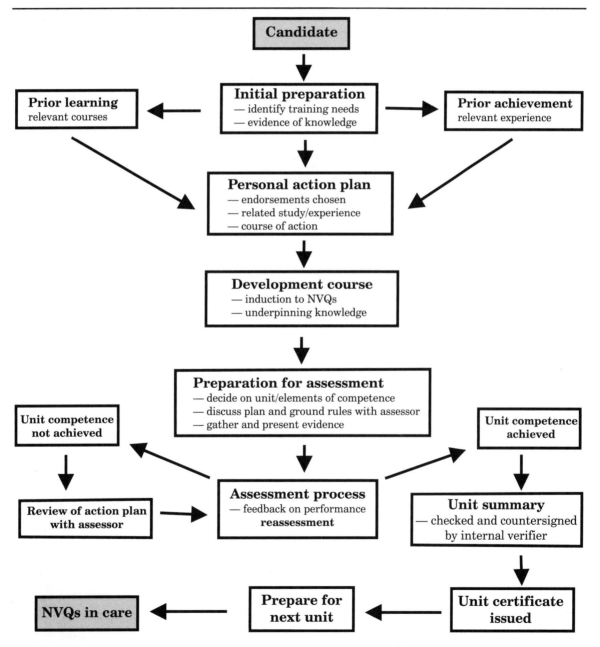

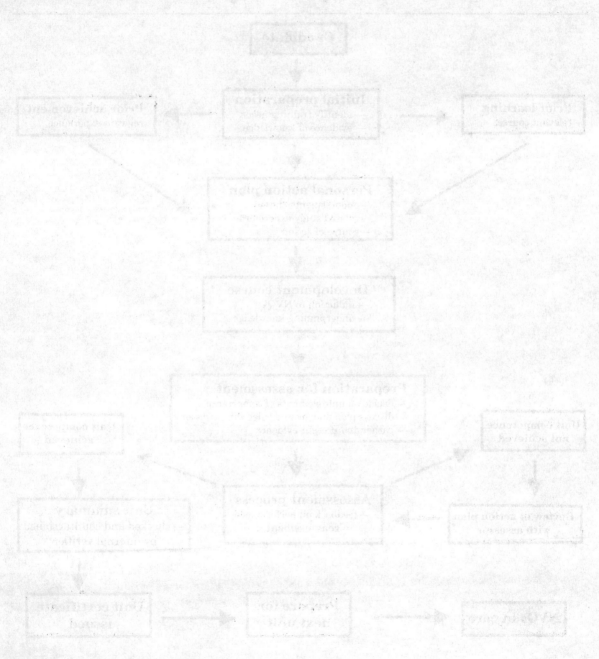

# Appendix B — Level 2 qualifications

## Mandatory units

O1   Foster people's equality, diversity and rights
CU1  Promote, monitor and maintain health, safety and security in the workplace
CL1  Promote effective communication and relationships
Z1   Contribute to the protection of individuals from abuse

## Option group A

CL2   Promote communication with individuals
CU5   Receive, transmit, store and retrieve information
NC12  Enable clients to eat and drink
W2    Contribute to the ongoing support of clients and others significant to them
Z6    Enable clients to maintain and improve their mobility through exercise and the use of mobility appliances
Z7    Contribute to the movement and treatment of clients and to maximise their physical comfort
Z9    Enable clients to maintain their personal hygiene and appearance
Z11   Enable clients to access and use toilet facilities
Z19   Assist clients to achieve physical comfort

## Option group B

CL5   Promote communication with those who do not use a recognised language format
CU3   Monitor and maintain the cleanliness of environments
CU4   Support and control visitors to services and facilities
CU10  Contribute to the effectiveness of work teams
N13   Prepare food and drink for individual clients
W6    Reinforce professional advice through supporting and encouraging the mother in active parenting in the first ten days of babies' lives
W8    Enable clients to maintain contacts in potentially isolating situations
X1    Contribute to the support of clients during development programmes and activities
Y1    Enable clients to manage their domestic and personal resources
Z5    Enable clients to maintain their mobility and make journeys and visits
Z13   Enable clients to participate in recreation and leisure activities

**Z15** Contribute to the care of a deceased person

**Z16** Care for a baby in the first ten days of life when the mother is unable

## To achieve award

**Candidates need to achieve nine units of competence:**

- four mandatory units plus up to five option units
- choose up to five units from option group A, if applicable to your work role
- where you have not chosen five units from option group A, then units from option group B must be chosen to make up five units in total.

# Appendix C — useful information

Action on Elder Abuse
1268 London Road
London SW16 4ER
Tel: 0181 679 7074

Age Concern:
    Scotland: 0131 288 5656
    Wales: 01222 371 821

Age Concern England
Astral House
1268 London Road
London SW16 4ER
Tel: 0181 679 8000
Fax: 0181 679 6060

Age Concern Welfare
15 Market Place
Devizes
Wiltshire SN10 OHT
Tel: 01380 727 767

Alzheimer's Disease Society
Gordon House
10 Greencoat Place
London SW1P 1PH
Tel: 0171 306 0606
Fax: 0171 306 0808

Arthritis Care
5 Grosvenor Crescent
London SW1X 7ER
The Arthritis Care/Wyeth Helpline
available 1–5 pm week days on
freephone service 0800 289 170

Association to Aid the Sexual and Personal Relationships of People with Disabilities (SPOD)
286 Camden Road
London N7 OBJ
Tel: 0171 607 8851

Bernard Sunley House
60 Pitcairn Road
Mitcham
Surrey CR4 3LL

British Association for Counselling
1 Regent Place
Rugby
Warwickshire CV21 2PJ
Tel: 01788 578 328

British Association for the Disabled
The Mary Glen Haig Suite, Solecast House
13–27 Brunswick Place
London N1 6DX
Tel: 0171 490 4919
Fax: 0171 490 4914

British Association for the Hard of Hearing (BAOH)
7–11 Armstrong Road
London W3 7DJL
Tel: 0181 743 1110

British Red Cross Society
9 Grosvenor Crescent
London SW1X 7EJ
Tel: 0171 355 454

Carers National Association
20–25 Glasshouse Yard
London EC1A 4JS
Tel: 0171 490 8818
Fax: 0171 490 8824

Counsel and Care
Twyman House
16 Bony Street
London NW1 9PG
Tel: 0171 485 1550
(Publishes fact sheets on elder abuse and provides help for older people and their carers)

CRUSE
Cruse House
126 Sheen Road
Richmond
Surrey TW9 1UR
Tel: 0181 332 7227

Deaf Blind UK
100 Bridge Street
Peterborough

Northants PE1 1DY
Tel: 0800 132 320
Tel: 01733 358 100 (voice and minicom)
Fax: 01733 358 356

Deaf Education Through Listening and Talking
PO Box 20, Haverhill
Suffolk CB9 7BD
Tel: 01440 783 687

Disability Income Group
Unit 5, Archway Business Centre
19–23 Wedmore Street
London N19 4RZ

Disabled Living Foundation
380–384 Harrow Road
London W9 2HU
Tel: 0171 289 6111
Fax: 0171 266 2922

Equal Opportunities Commission
Overseas House
Quay Street
Manchester M3 3HN
Tel: 0161 833 9244

Family Welfare Association
501–505 Kingsland Road
Dalton
London E8 4AU
Tel: 0171 254 6251
Fax: 0171 249 5443

Pauline Ford, Care of Elderly People
Royal College of Nursing
20 Cavendish Square
London W1M OAB
Tel: 0171 409 3333
(Provides guidelines for nurses on abuse and older people)

Friends of the Elderly
42 Ebury Street
London SW1 OLZ
Tel: 0171 730 8263
Fax: 0171 259 0154

General Welfare of the Blind
37–55 Ashburton Grove
London N7 7DW
Tel: 0171 609 0206
Fax: 0171 6074425

Guild Aid for Gentle People
10 St Christopher's Place
London W1M 6HY
Tel: 0171 935 0641

Hearing Concern
7–11 Armstrong Road
London W9 7JL
Tel: 0181 743 1110 Voice and minicom
National Helpline: 01245 344 600
e-mail: hearing concern@ukonline.co.uk

Help the Aged
16–18 St James's Walk
Clerkenwell Green
London EC1R OBE
Tel: 0171 253 0153
Seniorline Freephone: 0800 289 404
Fax: 0171 250 4474

Help the Homeless
Yeoman House
168–172 Old Street
London EC1V 9BP
Tel: 0171 336 7696
Fax: 0171 336 7721

Help the Hospices
34–44 Britannia Street
London WC1X 9JG
Tel: 0171 278 5668
Fax: 0171 278 1021

The Holiday Care Service
2 Old Bank
Station Road
Horley
Surrey RH6 9HW
Tel: 01293 774 535

International Voluntary Services
Old Hall, East Bergholt
Colchester
Essex CO7 6YQ
Tel: 01206 298 215
Fax: 01206 299 043

Methodist Homes for the Aged
Epworth House
Stuart Street
Derby DE1 2EQ
Tel: 01332 296 200
Fax: 01322 296 925

MIND (The National Association for Mental Health)
22 Harley Street
London W1N 2ED
Tel: 0171 637 0741

Mobility Trust
50 High Street
Hungerford

Berks RG17 ONE
Tel: 01488 686335 (Answerphone)
Fax: 01488 686 336

National Back Pain Association
16 Elmtree Road
Teddington
Middlesex TW11 8ST
Tel: 0181 977 5474

National Health Service Pensioners Trust
11–13 Cavendish Square
London W1M OAN
Tel: 0171 307 2506

National Library for the Blind
Cromwell Road
Bredbury
Stockport SK6 2SG
Tel: 0161 494 0217

National Listening Library
12 Lant Street
London SE1 1QH
Tel: 0171 407 9417

National Poverty Action Group
1–5 Bath Street
London EC1V 9PY

Occupational Pensions Advisory Service
11 Belgrave Road
London SW1V 1RB
Tel: 0191 233 8080
Provides guidance on the law relating to company or occupational pension schemes

Occupational Pension Registry
PO Box 1NN
Newcastle-upon-Tyne
NE99
Tel: 0191 225 6394
Offers to trace lost occupational pension schemes

Pension Investment Authority (PIA)
1 Canada Square
Canary Wharf
London E14 5AZ
Tel: 0171 538 8860
Regulates the sale of financial services to members of the general public

RADAR (The Royal Association of Disability and Rehabilitation)
250 City Road
London EC1V 8AF
Tel: 0171 250 3222

Relatives Association
5 Tavistock Place
London WC1H 9SN
Tel: 0171 916 6055
Advice and help for relatives and friends about the care of older people in health care homes

Royal National Institute for the Blind
224 Great Portland Street
London W1N 6AA
Tel: 0171 388 1266

Royal National Institute for Deaf People (RNID)
105 Gower Street
London WC1E 6AH
Tel: 0171 387 8033
Fax: 0171 388 2346

Talking Newspaper Association of the United Kingdom
90 High Street
Heathfield
East Sussex TN21 8JD
Tel: 0143 526 102

Thames Valley Medical
Medical Products for Rehabilitation
Chatham Street
Reading
Berks RG1 7HT
Tel: 0734 595 835

The Sympathetic Hearing Scheme
7–11 Armstrong Road
London W3 7JL
Tel: 0181 740 4447

# Equipment and services

HB, Equipment and services for people with disabilities
Health Publications Unit, No 2 Site
Heywood Stores
Manchester Road
Heywood OL10 2PZ

# Audio visual aids

BBC Enterprises Ltd
Woodlands
80 Wood Lane
London W12 0TT

Career Track International
Sunrise House
Sunrise Parkway
Linford Wood
Milton Keynes MK14 6YA
Tel: 01908 354 010

Concord Film Council
201 Felixstowe Road
Ipswich
Suffolk IP3 9BJ
Tel: 01473 76012/715754

Citizen Advocacy Information and Training
Unit 2K, Lerory House
436 Essex Road
London N1 3QP
Tel: 0171 359 8289

Oxford Educational Resources Ltd
PO Box 106
Kindlington
Oxford OX5 1HY
Tel: 01865 842 552
Fax: 01865 842 551

Pathway to Care
PO Box 3077
London NW1 8NW

Royal College of Nursing
20 Cavendish Square
London W1M OAB
Tel: 0171 872 0840

Video Arts Ltd
Dumbarton House
68 Oxford Street
London W1N 9LA
Tel: 0171 637 7288

# Index

## A
abnormalities in urine 272
abrasions 104
abuse
    forms of 137
    management of problems 138
    people at risk of 137
    preventive measures 139
Access to Health Records Act 1990 78
Access to Medical Record Act 1988 78
accidents
    action 107
    individuals at risk 105
    management of 107
    prevention of 108
acquired defence system (acquired) 114
act of respiration 171
act of swallowing 188
action at emergency situations 98
action research 46
action to be taken on discovery of smoke/fire (ARCE) 95
Administration of medication 284
administration of medicines
    legal aspects 287
admission
    effects on the client/patient 150
    factors leading to 146
    reasons for 147
admission for care 351
admission of elderly people for care 145
admission procedures 147
admission to institutions for care 17
admission, transfer and discharge 145
adult as a learner 386
adult learning
    factors which may influence 387
    motivation 388
advocacy 50
    definition 51
    forms 51
after care of wounds 130
ageing process and mental health 349
aggressive behaviour 357
AIDS (Acquired Immune Deficiency Syndrome) 114
Alzheimer's disease 350
anger 338
anorexia 340
anti-discriminatory practice 69
anxiety 147, 181
aphasia 168
appendix 49
application of cream and ointments 286
approaches to combat discrimination 70
areas of discrimination 70
aromatherapy 182
artificial eyes 166
aseptic technique 119
assault 35
assertiveness
    forms of 86
assertiveness skills 86
assessment 148
assessment of clients' needs 330
assessment of functional abilities 353
assessment of needs 309
attendance allowance 310
attitude 378

## B
Balance of Good Health 185
barriers to effective communication 83
    environmental 83
    language 83
    personal characteristics 83
    specific conditions 84
bath
    after 241
bathing 238
bathing specific areas 240
bathrooms 292
baths 239
battery 35
bed baths 240
bedrooms 291
behaviour 15, 367, 377
behavioural problems 367
    causes of 368
    forms of 368
    management of 368
belief system 65
beliefs 65
benefits of being assertive 87
benefits of NVQs 396
bereavement 337
Births and Deaths Registration Acts 1947 346
bleeding
    types of 102
bleeding — haemorrhage 101
blindness 163
blood pressure 279
body defence system (natural) 114
body lice 123
body temperature 267
brainstorming 26
breach of confidentiality 79
breathing
    cessation of 99
burns and scalds 101

## C
the confused elderly person 366
candidates' responsibilities 400
carbohydrates 186
care assistants 3, 28, 45, 75, 90
care environment 66
care establishments 8
care of catheter and drainage bags 222
care of clients with HIV/ AIDS and hepatitis B virus 126
care of mobility aids 259
care of residents in isolation 135
care of spectacles and prosthesis (artificial eyes) 166
care of teeth and mouth 235
    neglected care 237
care of the bowels 213
care of the dying 339
care of the elderly 17
care of the mouth, teeth and dentures 233
care plan 66, 149
care plan for clients with a 'temperature' 268
care plan for clients with hypothermia 270
care plans 330
Care sector consortium (CSC) 394
care study
    preparing 47
carers
    role of 52
carrying out a project 47
case studies 47
categories of elderly people 16
catharsis 31
catheter 222

413

changing 222
causes, sources and mode of spread of infection 113
characteristics of a normal urine 276
chemical burns 101
chest pain 173
Children's Act 1989 64, 66
choice 64
choking and cessation of breathing 174
Christians 343
chronic pain 251
claim of payment and benefits 310
cleanliness of care environment 313
client's room
    preparation of 147
clients with sensory deprivation 157
clients' needs 22
clinical activities 267
clothing 312
code of professional conduct 69
collecting body wastes 272
collection of payments and benefits 311
collection of specimen of faeces 274
collection of specimens 272
Commission for Racial Equality 71
communication 80, 358
    listening 81
community care 321, 330, 373
complaint code 36
computer information 76
confidentiality 53
confidentiality of information in care 76
confusion 15, 146, 315, 342, 352, 357
confusion and disorientation 351
consent for treatment 67
Consent for treatment 77
consent to treatment 371
constipation 210, 341
    prevention of 211
contact with family and significant others 153
contract of care 145
control of visitors 301
conversation 85
    termination of 85
coping mechanism 32
cough 172
counselling skills 29
Court of Protection 372
Court of Protection Order 311
critical essays 46
culture 66, 378

**D**

the depressed elderly person 363
Data Protection Act 1984 63, 77
deaf and blind people 165
    management of care 165
deafness 158
    forms of 158

management of problem 159
death
    after 344
    causes of 336
    forms of 336
decision-making in care 26
deep boring pain 252
defamation 35
dehydration 146, 194, 196, 340, 351
    prevention of 194
    signs and symtoms 196
delusion 364
dementia 350
dentures 235
depression 15, 315, 338, 342, 363
    causes 363
    effects of 364
    symptoms 363
diabetes 204
    complications of 205
    management of 205
    types of 204
diabetic diet 200
dietary constituents 186
dietary fibre 186
diets 198
digestive system 187
dignity 63, 238
Disabled Person's Act 1974 66
discharge arrangements 151
    procedure 152
discharge from the home 151
disclosure of information 77
discomfort
    with exercise or mobility 251
discomforts associated with breathing 171
discrimination 69
disinfectants 117, 293
    precautions 293
    types of 293
disinfection
    methods of 293
disorientation 15
diversional therapy 306
domestic and ancillary staff 91
drainage bag 222
    changing 223
    emptying 222
dressing 227
drink 193
drinking
    nature and purpose of 193
drive 377
dual registration 9
dust 294
duty of care 35
dying 336
    nature and purpose of 336

dying person
    psychological needs 342
dysarthria 167
dysphasia 341
dyspnoea 173, 341

**E**

the elderly person 14
ear 157
    functions of 157
ears 231
eating 184
effective communication 80
effective learning 390
effects of admission
    on relatives 150
effects of deprivation of needs 380
effects of discrimination 70
electronic tagging 299
employees' responsibilities 90
employers' responsibilities 89
enabling clients to eat 189
enemas 214
    purpose of 214
environmental hazards 106
environmental influences 22
environmental stimulation 361
epileptic seizure
    care after 112
    immediate care 111
epileptic seizures
    care during 111
    causes 111
    management of 111
equal opportunities and anti-discrimination 36
Equal Opportunities Commission 71
Equal Opportunities Commission Code 1985 66
Equal Opportunities Commission's Code 1985 10
equal opportunity 69
equipment
    safety of 289
equipment for personal use 289
escorts 317
essential attributes 5
essential skills 42
ethnic and cultural traditions 301
EU regulations 246
exercise
    provision of 251
exercise and diabetes 200
exercise and passive movement of limbs 250
experience 387
expressing sexual relationships 325
eye 163
eyes 231

# index

## F
face 231
factors influencing mobilisation 315
factors influencing old age 16
    physical state 16
    social state 16
factors influencing swallowing 188
factors which influence personality 67
factors which may influence role and function 4
faeces or stools 274
Fair Employment Act 1989 66
falls and accidents 105
false documentation 35
fats 186
faulty equipment 290
fear 338
fear and anxiety 342
fear of failure 378
financial support
    sources 310
fire extinguishers 94
Fire Precaution Act 1971 10
Fire Precaution Act, 1971 93
fire precautions 93
Fire Precautions Act 1971, Food Hygiene Act 1990 107
first aid 109
    aims of 97
fleas 123
fluid balance chart 195
food handling 119
forms of communication 80
forms of discrimination 70
forms of information 74
forms of learning 387
fracture 102
fractures
    management of 103
    See types of
framework for delivery of care 41
functions of care assistants 4
functions of the eye 163
furniture 312

## G
general and administrative records 74
general maintenance staff 91
getting clients out of bed 245
gifts from clients 36
gloves 133
good faith 36
grief 337
grooming 227
guidance for collecting specimens 275
guidelines for good health 200
guilt 338

## H
hair 229
hallucinations 364
handling and lifting techniques 248
handling and moving residents or patients 247
handling of food 203
handwashing 117, 229
head lice 123
Health and Safety at Work Act 1974 10, 89
Health and Safety at Work Act 1974/92 246
Health and Safety at Work Act, 1974 290
health education 320, 328
health education and promotion 319
health emergencies 99
health emergencies (first aid) 96
health promotion 319
health, safety and security 89
healthy diet
    basic guidelines 201
hearing aid
    care of 160
hearing aids 160
    troubleshooting 161
hearing Loss 157
helping the elderly to express sexuality 327
helping a client to eliminate 209
helping clients to mobilise 316
helping clients to relax 177
helping clients to sleep 179
helpless patients 190
hepatitis B virus
    modes of transmission 125
Hepatitis B virus 125
hoists 246
holistic approach to care 296
holistic concept of health 39
home equity plans 310
housing benefit 310
how adults learn 389
how to become a candidate 397
how to deal with information 75
how to promote effective communication 82
how to study 390
how to use the library 392
human ageing process
    biological aspect 14
    psychological aspect 15
    social aspect 16
human needs and motivation 377
hyperglycaemia 206
hyperpyrexia 269
hypoglycaemia 206
hypothermia
    prevention of 270

## I
identity 65
immobility and falls 351
immunity 124
    types of 124
immuno-deficiency virus (HIV) 114
inappropriate sexual activity 325
income support 310
incontinence 181, 256, 341
    effects on the person 217
    types of 218
individualised care programme 40
    stages of the process 40
infection
    care of client with 115
    causes of 113
    control of 117
    management of 117
    modes of transmission 113
    precautions 116
infectious diseases 345
infestations 121
inhalations
    administration of 175
    oxygen 175
    steam 175
insomnia 179
inspection and registration 8
intelligence 15
interpersonal relationship skills 84
interpreting services 83
inventory 288
isolation nursing 118, 131
    methods of control 131
isolation techniques 132

## J
Jews 343
judgement 350

## K
kitchen areas 291
kitchen staff 91

## L
last offices 344
    equipment 345
    procedure 344
laundry 292
learning 386
learning opportunities 391
legal aspects of confidentiality 77
legal requirement 23
legal rights 63
legislation 66, 118, 246
leisure activities 305
    management of 305
leisure and social activities 307
lice 122
lifting 245
    principles of 245
lifting and handling aids 246
linen 293
listening 29

living wills 36
loneliness 342
loss of pain and sensation 352
lying in bed 243

## M

maintaining a personal portfolio
    advantages 385
maintaining the safety and security of the care environment 117
maintenance of a safe environment 321
maintenance of stocks and equipment 288
making complaints 36
making it easier for clients to sleep 181
management of a special dietary programme 199
management of mental health problems 356
management of wounds 256
management responsibilities 89
manager 55
mandatory units 407
masks 133
massage 182
measuring pulse rate 268
measuring respiration rate 269
measuring temperature, pulse and respiration 267, 271
measuring weight 281
measuring weight and height 281
mechanism of elimination 209
medical and nursing records 74
medication 106
memory 15, 350
mental confusion 147
Mental Health Act 1983 23, 64, 66, 77
mental health problems in the elderly 348
methods of communication 81
methods of maintaining contact 153
methods of obtaining information 73
methods of storage and retrieving information 75
mineral salts 186
missing person 295 - 296
    preventative measures 298
    return of 298
    the search 297
mobile patients/clients 190
mobilisation
    purpose of 313
mobility 313
mobility allowance 310
model of care 39
models of care 54
modes of transmission of HIV 124
monitored dosage system 285
monitoring standards of care 37
mood 351

motivation 380
motivation for work 381
mouth 187, 233
    content of 234
    functions of 234
mouth care 340
moving and handling clients 245
muscles
    functions of 315
muscular system 314
music therapy 307
Muslims 343

## N

The National Health Service and Community Act 1993 66
nails (hands and feet) 229
nasal congestion (catarrh) 173
National Health Service and Community Care Act 1993 10, 330
national vocational qualifications 394
National Vocational Qualifications in Care (NVQs) 394
nature and purpose of breathing 170
nature and purpose of exercise 250
nausea and vomiting 340
needs 377
needs or problems 40
negligence 35
neurosis 349
new Health and Safety at Work Regulations (1992) 91
NHS and Community Care Act (1993) 34
night drainage bag
    attachment of 223
    removal of 224
normal immune system 124
notification of death 345
nursing care plan 41
nursing homes 8
Nursing Homes Act 1984 291
nursing process 39
nutrition 184, 255
nutrition for elderly people 185

## O

the overactive elderly person 367
observation 21
observation and reporting 148
observation skills 21
obstruction of airway 100
occupational therapy 306
oedema 195
organs of digestion 187

## P

The Patient's Charter (1990) 63, 66
pain 181, 251, 340
Parkinson's disease 350
pensions 310
people with dysarthria 167

people with mental health problems 168
personal affairs 312
personal and domestic resources 309
personal beliefs and identity 65
personal belongings 148
personal cleanliness 238
personal cleanliness: care of face, ears, eyes and prosthesis 231
personal development 382
personal financial affairs 309
personal grooming and dressing 227, 356
personal hygiene 341
personal hygieneand appearance 227
Personal portfolio 384
personal support 29
personality 67
phantom pain 252
physical well-being
    poor eye-sight 22
physiological needs 379
physiotherapy 307
portfolios
    organising 384
positioning 255
positions used in care 243
preparation for the role 6
preparation for workbased assessment 398
preparing clients for a journey or visit 316
presentation of project works, assignments 400
pre-sleep routine 180
pressure sore risk assessment 257
pressure sores 341
    areas commonly affected 253
    clients prone to 253
    predisposing factors 253
    recognition of 255
preventative measures 93
prevention of HIV/AIDS and hepatitis B 126
primary health care team 331
primary nursing 42
principles of care 122, 238
principles of elimination 208
privacy 63
    need for 238
problem solving 389
problems in maintaining social contacts 16
problems of advocacy 53
problem-solving 25
problem-solving and decision-making 24
problem-solving cycle 25
process of communication 81
profoundly deaf 159
project

carrying out 47
    presentation of 49
project work 46
    preliminary preparation of the report 48
promote health education 126
promoting clients' personal beliefs and identity 67
promoting quality of care 381
promotion of clients' rights 64
promotion of continence 217, 219
promotion of family contact 154
promotion of independence 358
promotion of personal grooming 228
prosthesis 232
protection of individuals from abuse 136
protective clothing 132
protective measures
    for epilepsy 112
proteins 186
psychological assessment 355
psychological needs 379
psychological well-being 22
psychosis 349
pulse 268
purpose of eating 184
pyrexia 269

## Q
quality of care 34

## R
Race Relations Act 1976 66
rapid eye movement 179
reality orientation 307
reasons for learning 388
reasons for rejecting learning 388
receipt of equipment 288
receiving telephone information 75
reception of client 147
recording of blood pressure 280
records 74
recovery position 98
recreational therapy 306
reference
    how to write a 49
register of patient 74
Registered Homes Act 1984 8
registered nursing and residential care homes 8
Registered Nursing Home Association 9
rehabilitation 149, 304
relationships 80
relatives 310
relaxation 176
religion 378
religious organisations 71
reminiscence therapy 362
repairs to clients' belongings 313
report of injuries 369
reporting 21
reporting skills 22
research 44
residential care homes 9
resources and opportunities for learning 391
respiration 269
respiratory infection 174
responsibilities under the Acts 71
rest 176
rest and sleep 343
rest, relax and sleep 176
restraint 67
rights
    of individuals in care 63
rigor 269
risk
    assessment of 43
risk of abuse 136
risk taking 148
risk-taking 43
role of care assistants 4, 26, 225, 258, 287, 306, 320, 327, 373
role of carers 339
role of health care assistants 78
role of the family 153
routes for measuring temperature 267

## S
safety of care environment 108
scabies 121
scalds of the mouth 101
security of personal belongings 311
self- 238
services and facilities in the community for the elderly 333
Sex Discrimination Act 1975 66
Sex Discrimination Act 1976 64
sexual health 328
sexuality 324
    purpose of 324
sexuality in later life 325
    benefits of 325
    factors influencing 326
sharp objects 119
sharp shooting pain 252
shaving 230
shock 99, 338
shopping expeditions 312
shower 239
showers 292
Sikhs 343
silence 32
sitting up in a chair 244
skeletal system 314
    function of 314
skill 19
skills 52
skin 254
    functions of 254
sleep 177
    factors interfering 179
    helping clients to 179
    lack of 178
    management of problems 180
    process of 178
    purpose of 177
    stages of 178
sleep, rest and relaxation 22
sluice and toilets 292
smoking 94, 174
social behaviour 351, 358
social needs 379
social skills 85
social well-being 22
sociological assessment 355
sore throat 173
sources of information 73
special diets 199
specific treatment programme 360
specimens
    purpose of collection 272
spectacles 166
spillage 118
spiritual needs 343
spiritual well-being 22
sputum specimen 274
    abnormalities 274
staff records 74
staff training 166
standard of care 34
standards and quality of care 34
standards of care
    monitoring 37
statutory bodies 71
sterilisation 117
stools or faeces 208
    common abnormalities 208
storage of food 119
strains and sprains 103
stress 31
study of elderly people 349
support for relatives 346
suppositories 215
    administration 215
suspicion 358
swallowing 188

## T
taking blood pressure 280
taking notes 389
task orientation 42
team building 54
team nursing 42
team work 54 - 55
telephone call
    making 75
telephone information
    receiving 75
testing the urine specimen 277
therapeutic diets 198

transfer 151
tube feeding 191
types of blindness 163
types of research 46

**U**
UKCC (United Kingdom Central Council for Nurses, Midwives and Health Visitors) 69
uniform 133
upbringing 378
urine 272
    procedure for collection of specimen 272
urine testing 276
use of special clothing, waterproof pads and pants 220
using counselling skills 29

**V**
validation therapy 362

valuables and other belongings 299
values 66, 378
visiting 300
visiting times 300
visitors 119
    support and control of 300
visits 153
    benefits to clients 154
    benefits to staff 154
    pre-admission 145
visits or journey to hospital 317
visits to theatres 307
visually impaired people 162
vitamins 186
vocational preparation 387
vocational preparation for adults 392
vocational training programme 392
voluntary services 333
vomit 275

abnormalities 275

**W**
wandering 295, 359
    reasons for 296
washing 228
waste disposal 134
water 187
weight loss 281
    management of 281
wet mops 294
when to study 390
work based training 393
workbased assessment
    procedures for 398
    purpose of 398
World Health Organization 348
wound care 300
wounds
    infection of 128
    types of 127
written reports 23